Optical Coherence Tomography and OCT Angiography
Clinical Reference and Case Studies

Darrin A. Landry, CRA, OCT-C
Amir H. Kashani, MD, PhD

BRYSON TAYLOR PUBLISHING

Publisher: Bryson Taylor Publishing

Author: Darrin A. Landry, CRA, OCT-C
        Amir H. Kashani, MD, PhD

Foreword: Gregory C. Hoffmeyer
Cover Design and Layout: Bryson Taylor Publishing
Edited by: Bryson Taylor Publishing

ISBN-13: 978-0-9983867-3-7
ISBN-10: 0-9983867-3-1
Library of Congress Control Number: 2016921611

BRYSON
TAYLOR

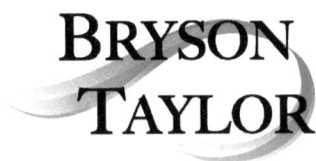

A MANAGEMENT & PUBLISHING COMPANY
199 NEW COUNTY ROAD SACO, ME 04072
www.BrysonTaylorPublishing.com

"Vision is the art of seeing things invisible."
Jonathan Swift

Contents

**SECTION
1**

**SECTION
2**

**SECTION
3**

Biographies

Amir H. Kashani, MD, PhD

Dr. Amir H. Kashani attended Johns Hopkins School of Medicine where he obtained his MD and PhD. He completed his ophthalmology residency at the USC Gayle and Edward Roski Eye Institute and fellowship in Vitreoretinal surgery at the top-rated Associated Retinal Consultants (Royal Oak, Michigan). He was awarded both the Heed and Michel's Fellowships (National Honors) during his training. Dr. Kashani is now a USC clinician-scientist with an active practice in both medical and surgical retinal diseases including diabetic retinopathy, retinal vein occlusions, age-related macular degeneration and retinal detachments among other common retinal diseases. In his research practice, Dr. Kashani is developing novel diagnostic and therapeutic methods to treat retinal diseases. His current work involves the use of advanced imaging spectroscopy and optical coherence tomography methods (such as OCT Angiography) to improve the diagnosis and treatment of retinal diseases. Dr. Kashani is a clinical investigator for a number of clinical trials. Most recently he is principal investigator for a clinical trial to test a novel stem cell therapy for severe vision loss from advanced dry age-related macular degeneration.

Darrin A. Landry, CRA, OCT-C

Darrin A. Landry has been an ophthalmic photographer since 1990, working primarily in retina practice. Prior to that, he served in the US Air Force as a surgical technician. In 2000, he founded Bryson Taylor Inc, a medical and management consulting company that specializes in ophthalmic education. Mr. Landry was part of an expert panel that devised the certification for optical coherence tomography for the Ophthalmic Photographers' Society. His list of clients includes private practices, academic institutions, clinical trial reading centers and biotechnology companies across the United States and in 14 countries in Europe and South America. Mr. Landry is the author of multiple peer-reviewed articles, as well as the textbooks *Retinal Imaging Simplified* and *Optical Coherence Tomography: A Clinical Atlas of Retinal Images*.

Preface

Optical Coherence Tomography (OCT) is one of the most fundamental imaging modalities in the field of ophthalmology. A basic understanding of OCT and its variations is critical for a number of people besides the clinician. These people include retinal technicians, ophthalmic imagers, medical students, medical residents and fellows. The ever expanding and rapidly changing role of imaging in the field of medical and surgical retina can present a challenge to those people who are just starting out in the field, or are in paramedical fields and are faced with a barrage of images that are not necessarily easy to interpret. In many cases, even veterans in the field can be overwhelmed by the multitude of imaging methods available to them. The goal of this book is to provide an easy and digestible primer for understanding of OCT images and related OCT imaging methods such as Enhanced Depth Imaging (EDI) and OCT Angiography (OCTA). These images are presented in the context of additional imaging modalities to aid the reader in making useful correlations.

Numerous authoritative texts exist to explain the pathology and pathophysiology of retinal diseases and it is not the goal of this book to compete with or mimic the classic textbooks of the field. Therefore, this book does not exhaustively discuss the pathophysiology of any particular disease process. Nor is this text intended to provide a comprehensive reference on the diagnosis and management of retinal diseases. For these kinds of references, the readers are referred to classic textbooks in the field such as Ryan's Retina series and Yanoff and Duker's Ophthalmology. In addition, Yannuzzi's Retinal Atlas provides excellent mutlimodal images of a wide variety of retinal diseases. These texts however are dense and targeted for the retinal specialist. It is our hope that less specialized readers can use our text to improve their ability to interpret and recognize patterns on OCT images, better understand the images that they are seeing and better understand how to image various pathologies. The diagnosis of retinal diseases in general requires a thorough clinical evaluation including detailed examination as well as ancillary testing such as OCT imaging. Therefore, the reader is advised to make careful clinical correlations before making a final clinical judgment about an OCT scan result or any imaging result.

Amir H. Kashani MD, PhD

Foreword

In 2003, years after the first retinal Optical Coherence Tomography devices started selling in the USA, I had the honor of co-directing *"The Art of OCT"* conference hosted by Duke Eye Center with Glenn Jaffe, MD. The workshop instructors consisted of my team of Duke ophthalmic photographers but we needed help, so I invited Darrin Landry, having met a few years prior as new Board of Education members for the *Ophthalmic Photographers Society*. We had almost 200 people attend our event in downtown Durham, North Carolina; OCT was still very, very new after all.

This was quite a while ago; Blackberries ruled, Facebook didn't exist, no Bluetooth, no texting for the most part, nothing went "viral" unless you caught it, and the Stratus OCT was the state of the art, Zeiss's third OCT iteration. Darrin was emerging as a leading instructor in the field of ophthalmic photography and soon mastered OCT, going on to teach technicians and physicians in both usage and interpretation. Darrin is a high energy, exceedingly well-prepared and insightful educator who obviously knows and enjoys what he is doing. He lectures quite clearly, in plain English, and with wit. I have seen him work directly with patients in the trenches; respectful, highly skilled, and very fast.

Flash forward to 2015, almost *20 short years* since the first production OCT launched; here we are with a new diagnostic imaging modality, OCT Angiography. Now what? Darrin made sure that his office in Portland was among the first private practices in the USA to receive a Zeiss Cirrus AngioPlex unit. I flew up there to help get him going, but by the time I arrived he had already unboxed the unit and started scanning patients with zero training, yielding good results. The next day we scanned about 40 patients, with astonishing results. You'll see.

Energized, Darrin started this book the week after he got his OCT-A, collecting cases and writing in a Stephen King-like flurry, but he needed a retina doctor's help to proof the cases and provide medical oversight. That's where Amir Kashani, MD comes in. I have not known Dr. Kashani nearly as long as I have known Darrin, first seeing his captivating OCT-A presentation at the AAO in Las Vegas 2015. I have given and attended a lot of OCT lectures over the past nearly two decades, but I was impressed with Dr. Kashani's eloquence and command, so much so that I thought to myself, "who the heck is this guy?" I am so glad he agreed to this effort.

It's really a thrill for me to introduce this work to you from my colleagues. I think you will find it quite helpful and perhaps a little surprising as to what OCT-A offers. Perhaps not unlike OCT's initial reception in the 1990s, *it's probably better than you think.* While using this reference, please keep a couple of things in perspective; one, this is a first edition introduction to new-frontier technology and two, there is no dye in most of these patients' eyes; and if there is (in regards to the OCT-A images), *it really doesn't matter.*

Enjoy.

Gregory C. Hoffmeyer
Sr. Clinical Relations Mgr., Global Retina-Glaucoma, Carl Zeiss Meditec

List of Abbreviations

AMD	Age-Related Macular Degeneration
BRAO	Branch Retinal Artery Occlusion
BRVO	Branch Retinal Vein Occlusion
CME	Cystoid Macular Edema
CRAO	Central Retinal Artery Occlusion
CRVO	Central Retinal Vein Occlusion
CSME	Clinically Significant Macular Edema
CSCR	Central Serous Chorioretinopathy
CWS	Cotton Wool Spot
DME	Diabetic Macular Edema
DR	Diabetic Retinopathy
DRL	Deep Retinal Layer (on OCTA)
ELM	External Limiting Membrane
ERM	Epiretinal Membrane
FA	Fluorescein Angiography
FAF	Fundus Autofluorescence
GCL	Ganglion Cell Layer
ICG	Indocyanine Green Angiography
ILM	Internal Limiting Membrane
INL	Inner Nuclear Layer
IPL	Inner Plexiform Layer
IR	Infrared
IRMA	Intraretinal Microvascular Abnormalities
MA	Microaneurysms
OCT	Optical Coherence Tomography
OCTA	Optical Coherence Tomographic Angiography
ONL	Outer Nuclear Layer
PCV	Polypoidal Choroidal Vasculopathy
PED	Pigment Epithelial Detachment
PVD	Posterior Vitreous Detachment
RD	Retinal Detachment
RPE	Retinal Pigment Epithelium
RS	Retinoschisis
SRL	Superficial Retinal Layer (on OCTA)
VMA	Vitreomacular Adhesion
VMT	Vitreomacular Traction

Introduction: OCT and OCT Angiography

Spectral Domain optical coherence tomography (SD-OCT) is one of the most commonly used imaging technologies in ophthalmic practices. It is capable of generating cross-sectional and en face representations of the retina and provides qualitative as well as quantitative data of retinal pathologies. [1]

In this book we will try to illustrate SD-OCT and SD-OCT Angiographic findings of various common (and some not so common) retinal pathologies with images from different OCT systems. As OCT technology is ever changing, the information provided in this book is presented using the most recent technology and information at the time of publication.

When OCT was commercially introduced in 2001, ophthalmic practice was dramatically altered. Here was an instrument that allowed for cross-sectional imaging of retinal layers, which up to this point could not be done without surgical biopsy and microscopic examination. Using a light source of 800nm that is capable of axial resolution of about 10 microns and axial depth of 2mm, the first system introduced to the ophthalmic market was a Time Domain system called the Stratus OCT (Carl Zeiss Meditec, Dublin, CA). [2] Since that time, many other companies have come forward with Fourier, or Spectral Domain technology, all of which are essentially a variation on a theme. Spectral Domain OCT technology uses a stationary spectrometer, which eliminates the need for a moving reference mirror that the Time Domain OCT systems use. This allows for faster acquisition of images (over 60,000 A-scans per second on some systems) [3], versus the 400 A-scans per second from the Stratus OCT [4] and increased sensitivity, resulting in improved image quality. Spectral Domain OCT (SD-OCT) systems offer better axial resolution of 5 microns, versus the Stratus OCT resolution of 10 microns. Spectral domain OCT also offers image stacking, which can be processed to produce 3-dimensional representations of retinal structures as well as 3- dimensional eye mapping. There are currently many manufacturers of Spectral Domain OCT [5] with more certain to join the market. Like fundus cameras, most OCT systems operate and produce images that are recognizable, with the differences being in database management, image manipulation, and image output. With this new wealth of information, physicians can make better-informed clinical decisions, better understand the pathophysiology of retinal diseases, and can visualize and quantify change within the retinal layers. OCT retinal thickness measurements have been, and continue to be used for many clinical trials related to retinal vascular diseases.

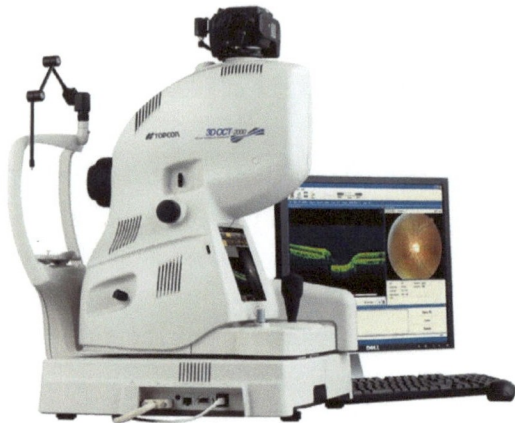

Topcon 3D OCT

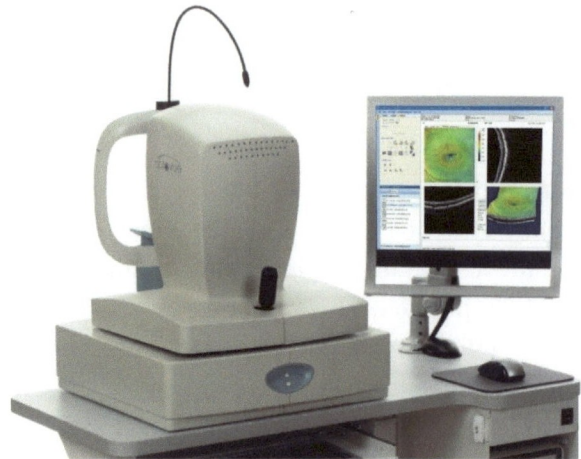

Optovue RTVue

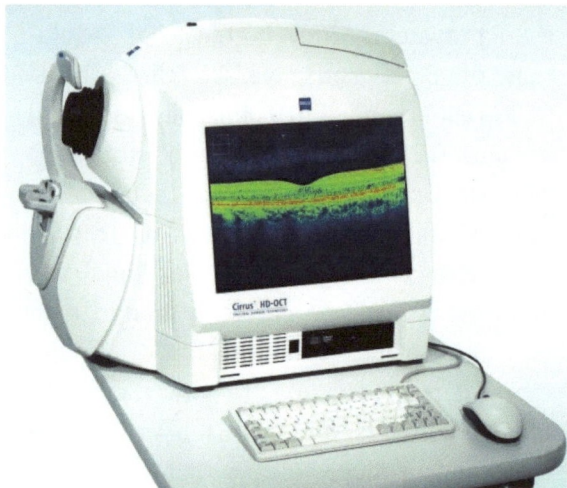

Zeiss Cirrus

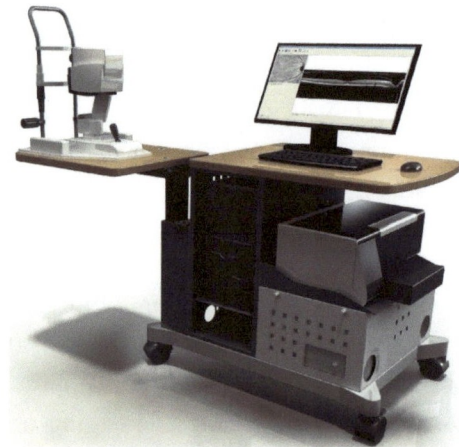

Heidelberg Spectralis

Some examples of OCT systems available in today's market

With new technology comes responsibility. OCT manufacturers are constantly producing systems that are more user friendly, both in hardware and software. What has not changed is the need for the OCT operator to understand retinal disease pathology, ocular anatomy, basic recognition of OCT findings and artifacts, and an understanding of how the OCT functions. The technician, or imager, who operates the OCT, must understand how retinal disease processes may affect a patient's vision. OCT systems, for the most part, rely on a patient's subjective fixation for alignment of the scan. Without physically moving the scan line, an operator relies on the system to scan directly through the fixation target, regardless of where the patient is actually fixating. In diseases that may affect central fixation, such as macular holes or macular degeneration, the patient may not be able to fixate on a central target. The patient with macular pathology involving the fovea may report that they can see the fixation light, but they may actually be fixating with an area of the macula, which may fall outside the fovea. This is a common problem, and may result in a scan not centered on the fovea. An operator that understands retinal disease should be able to recognize this, and remedy this by moving the scan pattern to scan properly through the fovea based on the anatomy. In most cases, a scan pattern that

is centered on the fovea is the desired and appropriate pattern for clinical diagnostic testing. Since the physician is typically not present at the time the imager is acquiring images it is the responsibility of the imager to identify and correct misaligned images. In some cases, where peripheral macular pathology is noted, it is also helpful for the imager to take the initiative to move the scan pattern and image the peripheral macular pathology, which may be of interest to the physician. Constant and close communication between the physician and imager is very essential.

Imagers must have a working knowledge of ocular and more specifically retinal anatomy. This greatly enhances their ability to provide appropriate scans.

References

1. Huang D, Swanson EA, Lin CP, et al. Optical coherence tomography. Science 1991;254:1178-81
2. Schuman JS, Puliafito CA, Fujimoto JG. Optical Coherence Tomography of Ocular Diseases. 2nd ed. Thorofare, New Jersey: SLACK Inc., 2004
3. Schmidt-Erfurth U, Leitgeb RA, Michels S, et al. Three-dimensional ultra-high resolution of optical coherence tomography of macular disease. Invest Ophthalmol 2005;123:1715-1720
4. Schuman JS, Puliafito CA, Fujimoto JG. Optical Coherence Tomography of Ocular Diseases. 2nd ed. Thorofare, New Jersey: SLACK Inc., 2004
5. Ophthalmic Optical Coherence Tomography Market: Past, Present, & Future, Optical Coherence Tomography News, Mar 29 2009

Pattern Recognition

Imagers must also have proficiency in pattern recognition. This is not to say that imagers should be able to diagnose findings on an OCT, but they should be able to recognize and identify normal layering of the retina represented on an OCT scan, as well as be able to identify abnormal structures, such as drusen and intraretinal fluid. This will allow the imager to differentiate pathological findings from OCT artifacts, which may degrade image quality. In some cases, it may be difficult to distinguish an artifact from true pathology but in many cases simple details such as appropriate ocular lubrication, fixation, and scan settings will allow the technician to acquire the best image possible.

Having a basic understanding of how an OCT system works also helps the imager understand how anatomy and disease pathology is represented on the OCT scan. OCT is essentially optical ultrasound and because it uses light instead of sound waves OCT provides much higher spatial resolution than ultrasound. OCT generates a cross-sectional image of the retina by measuring the interference pattern of light reflected from the retina with an internal reference beam. The resulting image represents the absorption, reflection and scattering of light by the retinal tissue. Tissue that absorbs light or scatters light away from the OCT detector will appear dark on OCT scans. Tissue that strongly reflects light will appear bright on OCT scans.

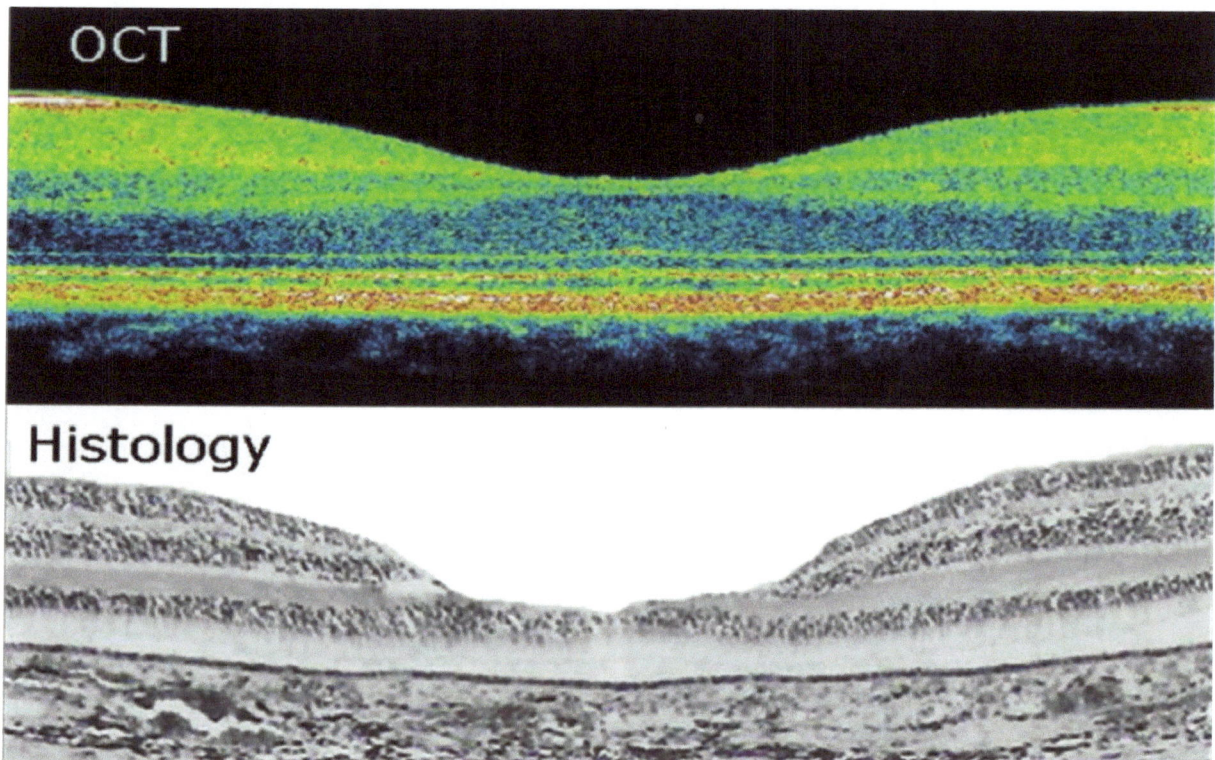

OCT provides a cross-sectional image that closely resembles a histological image of the retina

This knowledge will also be useful for the imager to recognize and remedy artifacts they may encounter as well. As with any imaging modality, communication between the ordering physician and the imager is crucial.

The key to a successful OCT scan is proper initial scan placement and repeatability of that scan. If a patient is being followed for a specific retinal disease, such as wet macular degeneration, proper scan placement at baseline is only half of what is necessary. Subsequent scans must be placed in the same exact location in order to recognize change from the baseline scan. More recent OCT systems have software that automatically aligns the scan with previous scan locations if the correct settings are selected. Older systems, specifically Time Domain technology, may not have this function, and therefore the imager must use anatomical landmarks to repeat the line scan. This is where proper training is important. After all, OCT scanning should be a dynamic, and interactive process. Accepting the first scan produced by the system is often not adequate. The imager, armed with knowledge of disease pathology, ocular anatomy, and a basic understanding of how the OCT system works will be able to produce quality, repeatable scans that are clinically viable.

The physician places an immense amount of responsibility in the hands of the imager. The image produced will, in many cases, determine the diagnosis and may dictate clinical treatment.

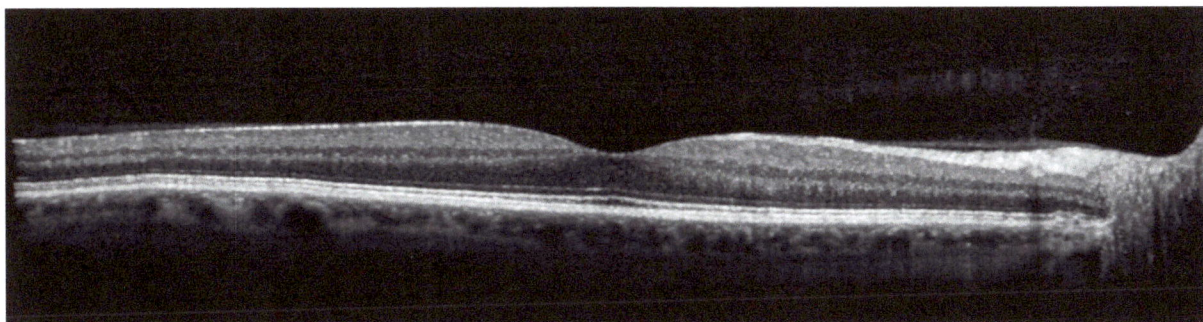

Normal retina in black and white and color

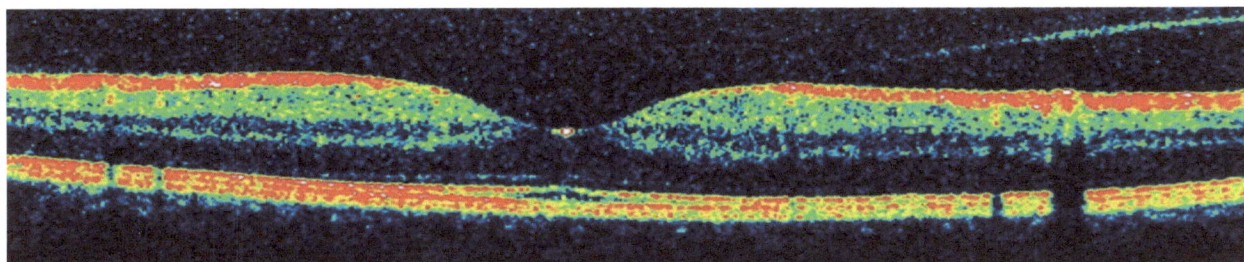

Anatomy of the OCT image

As mentioned previously, OCT is a standard clinical imaging tool that when performed properly can provide invaluable clinical information for the physician. In order to perform a proper scan, the technician must understand how OCT works, be able to identify ocular anatomy, and understand retinal pathophysiologic disease process. All of these are key to providing relevant information to the clinician and will assist in better clinical and treatment decisions. One of the tools a technician should employ is the ability to descriptively interpret an OCT scan. Technicians are not responsible for diagnosing disease based on OCT, but can better their technique by understanding how to descriptively interpret the scan. This facilitates communication between colleagues as well as with physicians. Before submitting the image to the physician through printed or digital image management systems, the technician needs to review his or her work to ensure a proper scan was obtained and the relevant sections are displayed. Being able to recognize how retinal disease manifests on an OCT is one of the best ways to make certain a scan is accurate. In some cases, physicians may be reviewing PDF prints of pre-selected B-scans and it is especially important in these cases for the technician to ensure that the appropriate sections are represented. It is always good practice to upload the complete OCT cube so that physicians can review the full data set. Physicians should be reviewing the full OCT image cube at a workstation to avoid missing relevant pathology.

OCT images can be displayed in pseudo-colors or in gray-scale according to the optical density of tissue. In the case of gray-scale images, borders of retinal layers may be easier to distinguish without the blooming effect that false color may provide. Dense tissue has a higher reflectivity, and will be illustrated in color as red or white. Less dense tissue, such as neurosensory retina, is represented as yellow or green, and even less dense tissue and fluid is represented as black. In gray-scale images highly reflective tissue is represented as white and less reflective tissue is increasingly black. Understanding and recognizing the layers of the retina seen on OCT will help the imager to distinguish pathology and recognize artifacts from true disease.

Vitreous

Internal limiting membrane
Nerve fiber layer
Ganglion cell layer
Inner plexiform layer
Inner nuclear layer
Outer plexiform layer
Outer nuclear layer
External limiting membrane
Inner/outer segment/Ellipsoid
Retinal pigment epithelium
Bruch's membrane
Choriocapillaris/choroid

Sclera

Fovea

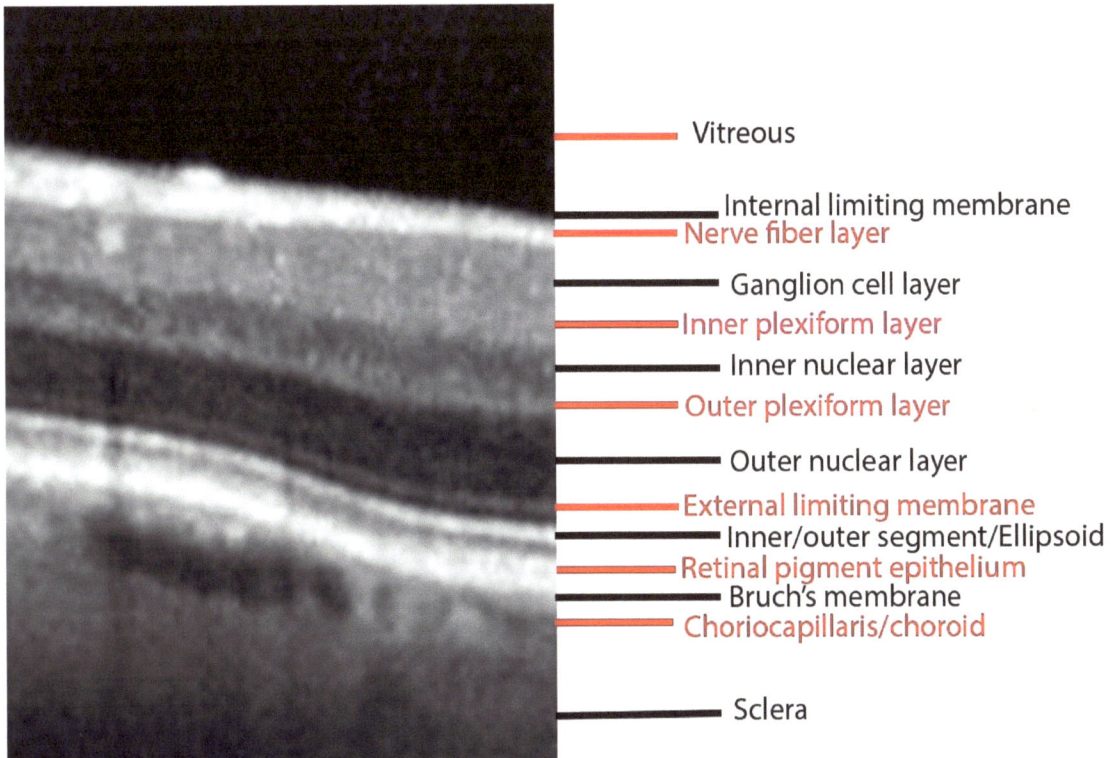

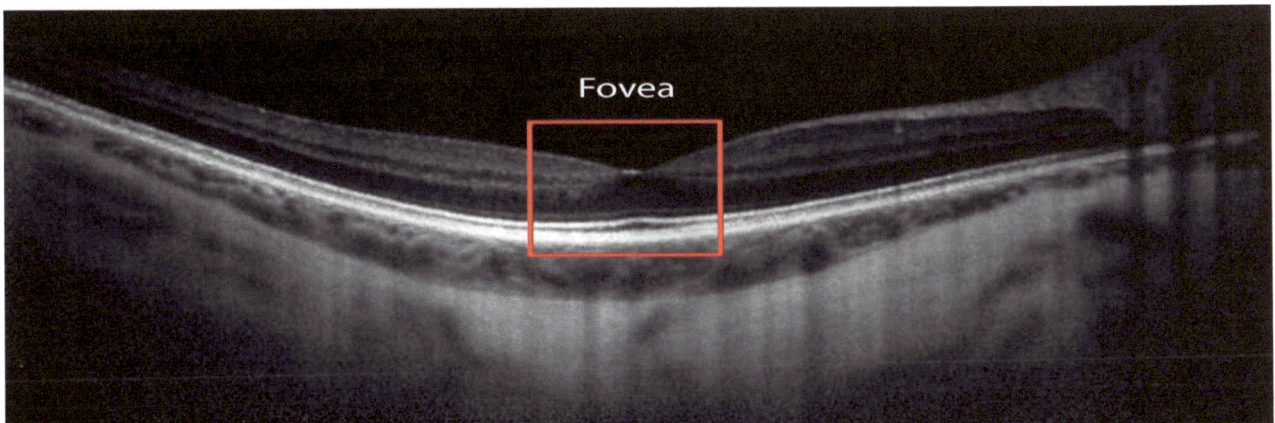

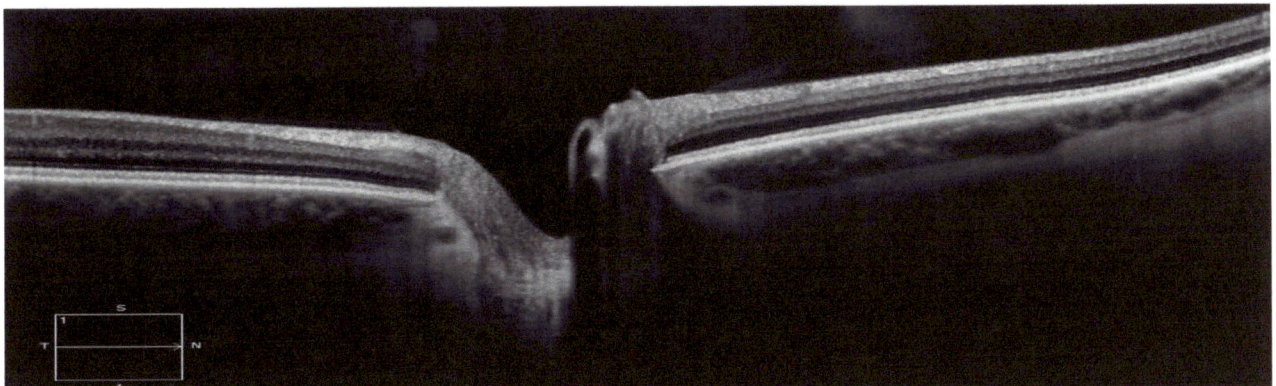

Normal optic nerve on OCT

Knowing all layers of the retina may not be necessary when it comes to descriptive interpretation for the imager. Retinal diseases can affect any layer of the retina but OCT changes generally fall into four categories. These are changes in the vitreoretinal interface, changes in the intraretinal tissue, changes in the subretinal space and lastly changes in the choriocapillaris and choroid.

Understanding a patient's retinal disease pathology is extremely helpful for the imager. A patient who has macular disease, such as macular degeneration or a macular hole, may not be able to fixate properly. Most OCT devices rely on subjective fixation to localize the scan and limit movement artifact. If the patient does not fixate centrally, due to a central visual defect, the OCT may scan parafoveally, or outside the pathologic fovea. The simple fix is to have the patient fixate subjectively, and then physically move the scan to identify the fovea. *(Images 1 and 2)* In order to execute this properly, the technician must be able to recognize retinal anatomy. This particular issue will be revisited as it pertains to specific retinal disease throughout this book.

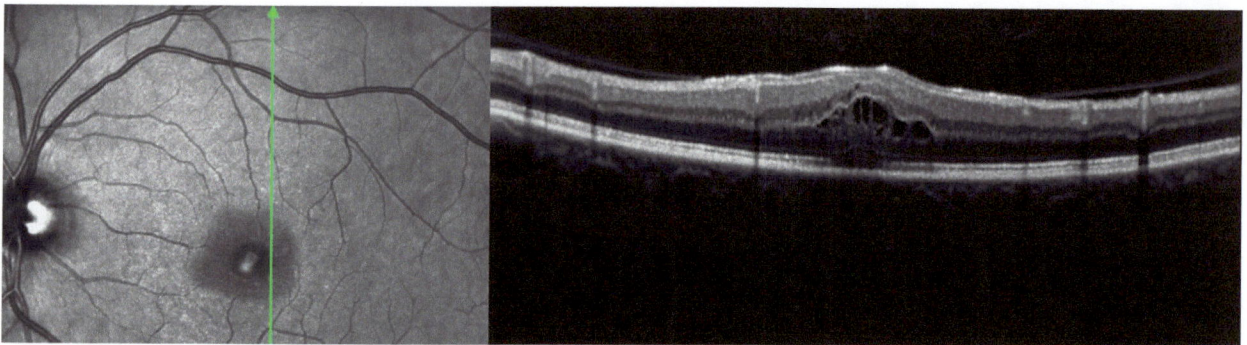

1. OCT image scanned temporal to the fovea, through subjective fixation

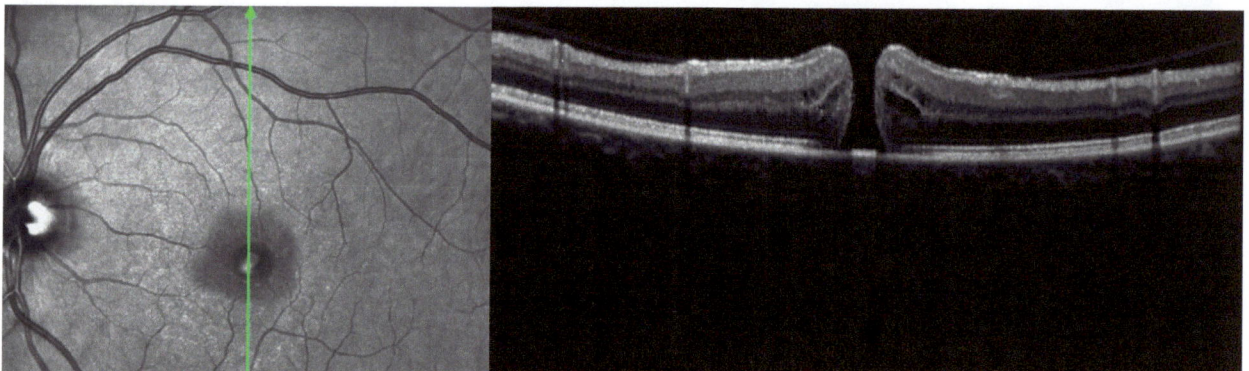

2. OCT image scanned through the fovea, after the user moved the scan

Moving the Scan

To compensate for patient's eye movements, and to ensure that subsequent scans are in the same exact location as original scans, most Spectral Domain OCT
systems have software that "tracks" eye movement, using retinal landmarks (e.g. blood vessels) to place the scan pattern in the same location as previously designated by the user. The system does not interpret pathology, so if an initial scan is performed in the wrong area, subsequent scans will produce the same wrong image.

On most OCT systems the scan pattern may be manually moved either using the mouse or keyboard. This can be done with any type of scan.

In the following example, note that the original scan was properly placed through the fovea, and set as a reference. The second image shows the same patient but now fixating nasally. The software recognizes the retinal landmarks from the previously referenced scan and, despite eccentric fixation, scans the exact same location.

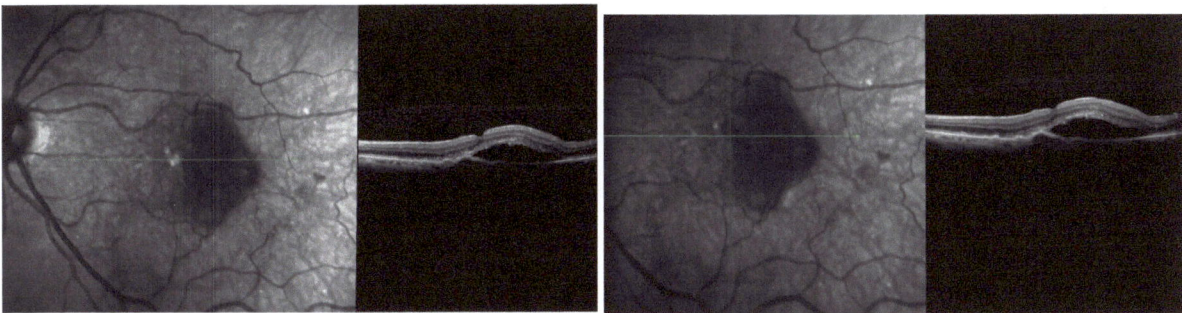

Original scan (left) with follow up scan using the reference set on baseline (right)

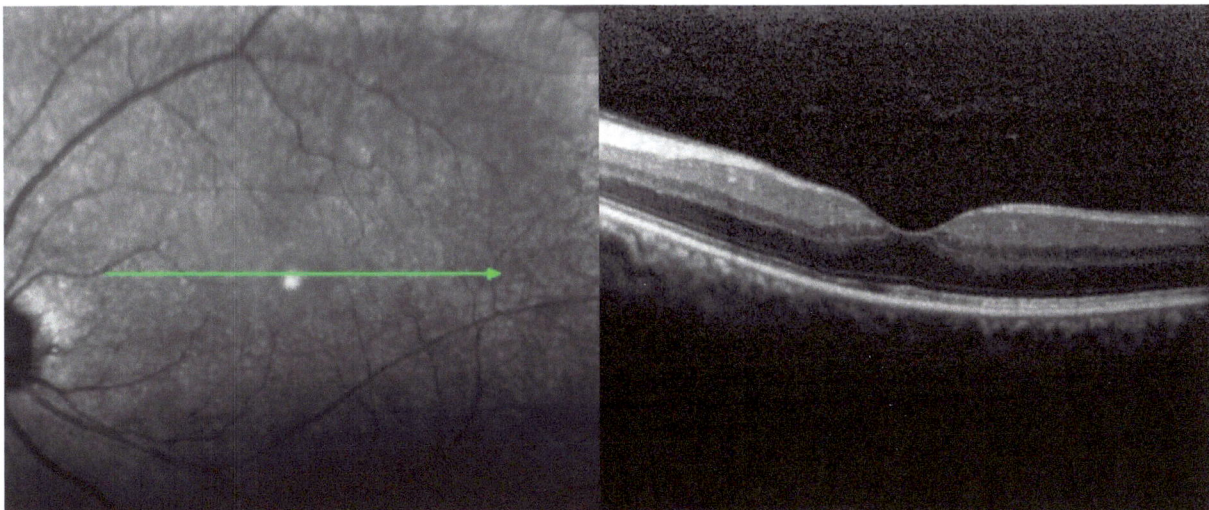

Anatomical structures are not always standard. In this scan, note the location of the fovea, which is higher than normally seen.

Pathology may not be in the linear scan area in one scan, but may be in another. Raster scans are appropriate for pathology that might be missed with a single scan line. Changing the angle of the scan can also reveal pathology. In most cases, a raster scan of the macula should be done to avoid missing relevant pathology.

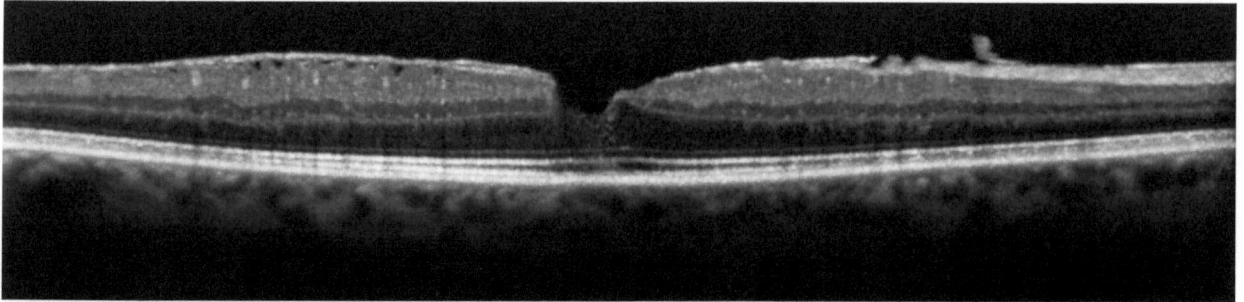

In this horizontal line scan, there is evidence of foveal irregularity, but no clear hole

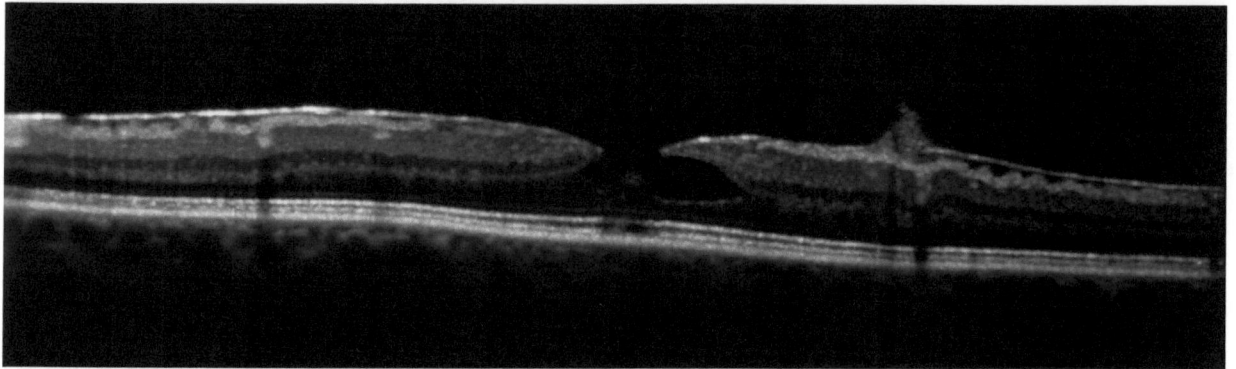

Vertical scan of same patient reveals partial thickness macular hole

Certain pathologies can also present a challenge to obtaining a quality image. Highly myopic patients have longer eyes, so the scan beam "focus" may not reach the retina in these cases. Most OCT software have a setting for normal, long and short eyes. This "pushes" the scan "focus" window into the appropriate plane for the length of the eye.

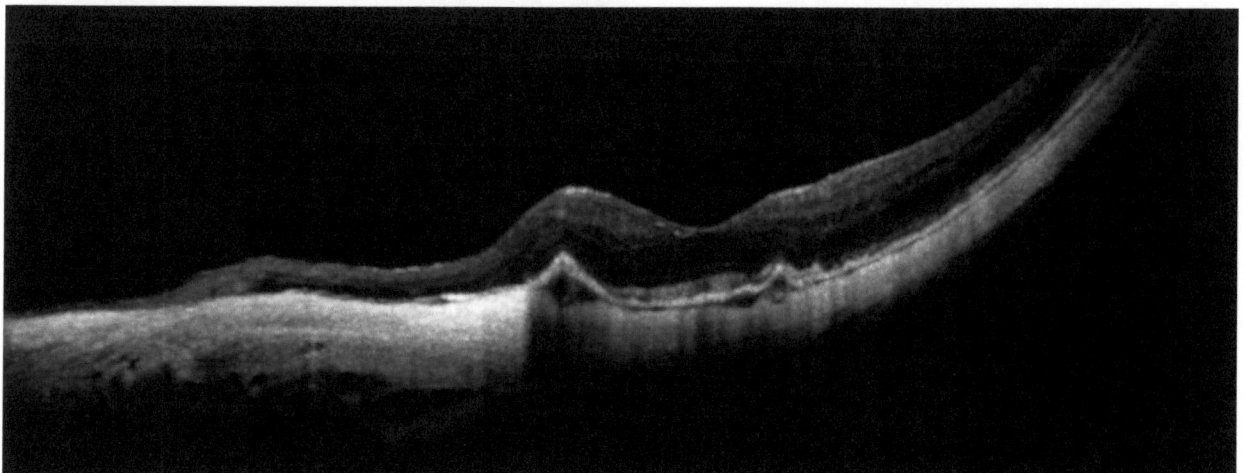

Typical curved scan of a myopic eye

In the case of patients who have trouble reaching the chinrest and forehead bar, switching to a "long eye" setting allows for scanning of an eye that is further away from the objective lens than normal.

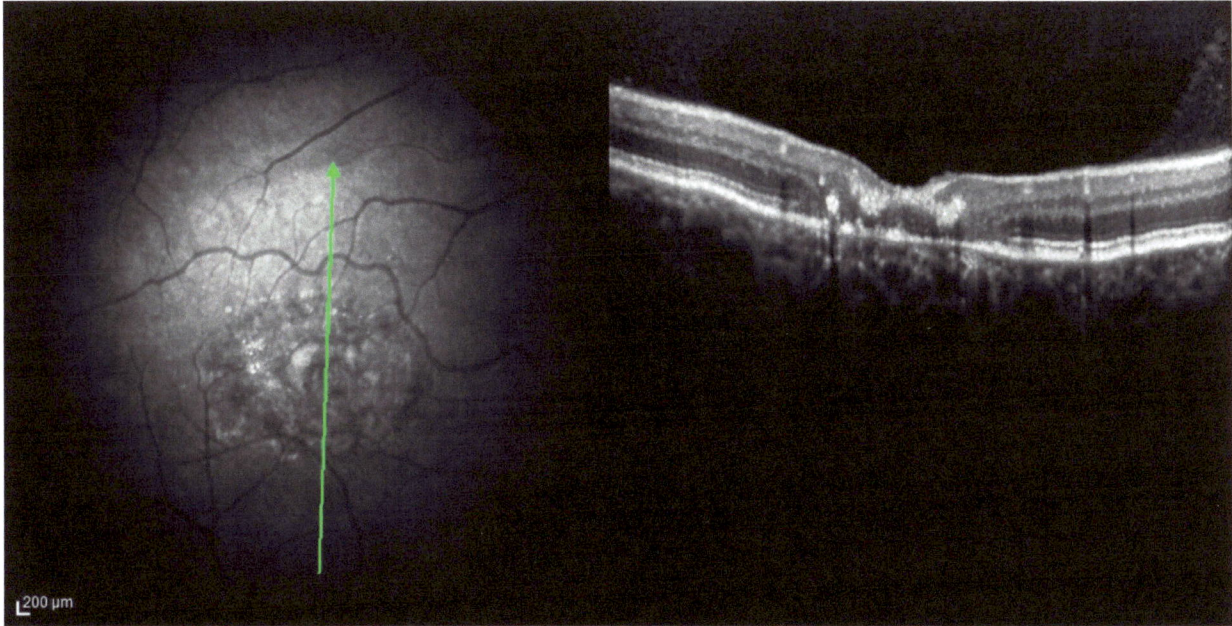

High myopic patient scan in the "long eye" setting. Note the vignetting of the infrared fundus image, which is the iris, due to the objective lens being farther from the eye.

OCT Artifacts

As was discussed, OCT uses light to produce an image, which inherently presents opportunity for artifacts. These artifacts are defined as interference with the normal pathway of light; either when entering the eye or returning from the eye. Any structure that can interfere with light can cause disruption or absence of information. The system has some software algorithms to combat some of the more common interfering anomalies, however, it is important that the imager understands the source of the artifact and identifies the resulting data as artifact.

When light enters the eye, it passes through the tear film, cornea, anterior chamber, lens or intraocular lens implant, and vitreous before it strikes the anterior surface of the retina, the internal limiting membrane. Opacity in any of those layers can cause disruption of the OCT light signal.

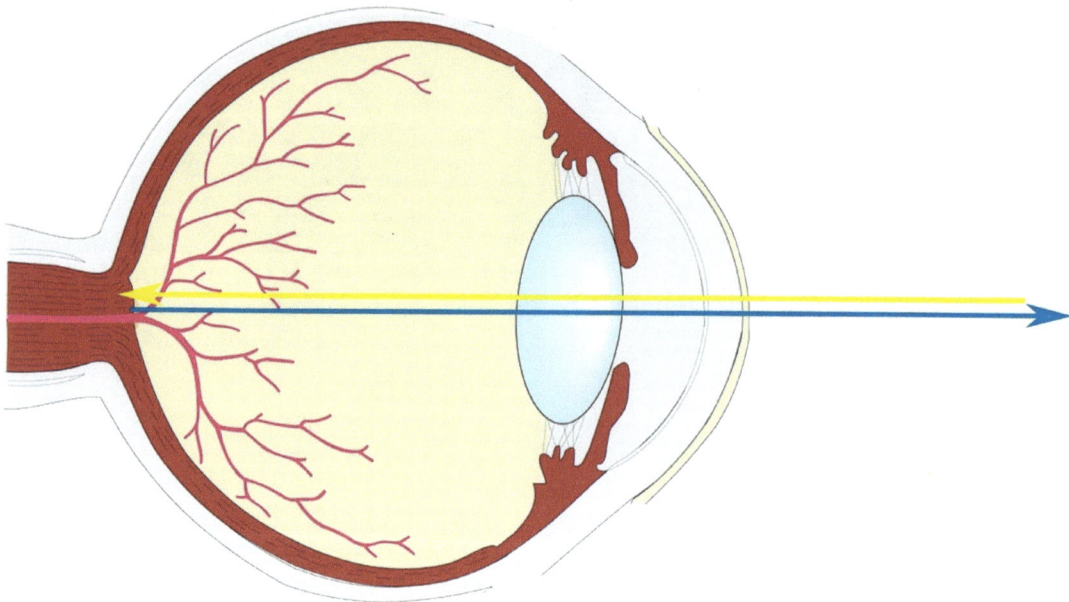

Light enters the eye (yellow arrow) and exits the eye (blue arrow), encountering structure and pathology along the pathway

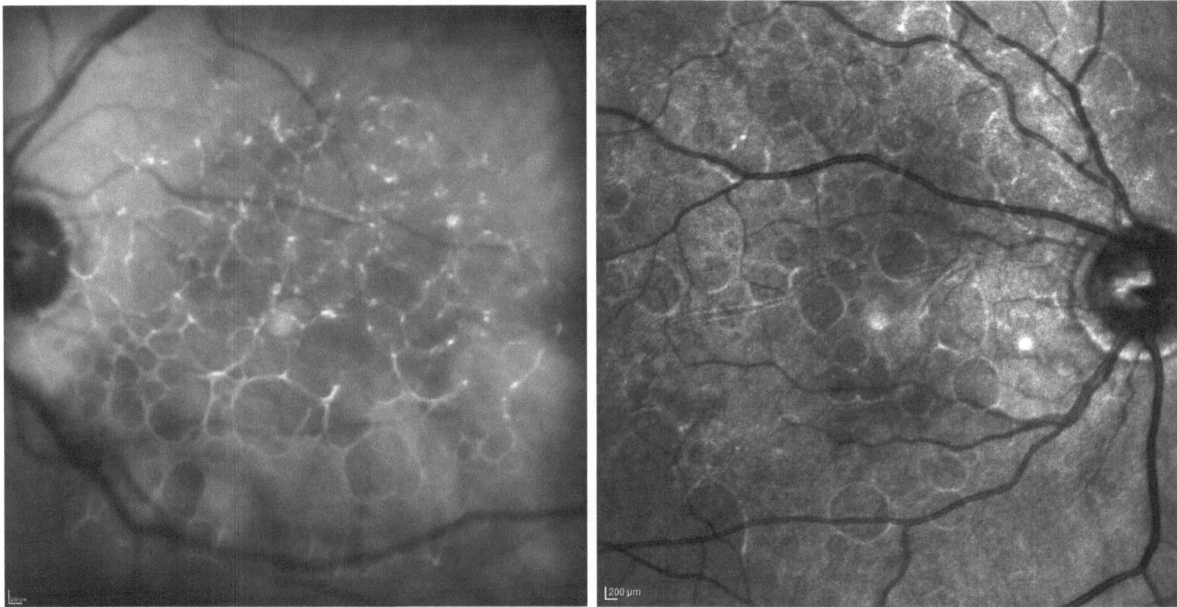

Drying of the tear film will result in white mosaic patterns on the infrared fundus image

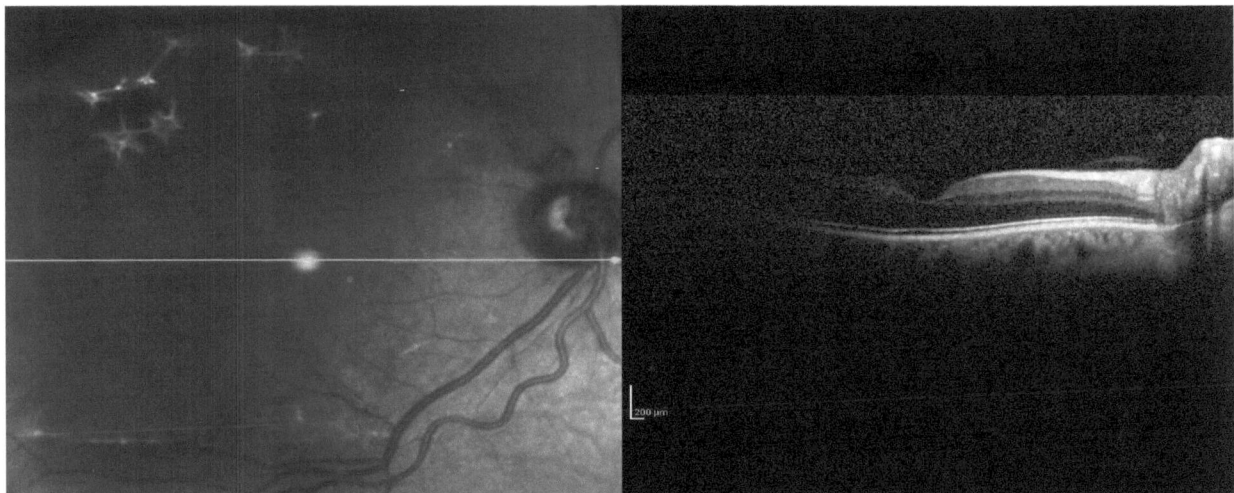

Signal loss temporally due to lens changes in a patient with a cataract. Also note the white reflections on the IR image from corneal drying

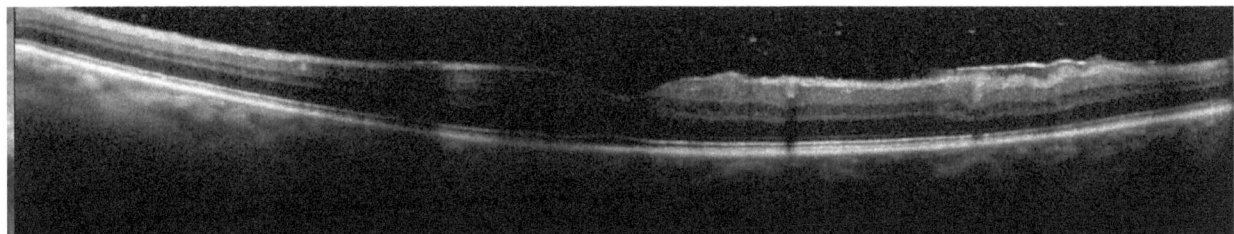

Vitreous hemorrhage or opacity can also block the light signal

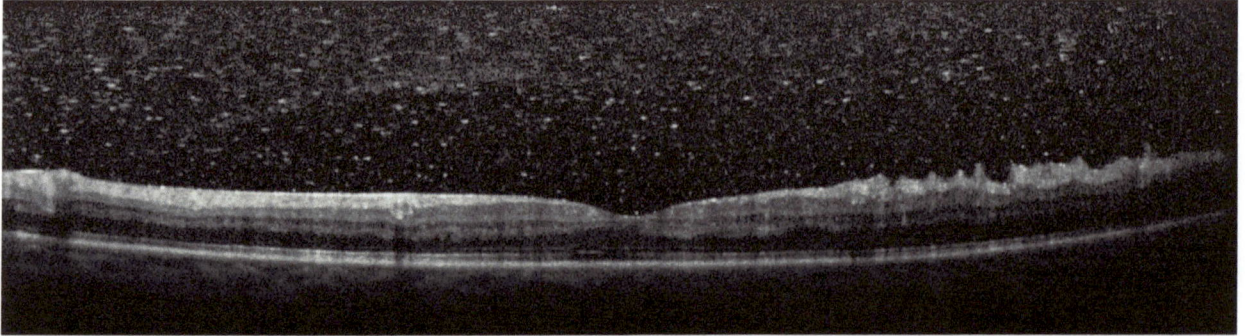

Vitreous hemorrhage or debris seen on the OCT B-scan

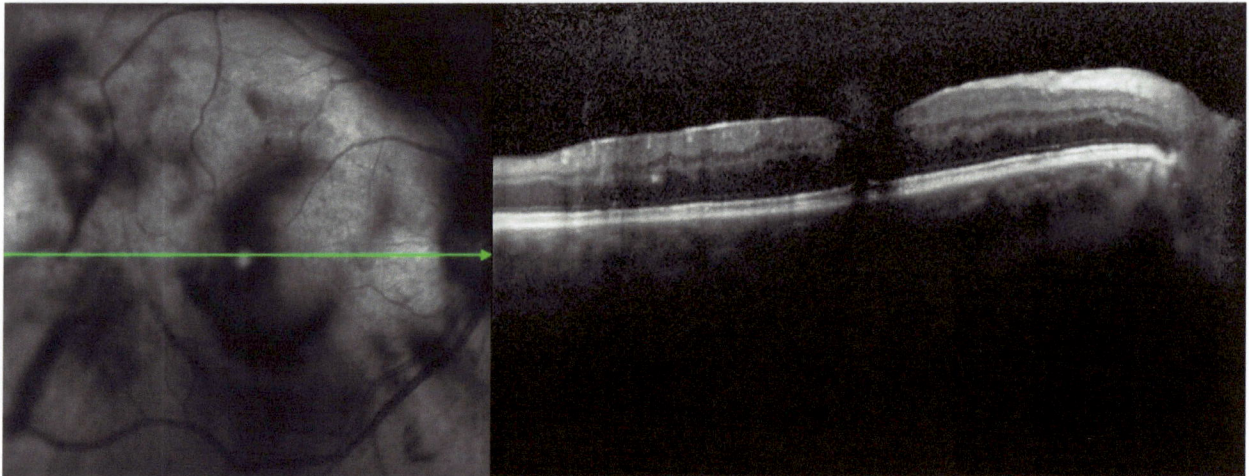

Vitreous hemorrhage can obscure detail in the retina by casting shadows. Having the patient move their eye can move the hemorrhage long enough to complete the scan, as below.

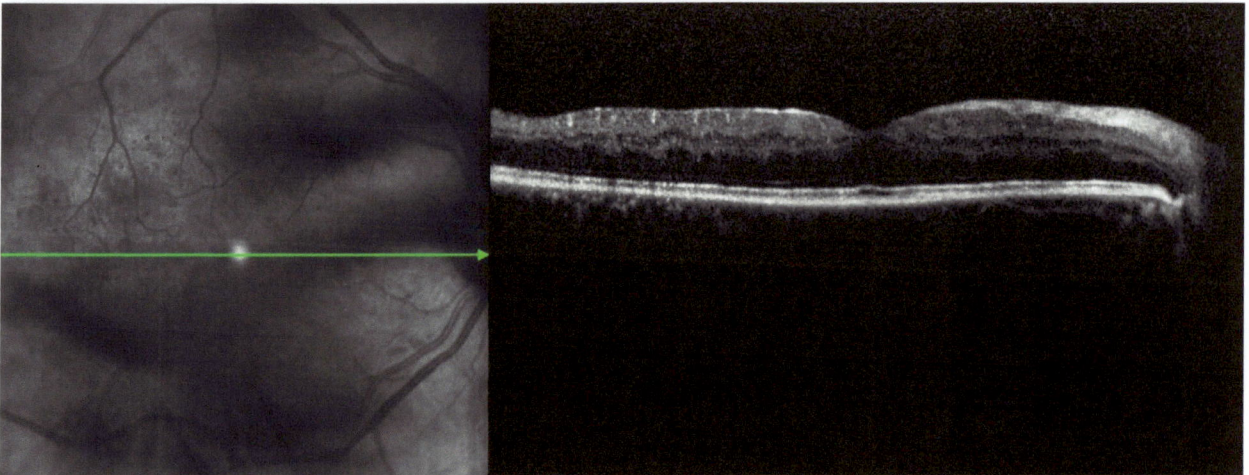

Oversampling, or averaging, is a software algorithm that combines multiple scan images from the same scanned area to produce a composite image. In most cases, it is a useful tool to work around regions with diminished signal.

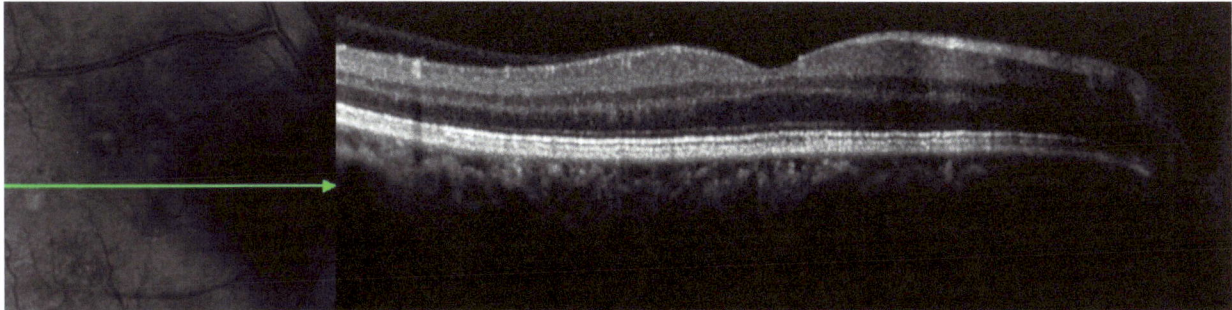

The nasal (right) aspect of this image is degraded due to vitreous hemorrhage

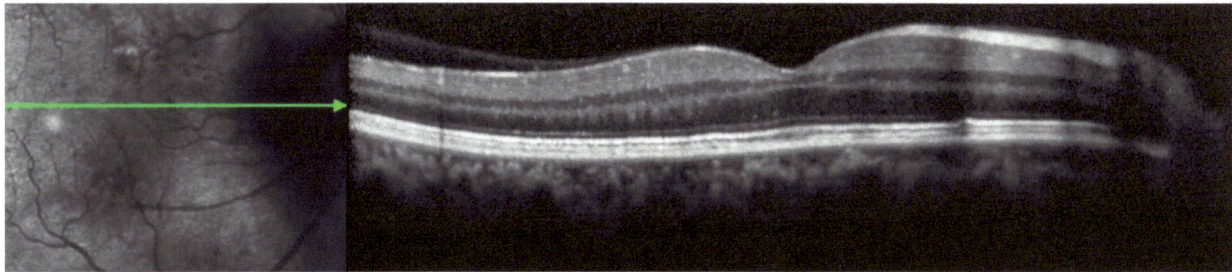

Same image using oversampling. Note the detail in the same area that was blocked previously

In some cases, due to multiple scans taken during slight eye movement, oversampling can "fill in" data from surrounding normal areas.

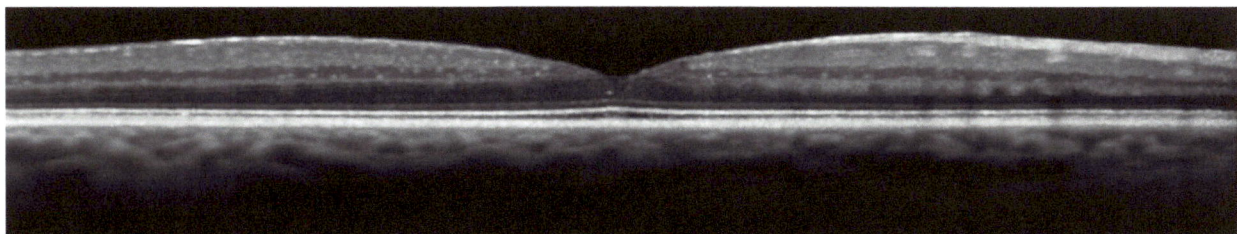

In this case, oversampling produces a normal appearing fovea

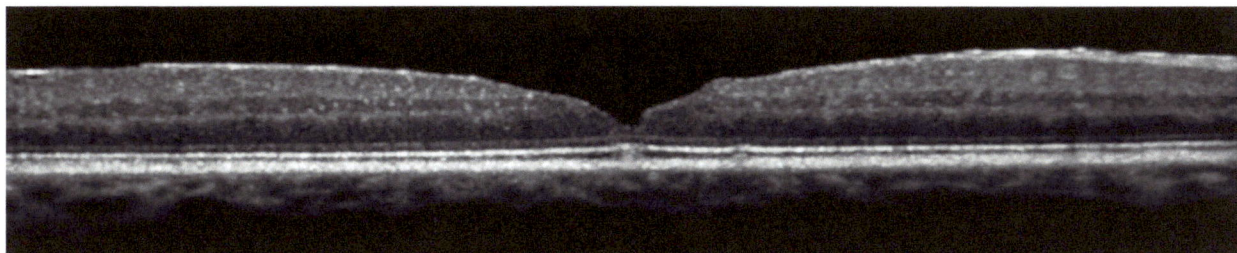

The same patient is scanned without oversampling, and a partial hole is revealed

It is also important to recognize anatomy that will normally cause artifact, such as posterior shadowing from blood vessels.

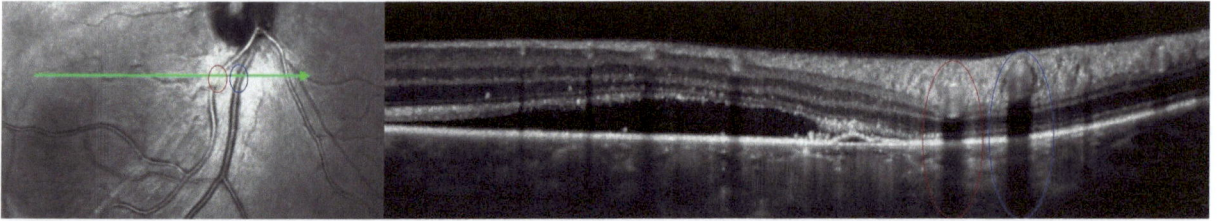

In this example, the artery is circled in red and vein in blue. Note the shadowing posterior to the vessels on the OCT image, due to loss of light signal once the light meets the vessel.

OCT systems are very susceptible to eye movement, as well as outside interference as demonstrated in the examples below:

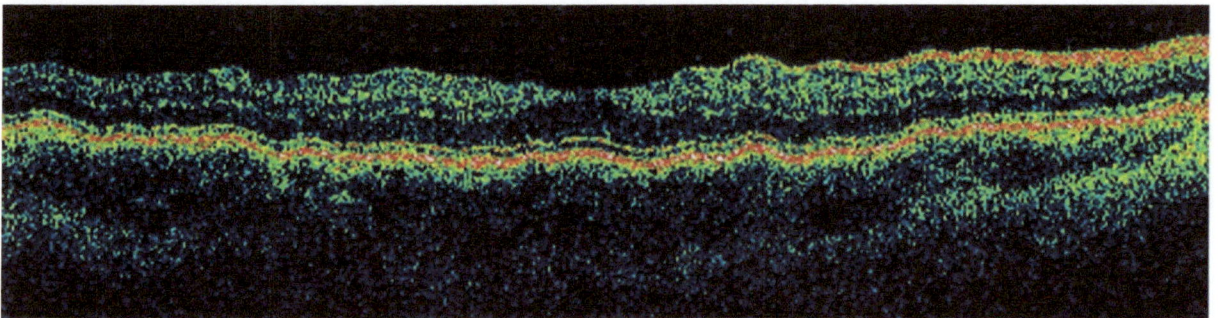

Building HVAC system under the floor in the OCT room can cause movement artifact. Note the "ripple effect" throughout the retinal layers.

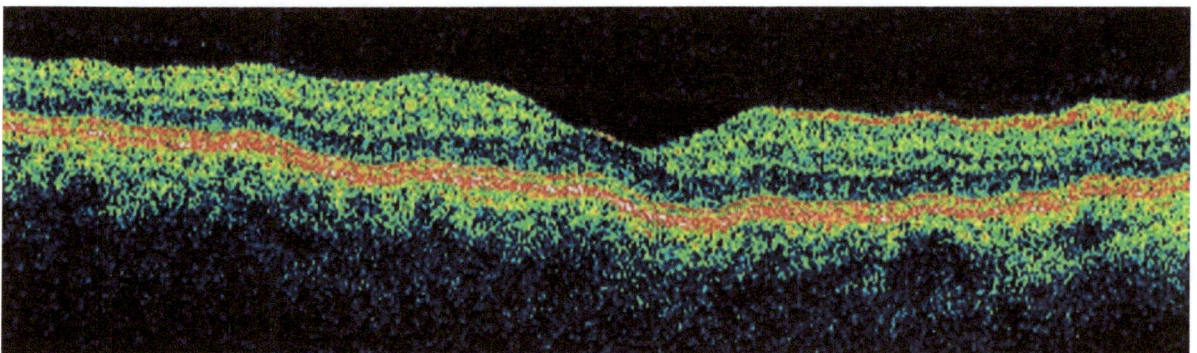

Patient with nystagmus

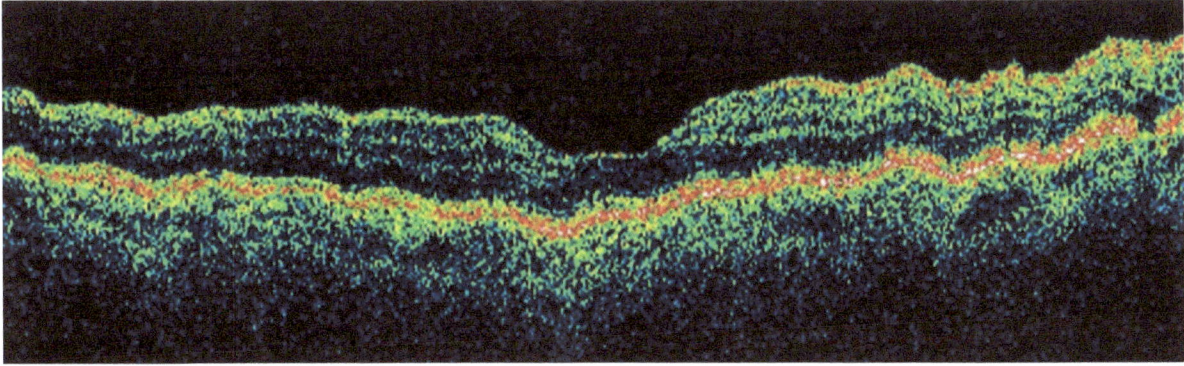

Patient with head tremor

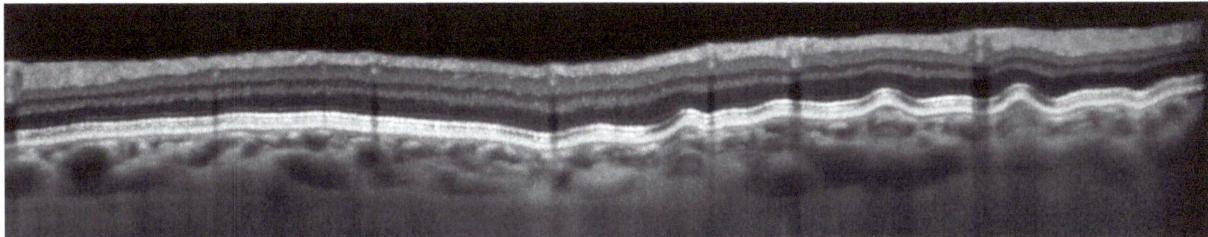

Choroidal folds

Enhanced Depth Imaging and Full Depth Imaging

Because OCT imaging systems have a limited depth-of-field, approximately 2-2.5 millimeters depending on the system, the decision to image either the anterior or posterior retinal tissue needs to be made. Anterior retinal imaging, which is to say the focus window lies from the vitreo-retinal interface to the choriocapillaris is done in the default setting of the OCT. Choroidal imaging, from approximately the RPE to the choroidal-scleral junction can be done using the Enhanced Depth Imaging (EDI) function on the OCT. This moves the window of focus posteriorly, which results in a higher resolution and more detailed image of the choroid while at the same time, imaging of the anatomy anterior to the RPE will be degraded. To create one image that captures the total of retinal tissue in focus, a technique called Full Depth Imaging (FDI) can be employed. This is done by setting the over-sampling size high, and scanning half the samples in standard mode, then the remaining samples in EDI mode. This technique will result in a larger window of focus, i.e.; from 2.5 to 5 millimeters.

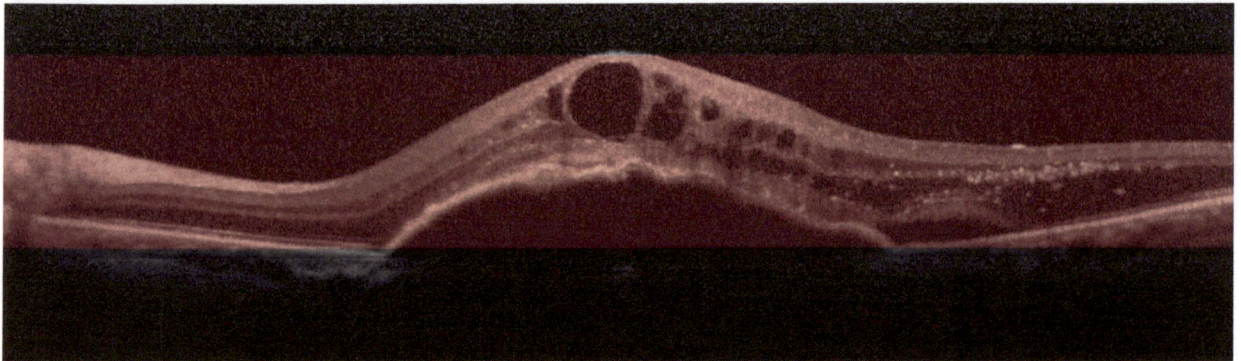

OCT B-scan using normal OCT settings. The focus is from the vitreo-retinal interface to the choriocapillaris (highlighted in red), with degraded image quality posteriorly.

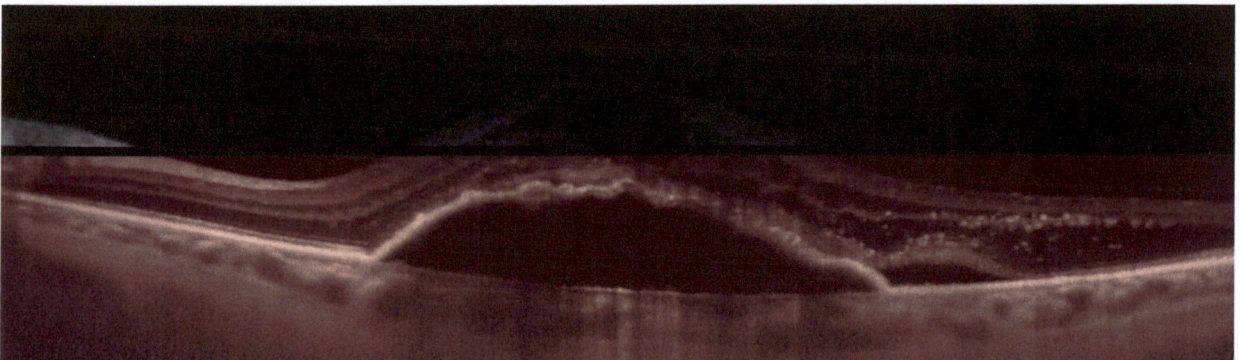

OCT B-scan using Enhanced Depth Imaging. The focus is shifted to the sub-RPE and choroidal-scleral junction, with degraded image quality anteriorly.

19

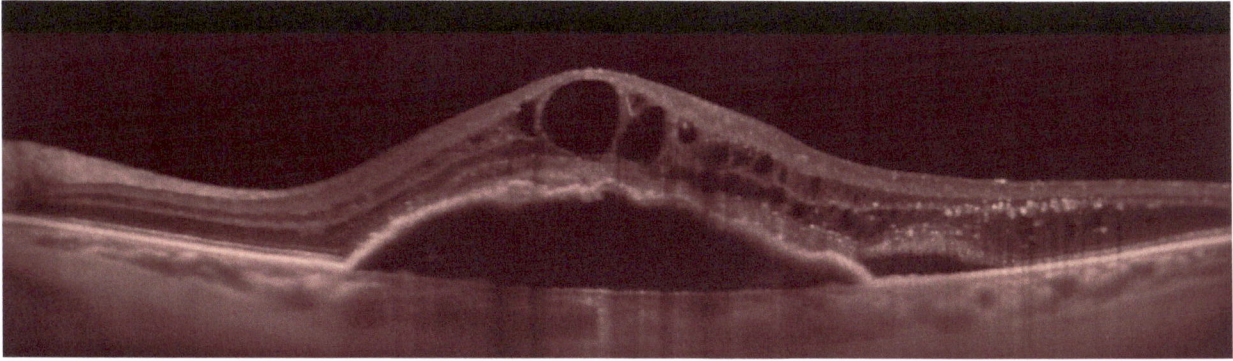

OCT B-scan using Full Depth Imaging, which combines standard and EDI imaging, rendering the entire retinal structure, from the internal limiting membrane to the choroidal-scleral junction in focus.

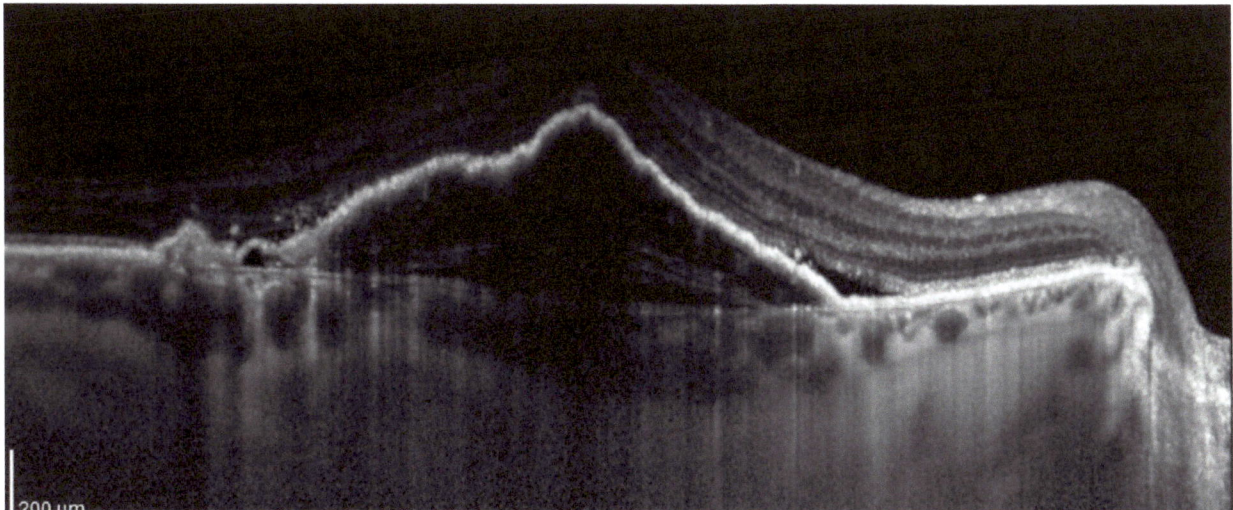

Enhanced Depth Imaging of RPE detachment (above) and Full Depth Imaging of same patient (below)

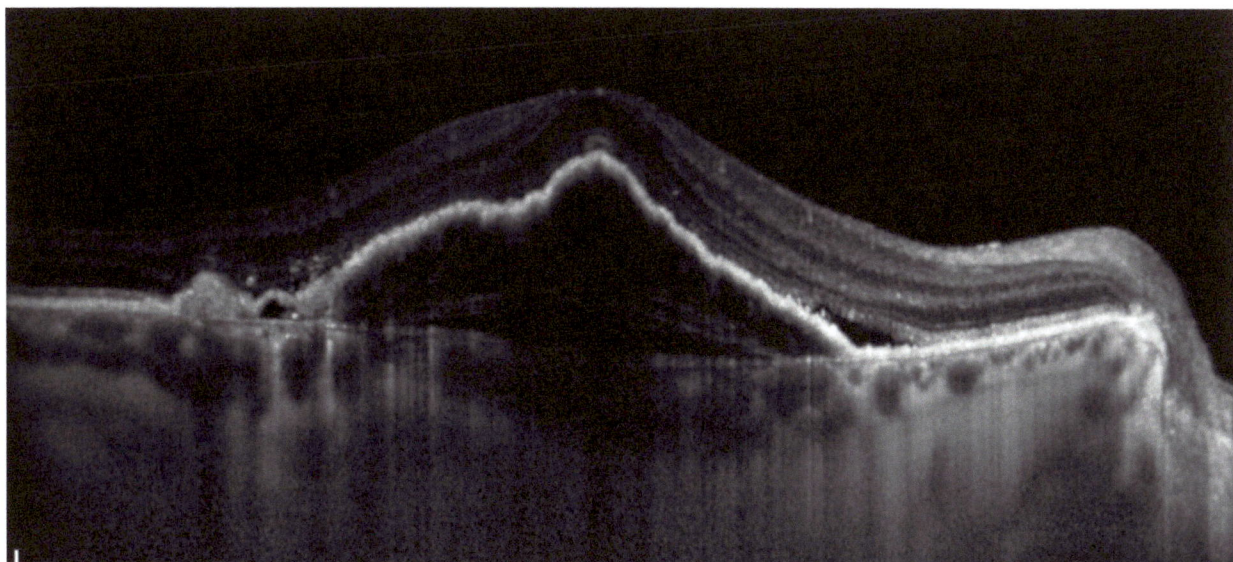

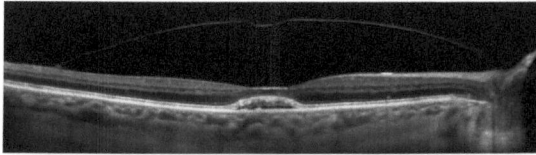

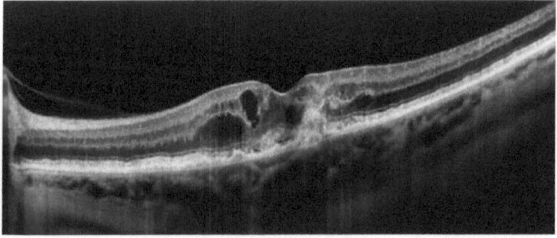

Examples of Full Depth Imaging

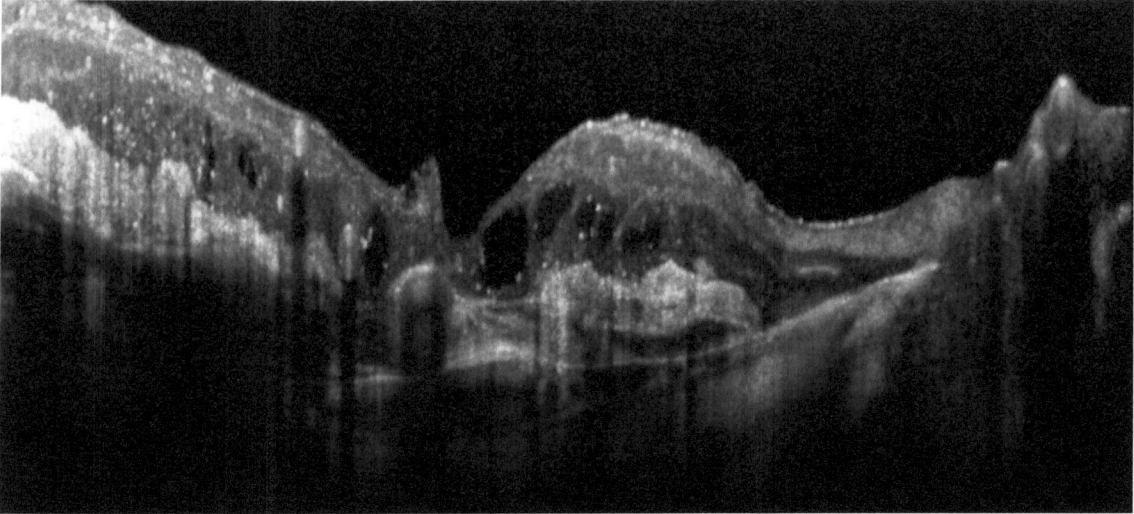

Standard focus on B-scan OCT of advanced neovascular AMD

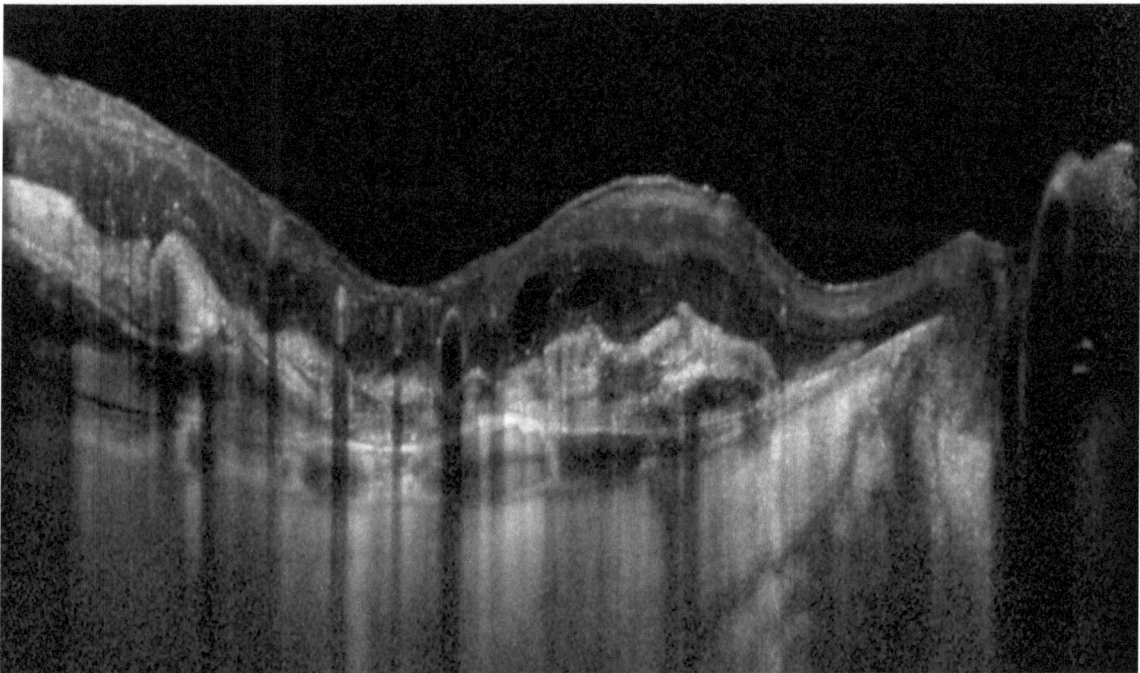

Full Depth Imaging of the same patient with advanced neovascular AMD

There are multiple options available for line B-scans, and until the imager is more comfortable with recognition of both anatomy and patterns of pathology, it is recommended to not restrict the scans to a single line, but utilize the scan protocols available.

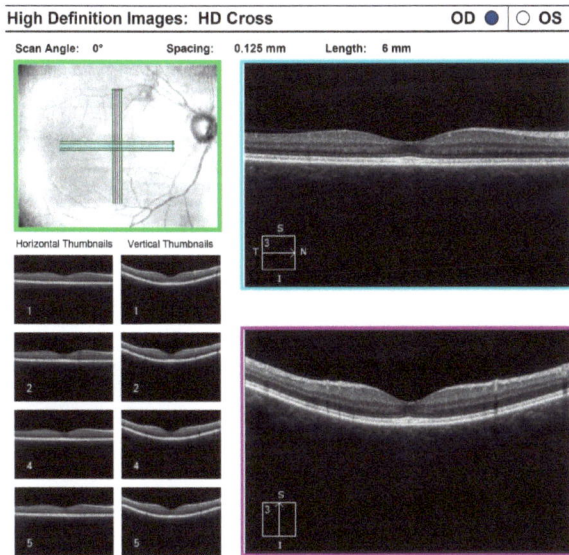

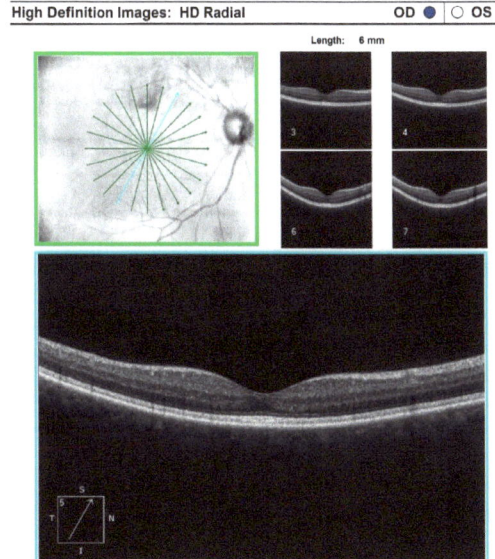

Examples of line B-scan options

Volumetric OCT

Volumetric OCT is a scan and analysis protocol that is particularly useful for following progression or regression of intraretinal fluid as well as sub-retinal fluid. Disease pathologies that manifest themselves with intraretinal fluid, such as cystoid macular edema, diabetic macular edema, vein occlusions, etc., present as excellent subjects for baseline and follow up volumetric analysis. Volumetric protocols include macular cubes and raster scans, which utilizes multiple scans over an area of the retina. In most systems, over sampling of line scans in the raster occurs (more about over sampling later), although when viewing the individual B-scans within a volume scan, they may appear grainy. This is due to the fact that most volumetric scans use line B-scans with less data points to produce a faster volume scan that is spread over a larger area.

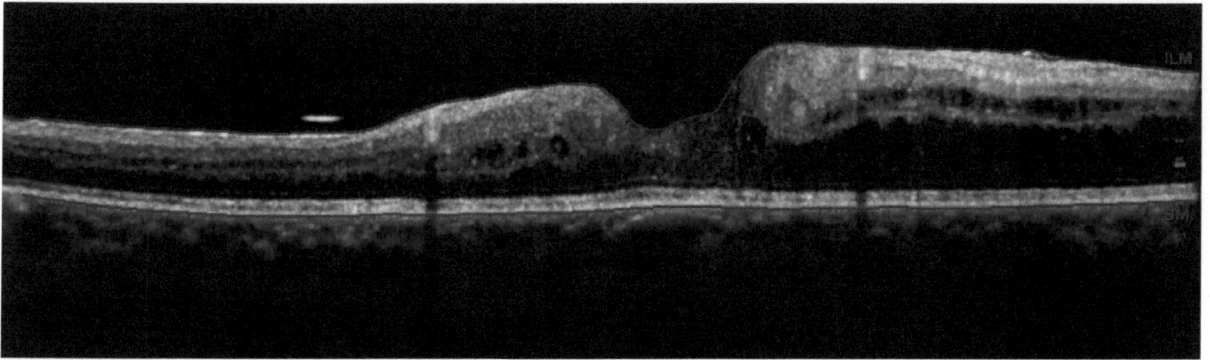

The boundary lines (in red) are at the internal limiting membrane and Bruch's Membrane

Volumetric OCT is particularly useful for following the volumetric change in retinal tissue on subsequent visits, and especially after treatment of intraretinal fluid. The software will not only show false color and numerical volumetric measurements, but can also display change analysis between images, represented in both color and numeric values. Normal foveal and retinal thickness varies by age, race and gender as well as by type and generation of OCT technology that is used. Caution is required in comparing thicknesses between and among subjects and devices.

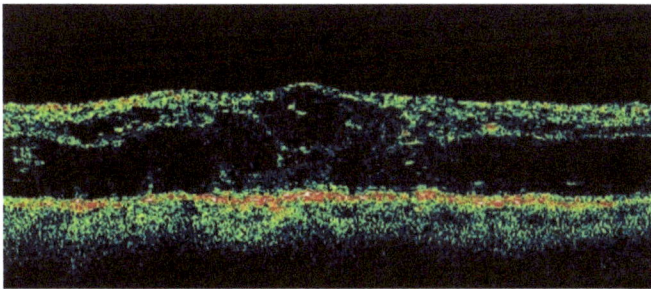

Pre treatment

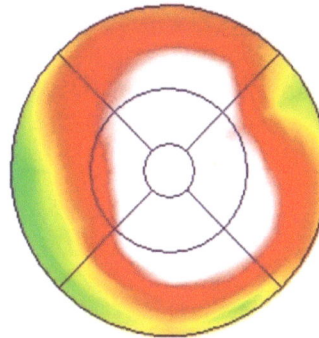

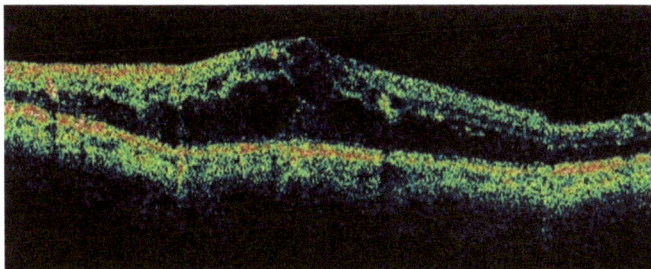

First treatment session

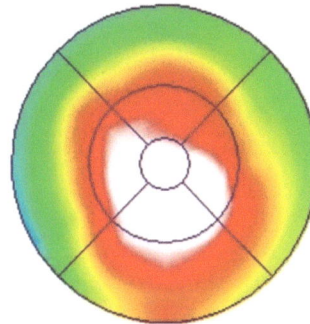

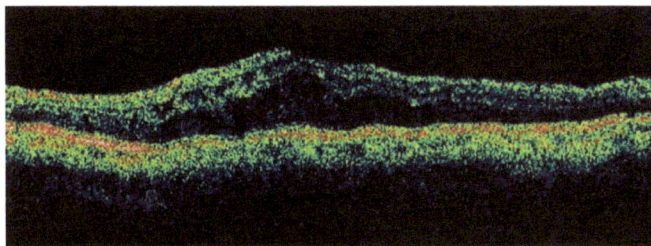

Second treatment session

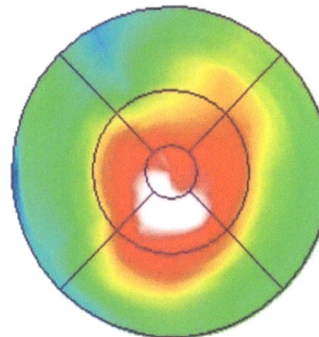

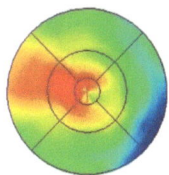

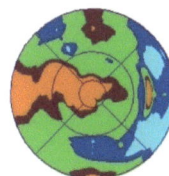

	Foveal Thickness	
OD	Total Macular Volume	
	Foveal Thickness	338+/-27 microns
OS	Total Macular Volume	7.83 mm²

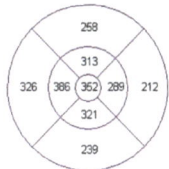

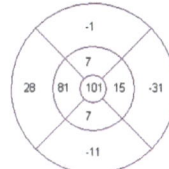

0 100 200 300 400 500 µm

-60 -40 -20 +20 +40 +60µm

Patient/Scan Information	
Scan Type	Fast Macular Thickness Map
Scan Date	6/14/2006 - 11/17/2005
Scan Length	6.0 mm

Pretreatment

Post treatment change analysis

It is important to evaluate the individual line B-scans that make up the volumetric OCT. Some pathology may mimic thickened or atrophic retina, and segmentation algorithms may be inaccurate. For example, here is a B-scan OCT of an epiretinal membrane that spans the fovea:

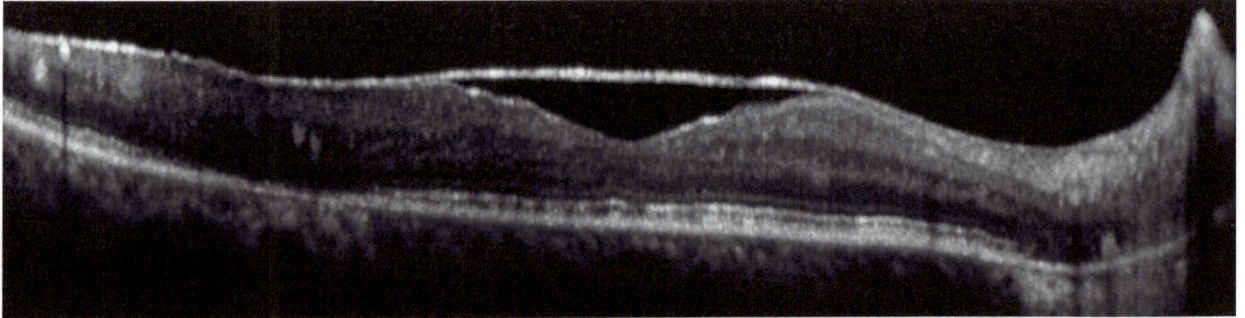

The corresponding volumetric OCT falsely reads the epiretinal membrane as the anterior aspect of the retina, and therefore interprets the retinal tissue as thicker than it actually is:

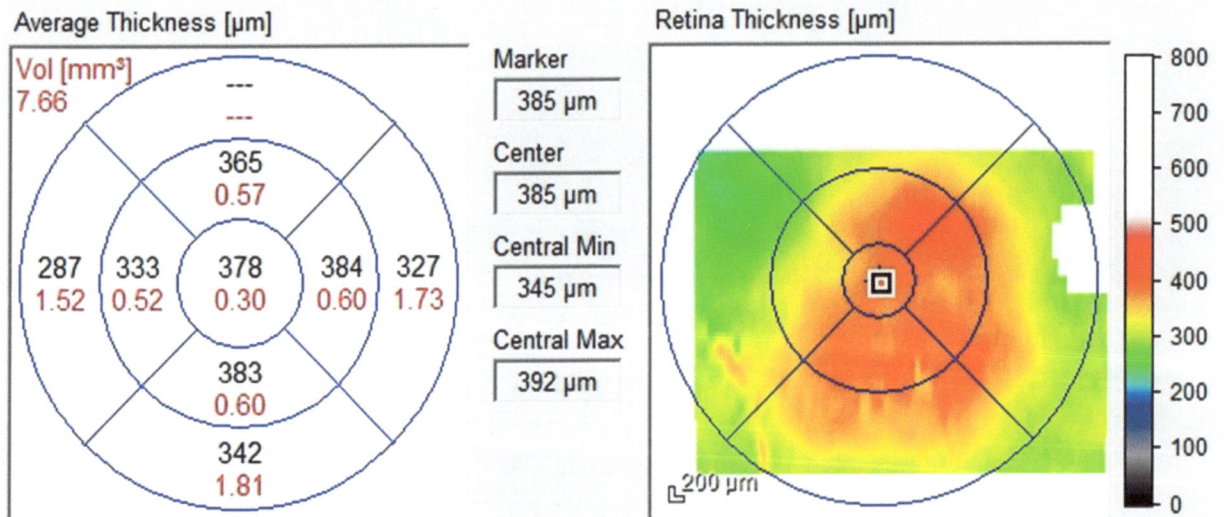

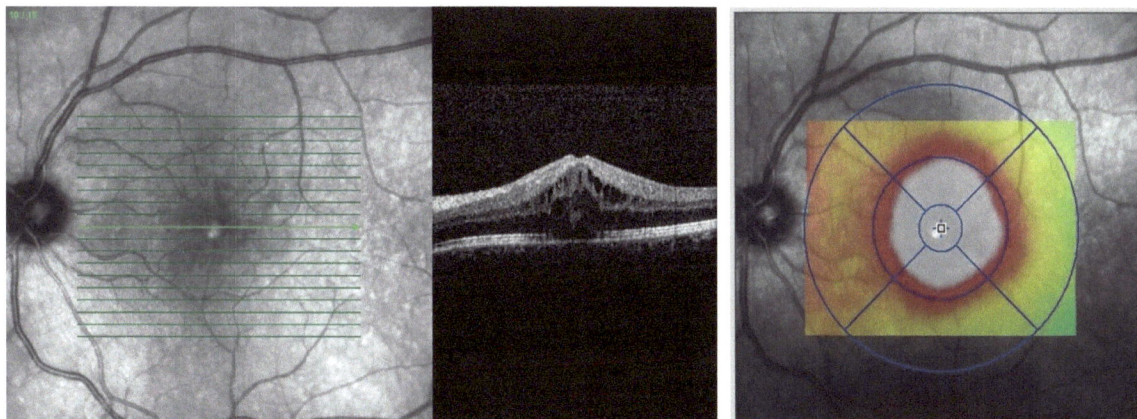

A raster scan (on the left), which uses a linear pattern of B-scans either horizontally or vertically, produces a color display (on the right) representing retinal tissue volume.

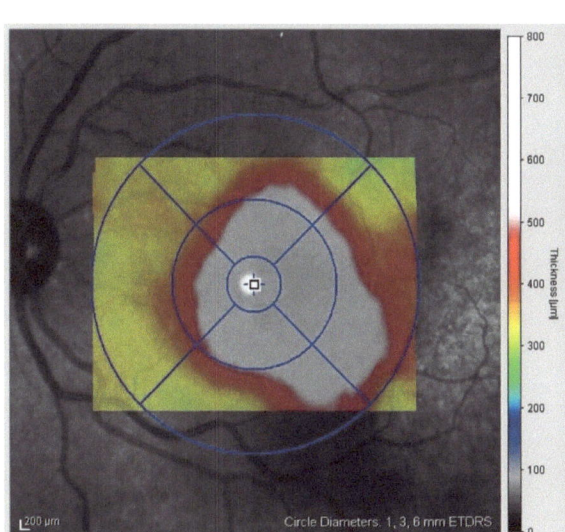

Macular edema pretreatment

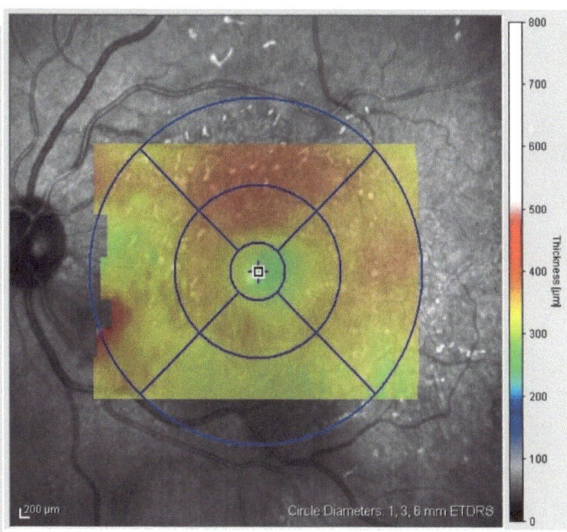

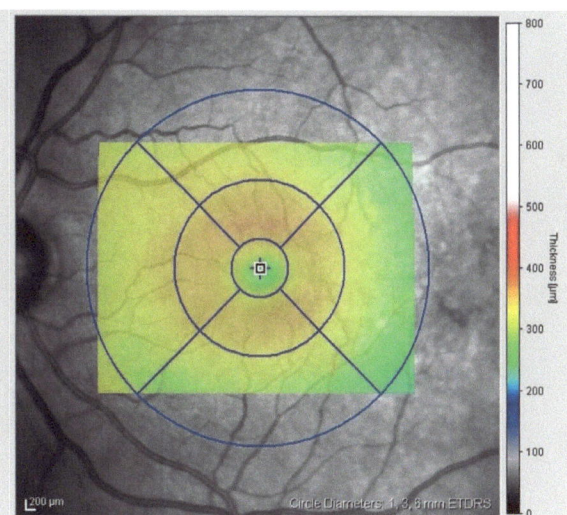

Post treatment

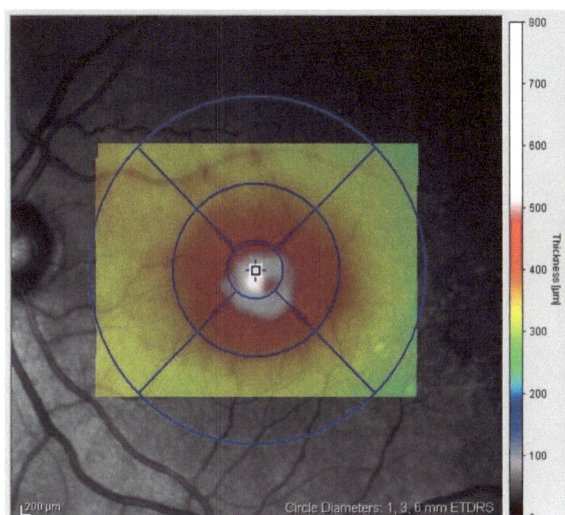

Macular edema pretreatment

Post treatment

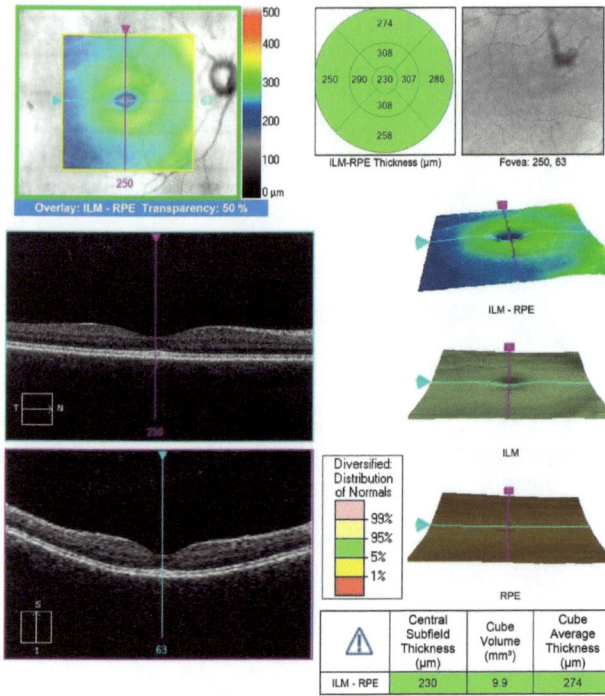

Normal macula thickness analysis with volumetric and B-scan OCT

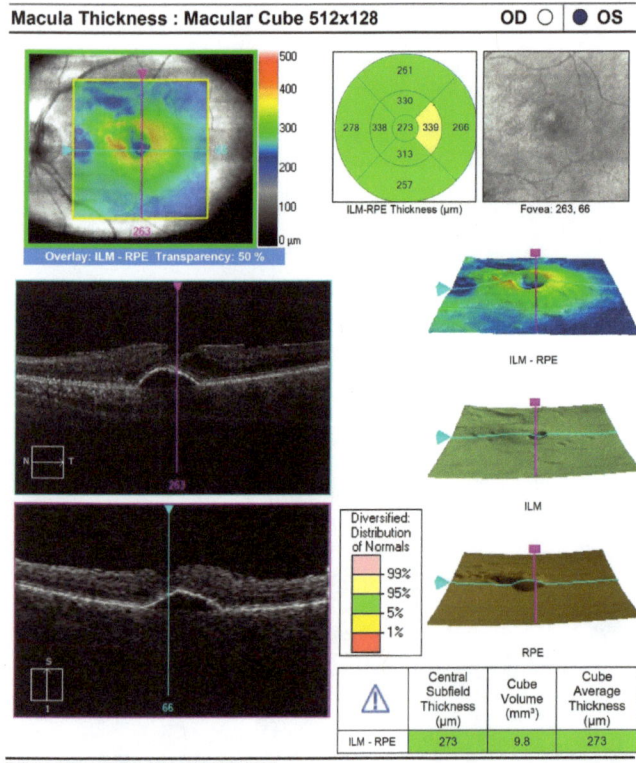

Macula thickness analysis with volumetric and B-scan OCT of RPE detachment

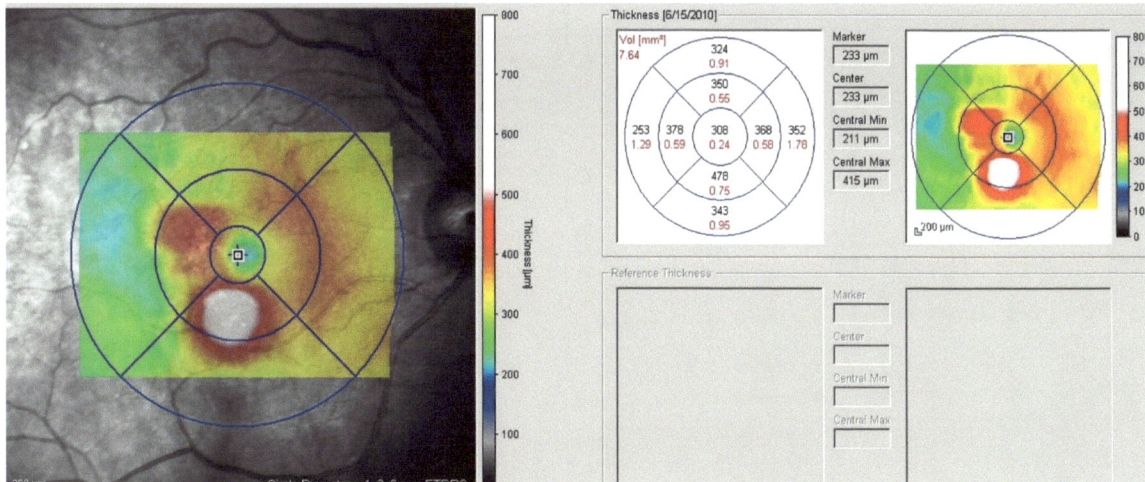

Volumetric OCT of an inferior RPE detachment

Macula Thickness : Macular Cube 512x128   OD ●   ○ OS

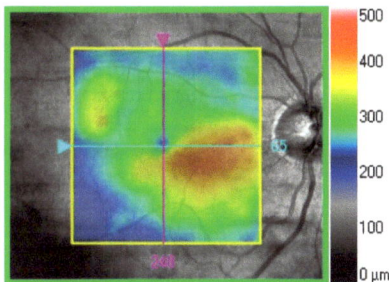

Overlay: ILM - RPE Transparency: 50 %

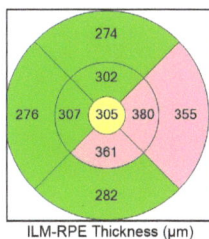

ILM-RPE Thickness (µm)

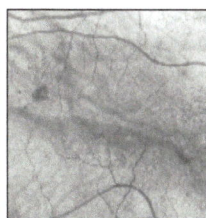

Fovea: 248, 65

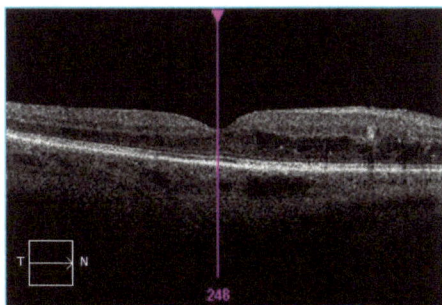

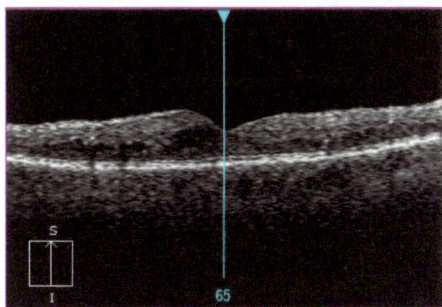

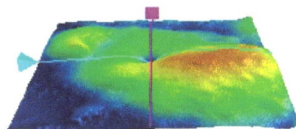

ILM - RPE

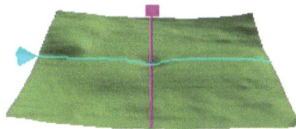

ILM

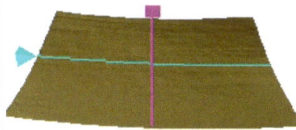

RPE

Volumetric and B-scan of BRVO

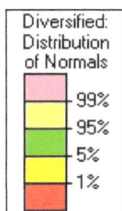

Diversified: Distribution of Normals	
▮	99%
▮	95%
▮	5%
▮	1%

⚠	Central Subfield Thickness (µm)	Cube Volume (mm³)	Cube Average Thickness (µm)
ILM - RPE	305	10.7	296

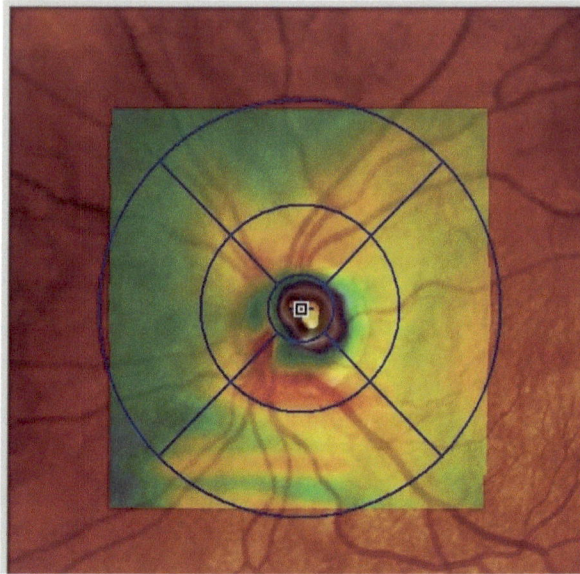

Normal volumetric OCT of optic nerve head

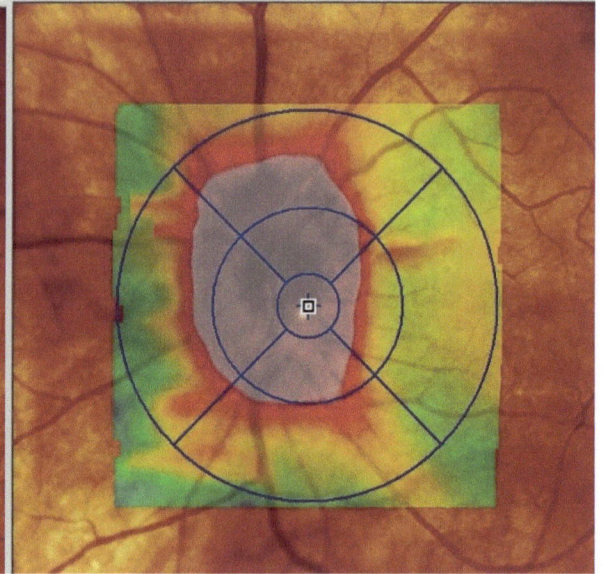

Volumetric OCT of optic nerve head with papilledema

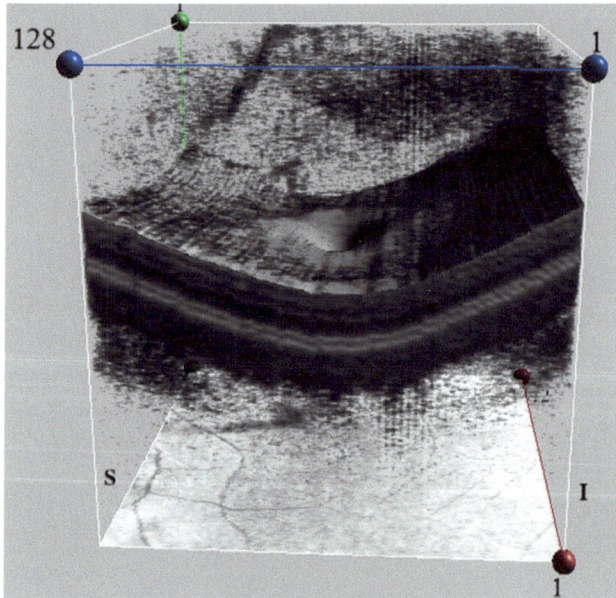

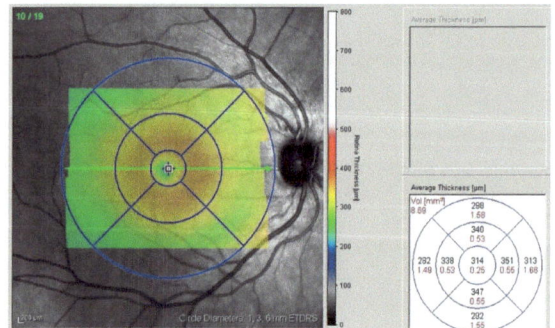

3 Dimensional rendering of normal OCT with volumetric OCT

OCT Angiography

Optical Coherence Tomographic Angiography (OCTA) was introduced commercially in 2015, and the Zeiss Angioplex system was the first FDA approved device to market in the US.

This technology is based on spectral domain OCT; both the acquisition and the analysis process are different than OCT in a few key aspects which allow for the detection of movement within the tissue. Since red blood cells are the only moving objects within retinal tissue, OCTA images nicely highlight the blood vessels in the vast majority of cases. OCTA scan patterns are similar to standard OCT patterns except that OCTA patterns require multiple B-scans (often 3-4) to be repeated in the same location so OCTA patterns may take a few seconds longer. The variation in the phase and/or the intensity of the backscattered light is then determined based on the comparison of the multiple B-scans in each section. Since moving red blood cells cause the most variation in the phase and intensity of backscattered light, blood vessels appear the brightest on OCTA images and static tissue (retina) appears dark.

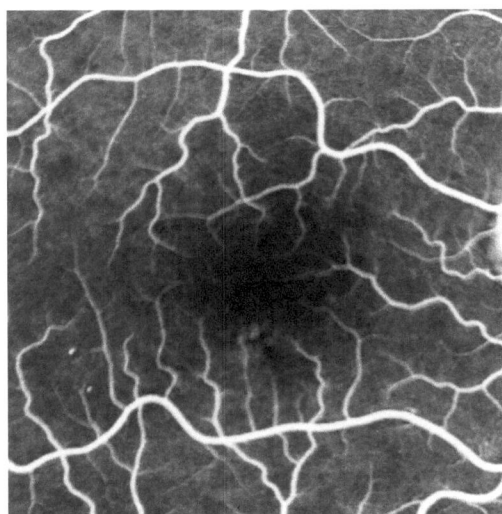

Macula on fluorescein angiogram

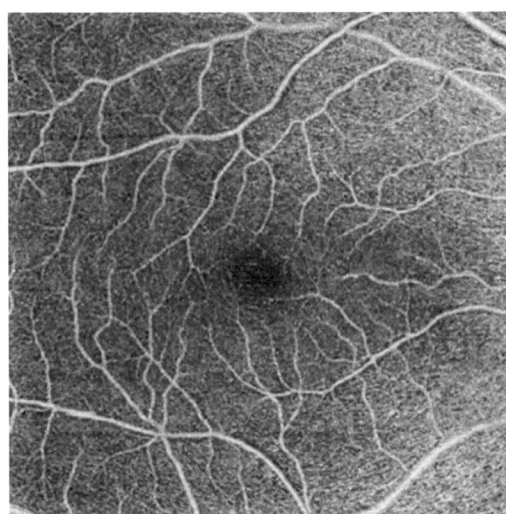

Macula on OCTA

The analysis software also allows for color depth encoding, which assigns different colors to the moving particles (blood vessels) depending on the depth in which they present in the retina. For instance, normal superficial retinal vessels may be coded in red, while deeper retinal vessels are green, and vessels found in the normally avascular tissue space (between the outer plexiform layer and the RPE) are assigned a blue color. It is important to keep in mind that the automated segmentation algorithms can be frequently incorrect. Therefore, the color coding can be misleading. Nevertheless, the general information contained in OCTA images usually reveals useful information about the vascular anatomy if the user can watch for and take into account the segmentation errors. The simplest way to think about OCT and OCTA is that *OCT reveals _neural_ structure, while OCTA reveals _vascular_ structure*.

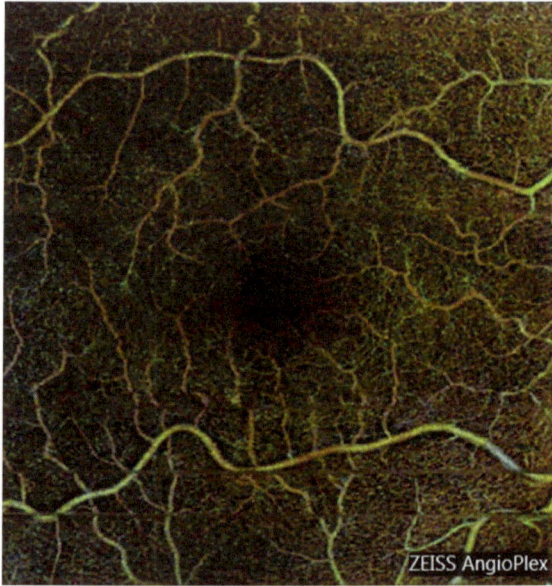

Normal macula on color depth encoding

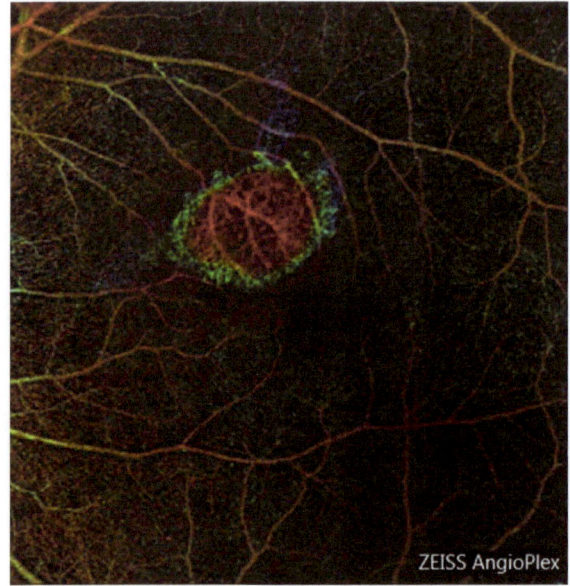

CNV on color depth encoding

OCTA allows for visualization various levels of the posterior pole, from the vitreoretinal interface to the choroidal-scleral junction. To accomplish this, OCTA images are viewed via en-face imaging, which is view-

ing the tissue in multiple "coronal" slices. This is essentially the same orientation as standard fundus photographs are taken and presented.

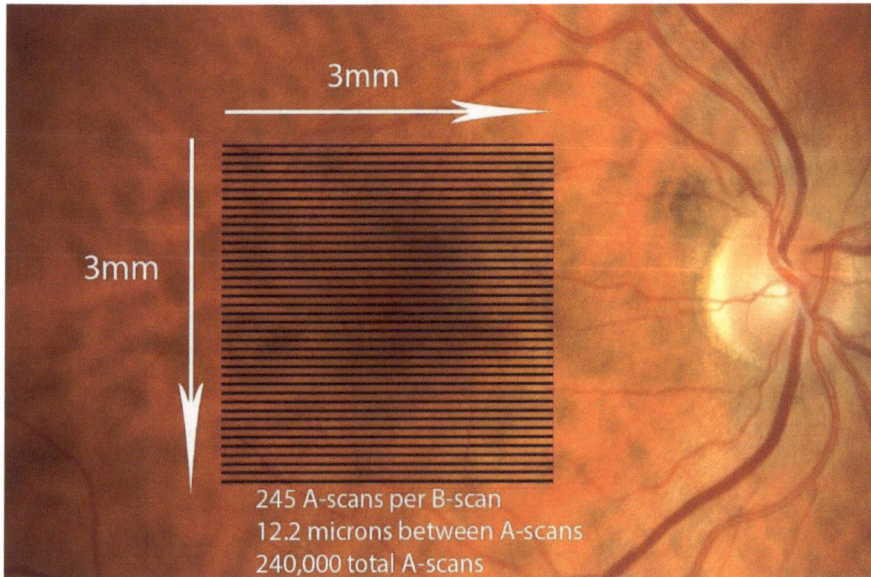

3mm

3mm

245 A-scans per B-scan
12.2 microns between A-scans
240,000 total A-scans

Sample scan pattern uses 245 A-Scans per 3mm B-scan "slice" and results in 240,000 total A-scans. Patterns may vary from device-to-device.

Another advantage of OCTA is that it allows visualization of the deep retinal plexus, which was not resolved on fluorescein angiography. In standard fluorescein angiography, the superficial and deep retinal vessels are imaged together and cannot be differentiated. Because we can image the tissue layer en face with OCTA, we can separate superficial from deep retinal vessels, to examine where impairment in perfusion is greatest.

OCT and OCT angiography of the retina imaged in cross-section B-scan (left) and en face (right) imaging. The red arrows indicate the segmentation borders of the designated slab that is displayed "en face" in the right panel. It is important to realize that the en face OCTA images are highly dependent on the segmentation scheme that is used, so the users should be familiar with and concurrently review the corresponding B-scans with the segmentation lines for every OCTA that is viewed. The segmentation schemes will likely vary from vendor to vendor, so OCTA images from one device are not likely to be directly comparable to another device from a different vendor. Also, OCTA images in subjects with diseases that distort the retinal anatomy are subject to mild or severe segmentation artifacts which may create erroneous or unusual depth encoded images and slabs. Therefore, it is up to the viewer to carefully review the segmentation patterns and ensure the accuracy of the en face OCTA projections. Nevertheless, OCTA images provide a wealth of information about the retinal vasculature that was not previously available.

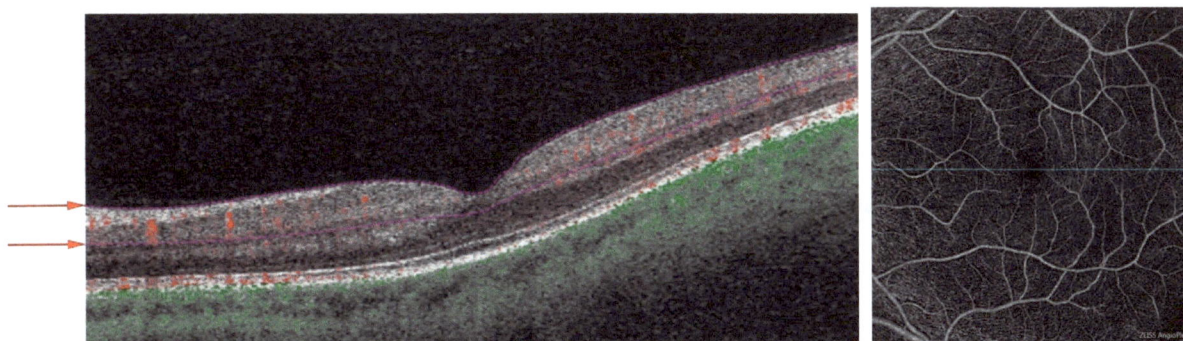

Superficial Retinal Layer is defined as the layer extending from the internal limiting membrane to approximately the inner aspect of the inner plexiform layer. This segmentation scheme is representative of the Zeiss AngioPlex device. Each manufacturer may have different and unique segmentation schemes, which may result in varied displays.

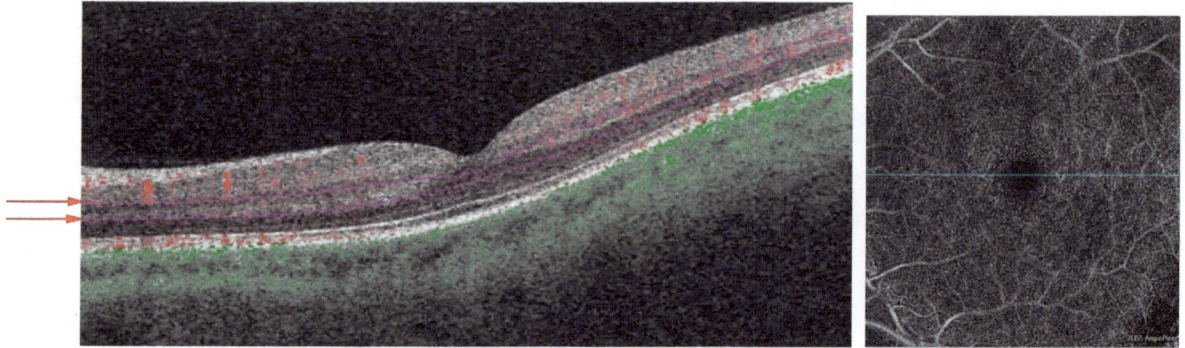

Deep Retinal Layer is defined as the layer extending from approximately the inner plexiform layer to inner edge of the outer nuclear layer. This segmentation scheme is representative of the Zeiss AngioPlex device. Each manufacturer may have different and unique segmentation schemes, which may result in varied displays.

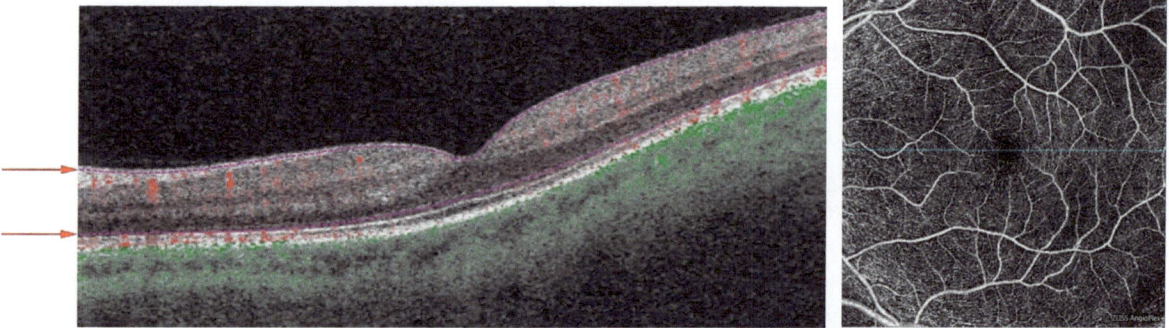

Full Thickness Retinal Composite is defined as the layers extending from the internal limiting membrane to the outer edge of the outer nuclear layer. This segmentation scheme is representative of the Zeiss AngioPlex device. Each manufacturer may have different and unique segmentation schemes, which may result in varied displays.

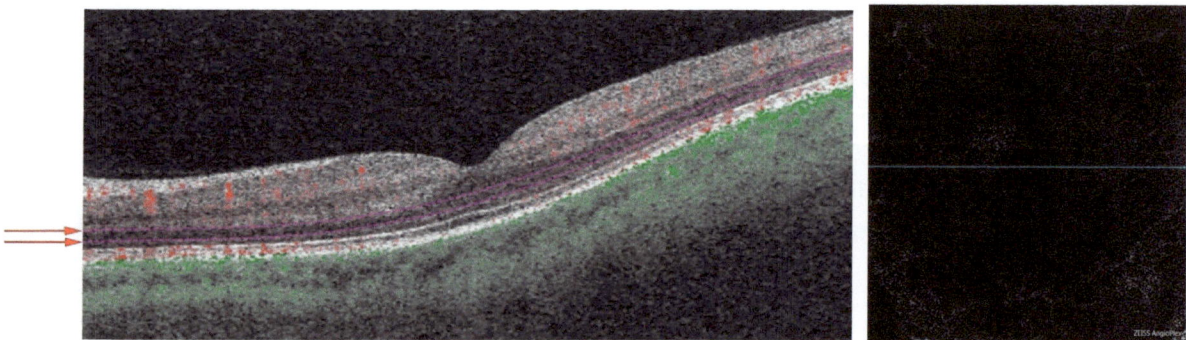

Avascular Layer is defined as the layer extending from approximately the inner edge of the outer nuclear layer to the outer edge of the outer nuclear layer. This segmentation scheme is representative of the Zeiss AngioPlex device. Each manufacturer may have different and unique segmentation schemes, which may result in varied displays.

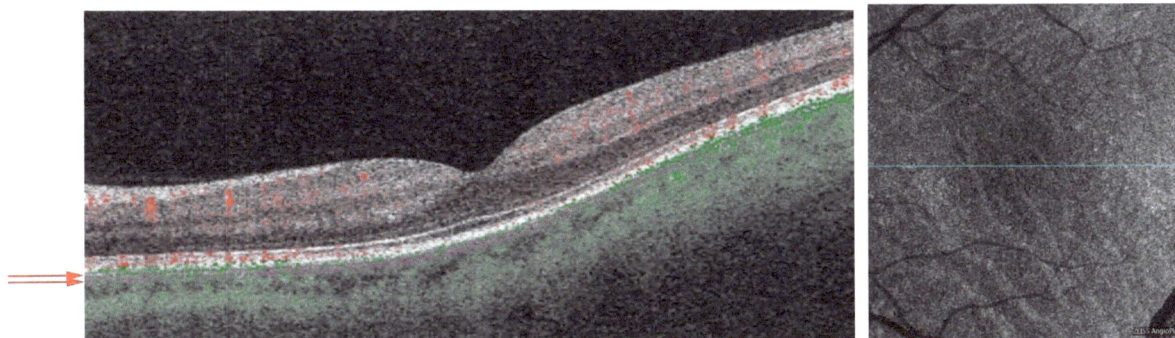

Choriocapillaris Layer is defined as the layer immediately below the RPE between the two red arrows and is approximately 25 microns in thickness. This segmentation scheme is representative of the Zeiss AngioPlex device. Each manufacturer may have different and unique segmentation schemes, which may result in varied displays. En face OCTA images of this layer are often confounded by shadows of the overlying retinal vessels, termed *projection artifact* (right).

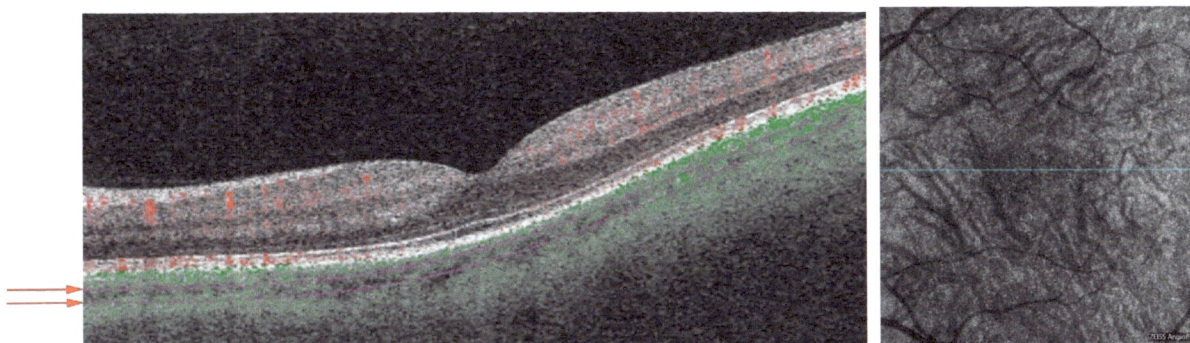

Choroidal Layer is defined as the layer extending from the outer edge of the choriocapillaris through the choroid and is approximately 60 microns in thickness. This segmentation scheme is representative of the Zeiss AngioPlex device. Each manufacturer may have different and unique segmentation schemes, which may result in varied displays.

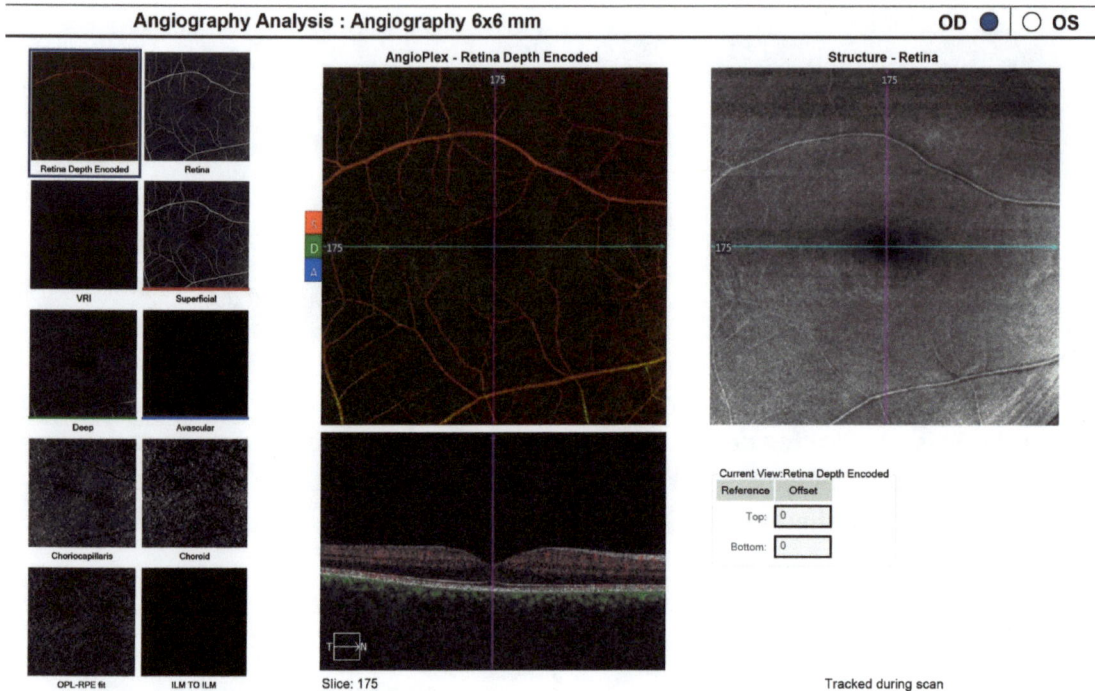

OCT angiography analysis of normal eye

As explained, OCTA allows for visualization of moving particles. The disadvantage is that intraretinal and subretinal fluid is generally not recognized by the OCTA analysis protocols. The fluid is obvious on the accompanying OCT image, which is why we cannot rely on one imaging source. In addition, OCTA detects most movement in the blood vessels but it is possible that blood movement can be too slow or too fast for OCTA to detect. In these cases, OCTA images will show the vessels as black. It is for this reason that areas of OCTA images, which are black, are called areas of "impaired perfusion" rather than "nonperfusion." The latter term is generally not correct and should be avoided.

At this point, it takes approximately 4-6 seconds to acquire the images necessary for an OCTA. For some patients it may be difficult to maintain fixation, and movement of the eye can cause artifacts just as it would on OCT images. In general, anything that causes an artifact on OCT images will also cause an artifact on OCTA images. Because OCTA images take slightly longer to acquire than SD-OCT images, movement is a more common source of artifacts in OCTA images. Movement is displayed in the processed image as a horizontal band appearing dark or blurred. Establishing a comfortable position for the patient, as well as educating them on the necessity to fixate will help to reduce these artifacts.

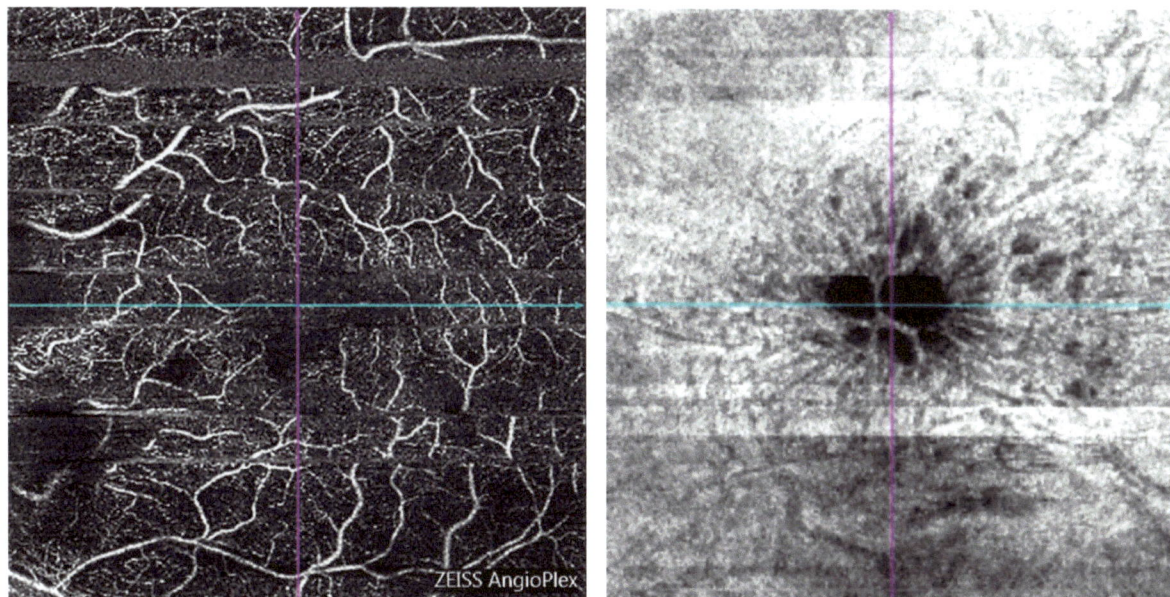

Examples of motion artifacts on OCTA and the accompanying en face image

Another common artifact on OCTA images are projection artifacts. These are very similar to the shadows cast by vessels on OCT images. Projection artifacts represent vessel patterns that are projected from anterior retinal layers to posterior layers. Projection artifacts make it appear that there are retinal vessels where there are none. It is important to pay careful attention to the pattern of OCTA findings in deeper retinal layers in order to determine if they are projection artifacts from overlying layers or truly vessels within the layer of interest. The projection of retinal vessels into the deeper levels can be minimized within the software after acquisition, but this is not perfect and user interpretation is typically required.

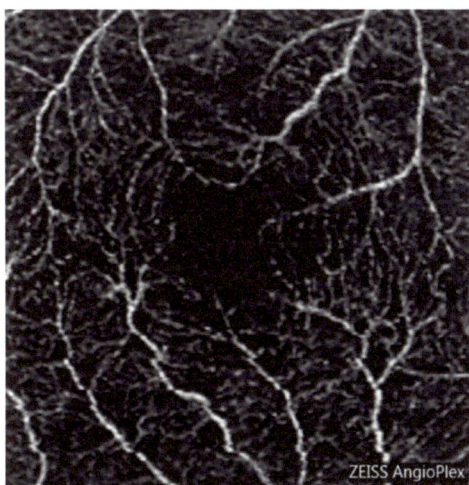

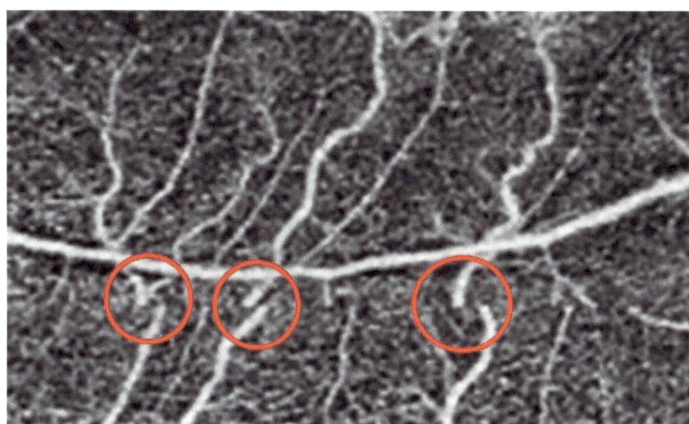

Motion can also cause vessels to appear broken or distorted

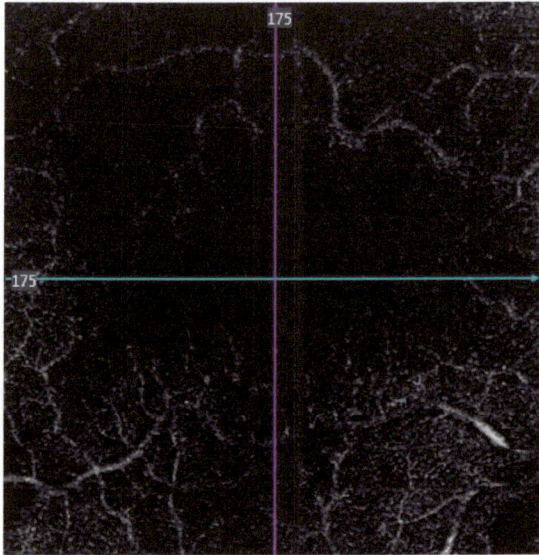

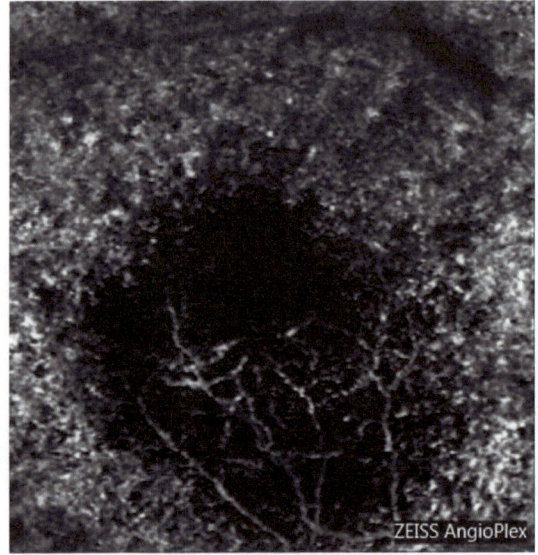

Superficial retinal vessels seen in the avascular and choriocapillaris level due to projection artifacts

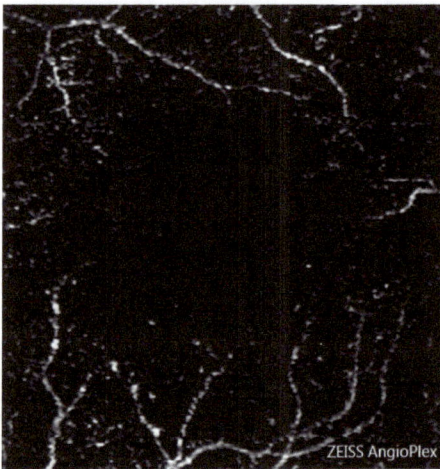

Projection artifacts in the avascular layer with corresponding B-scan. Note the pink dotted line in the B-scan, which indicates the retinal layer from which the OCTA is derived.

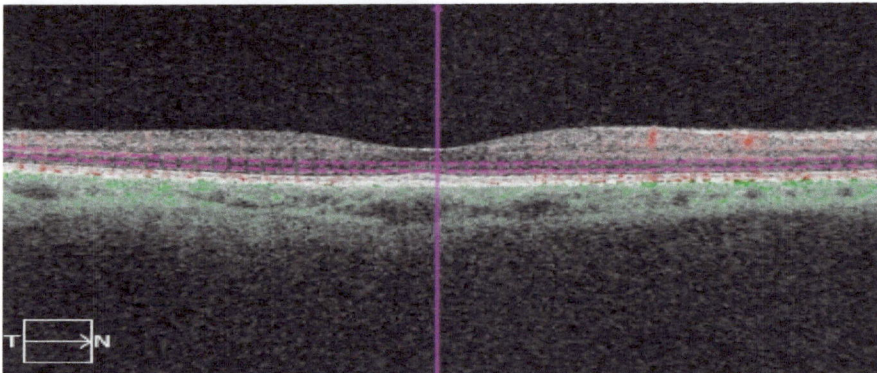

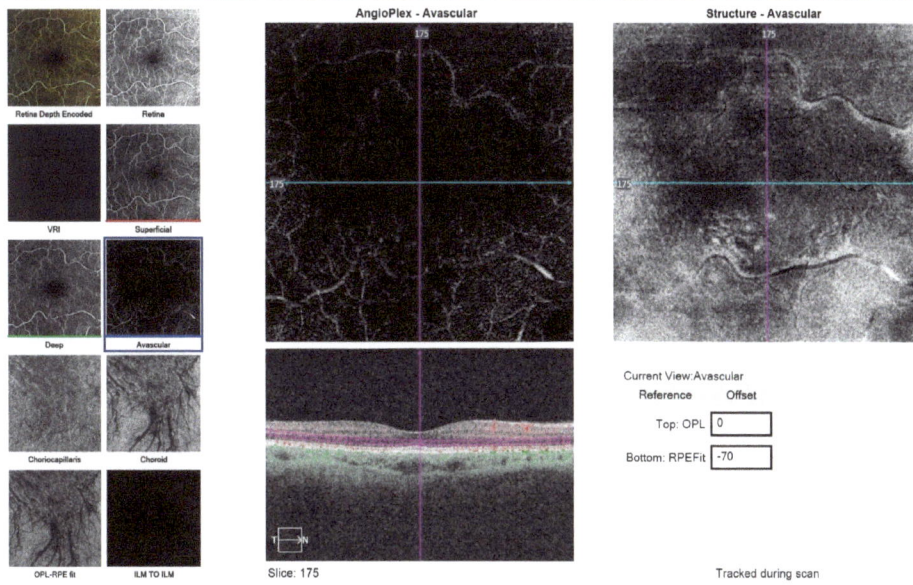

Superficial retinal vessels are seen as projection artifacts in the avascular layer.

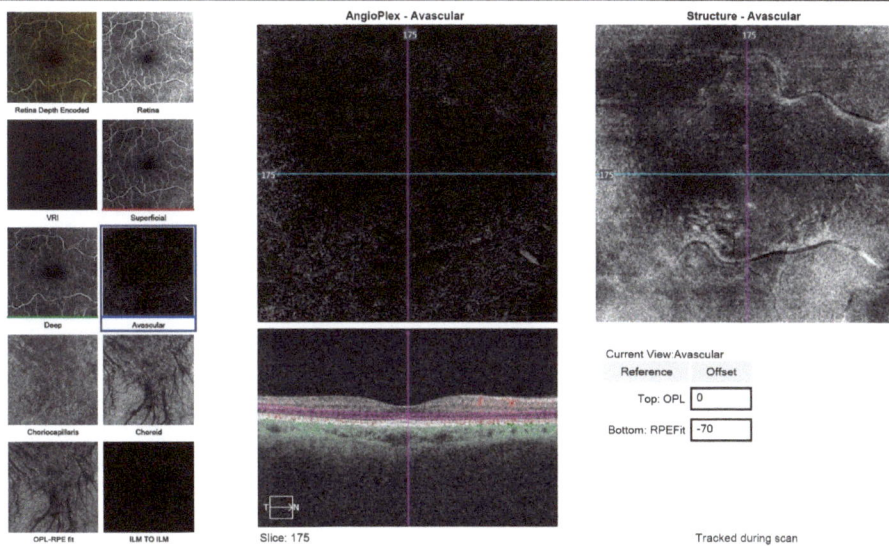

The same analysis after the removal of the projection artifacts - (may not be available on all models).

Atlas of Images and Disease Pathology

Vitreous Pathology

The vitreous is the clear substance that fills the posterior cavity of the eye (extending from the lens to the retina). It is made up of 99% water and accounts for the majority of the total volume of the globe. The vitreous is attached to the retinal surface, and eventually detaches from the retina in most people, due to the breakdown of vitreous gel in aging. This process is called posterior vitreous detachment or PVD.

Vitreomacular Traction

In some cases, the vitreous may not completely separate from the retina and this condition causes "pulling" on the retina, which is commonly referred to as vitreous traction or vitreomacular traction (VMT). Vitreous changes can be very difficult to visualize on clinical examination but are often demonstrated in excellent detail on OCT. Vitreous traction is implicated in many retinal diseases.

It is important to differentiate vitreomacular traction (VMT) from vitreomacular adhesion (VMA), which refers to the normal attachment of the posterior vitreous to the retina, and simply refers to the attachment between the retina and vitreous without mechanical traction, or pulling on retinal tissue. Therefore VMA typically does not cause any notable distortion of the retinal anatomy.

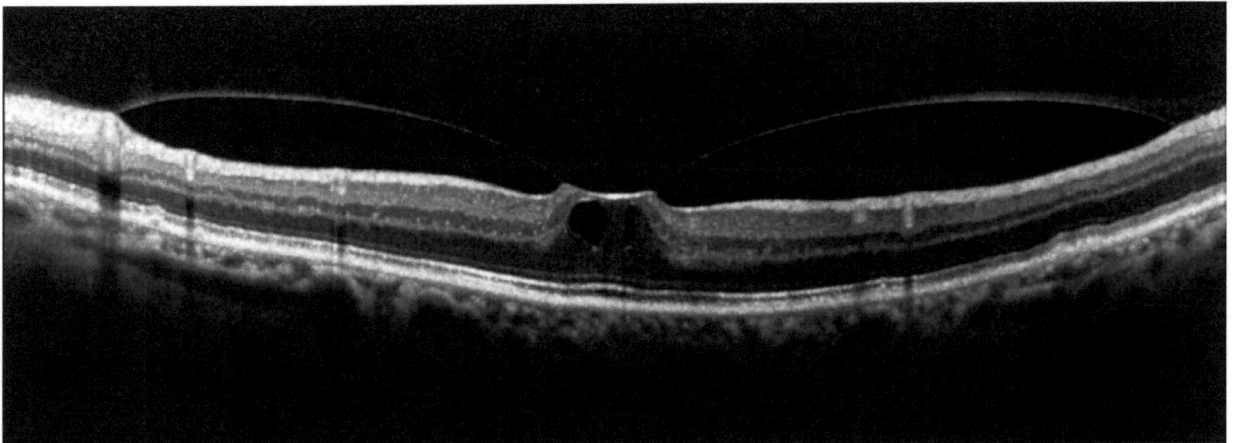

B-scan OCT demonstrating vitreomacular traction on the fovea and distortion of the underlying retinal anatomy. There are cystoid spaces within the retina that are consistent with VMT. Also note the vitreous attachments in far right and left sides of the image.

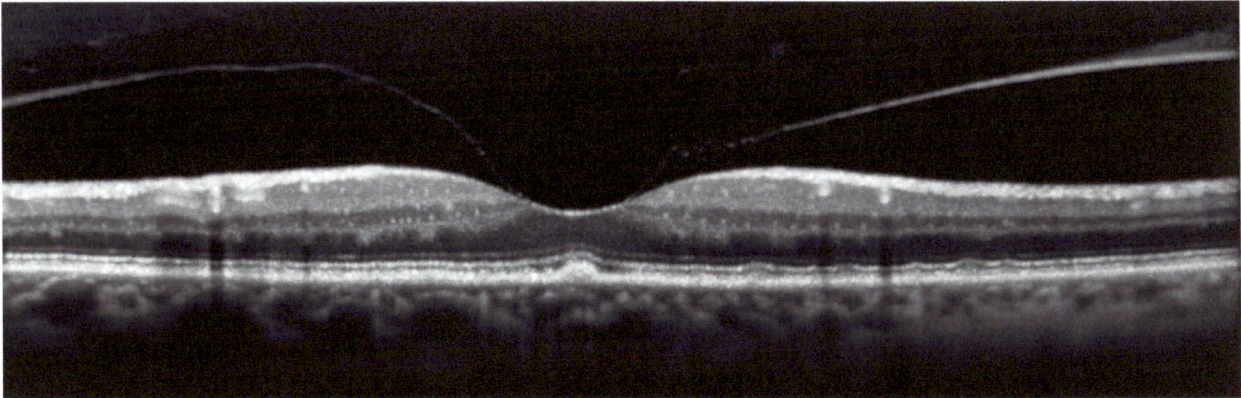

B-scan OCT demonstrating vitreomacular adhesion without any distortion of the underlying retinal anatomy

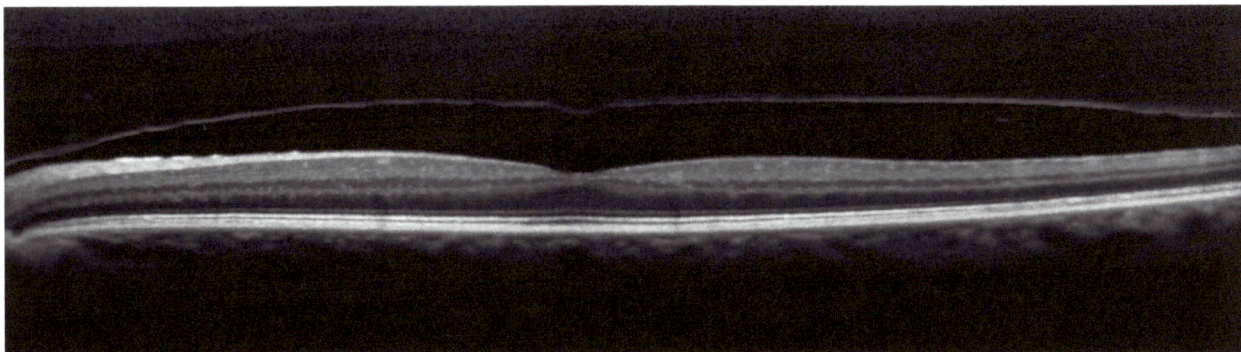

B-scan OCT demonstrating a partial posterior vitreous detachment. The bright line in the vitreous represents the posterior aspect of the vitreous (or posterior hyaloid). The downward trajectory of the posterior vitreous as it approaches either extreme of the image suggests that it is still attached in the regions just outside the field of view of this image. Therefore, in general, a low-lying separation of the posterior hyaloid over the macula does not necessarily mean that the vitreous is completely separated throughout the eye.

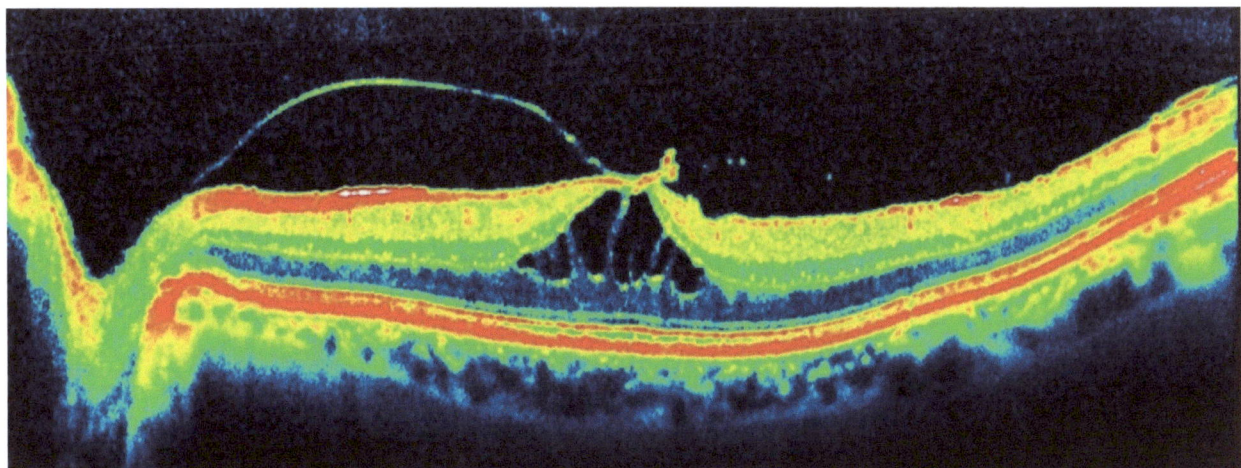

Pseudocolored B-scan OCT of vitreomacular traction with intraretinal edema

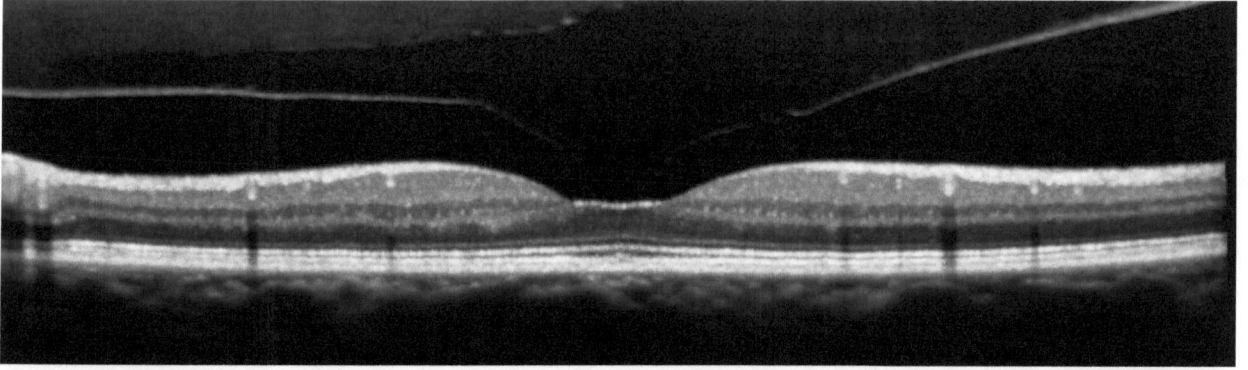

B-scan OCT demonstrating vitreomacular adhesion without any distortion of the underlying retinal anatomy

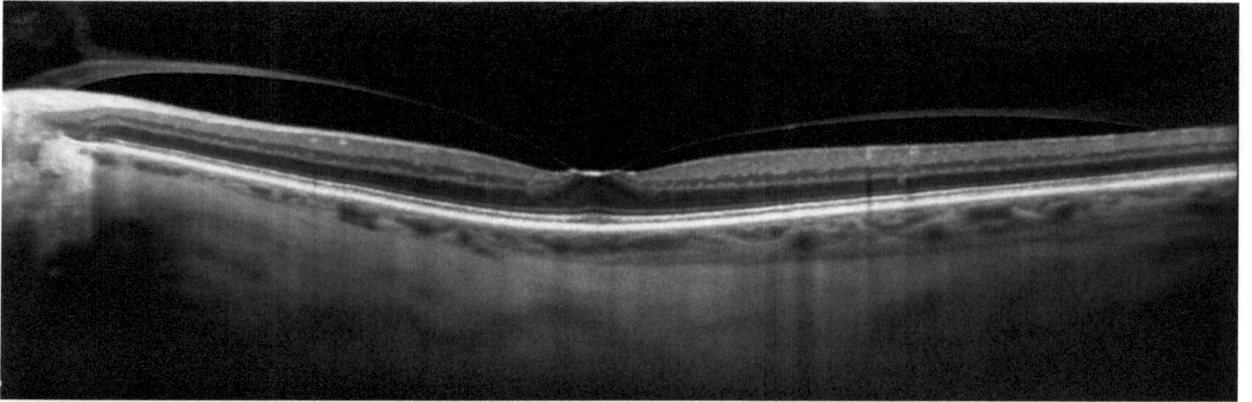

B-scan OCT of a case of VMT. The foveal depression is almost completely blunted, and the posterior hyaloid is still attached at the disc and the temporal macula.

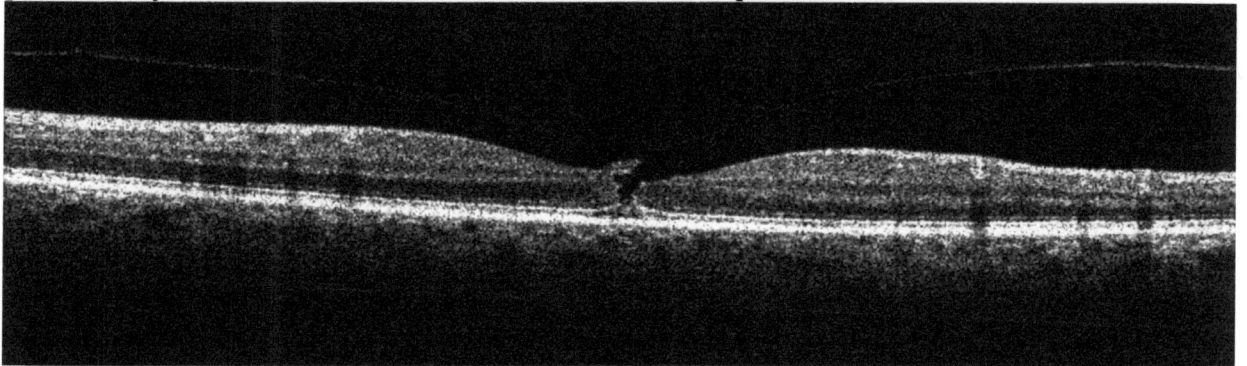

B-scan OCT showing VMT and likely full thickness macular hole. The full extent of the retinal defect is not illustrated on this image but the vitreous attachment to the edge of the retinal defect is apparent.

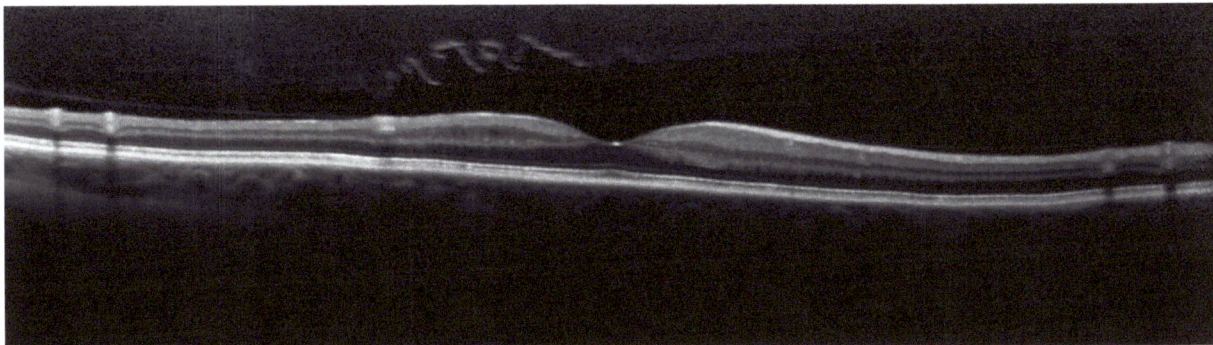

B-scan OCT demonstrates undulating white lines in the vitreous, which mimic the appearance of the posterior hyaloid but in this case are consistent with vitreous syneresis. The posterior hyaloid is visible as the faint white line that is just above the retinal surface and is most easily visible at the edges of the image. Therefore, this image is consistent with VMA. Interpretation of vitreous changes requires very high resolution and good quality images so that vitreous syneresis is differentiated from posterior vitreous changes. Clinical examination and correlation are also important.

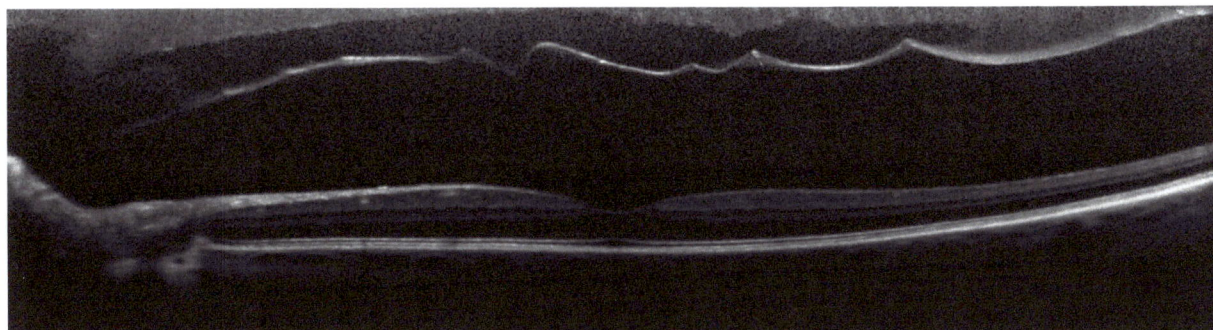

B-scan OCT demonstrates separation of the posterior hyaloid over the entire macula but the downward trajectory of the posterior hyaloid on the left side of the image suggests that it may still be attached at the nerve. This image is consistent with partial posterior vitreous detachment. Note the variations in the intensity of the internal vitreous contents just above the posterior hyaloid.

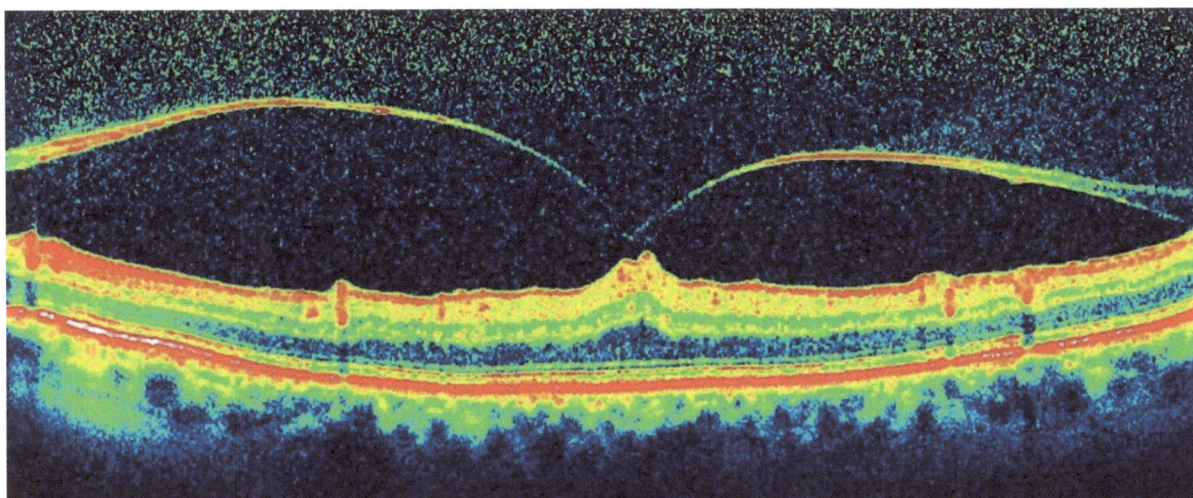

B-scan OCT of vitreomacular traction with attachments temporally, nasally and centrally

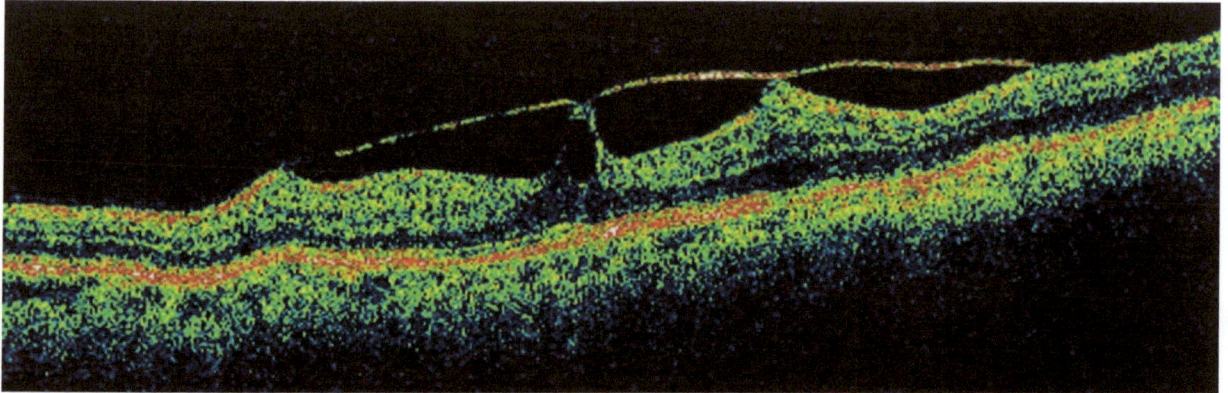

B-scan OCT shows vitreomacular traction with multiple attachment points between the posterior vitreous and the retina

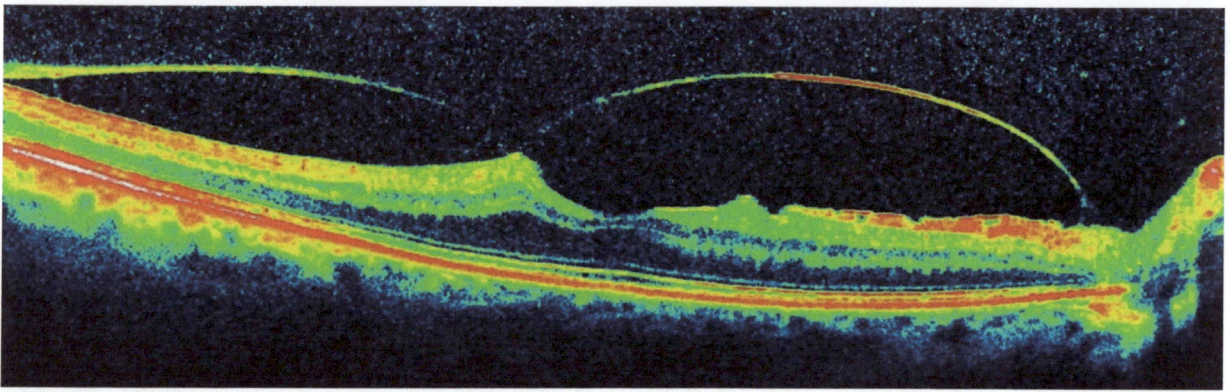

Vitreomacular traction is evident on this B-scan OCT in the temporal foveal region. There is normal vitreomacular adhesion (VMA) in the far left and right of the image.

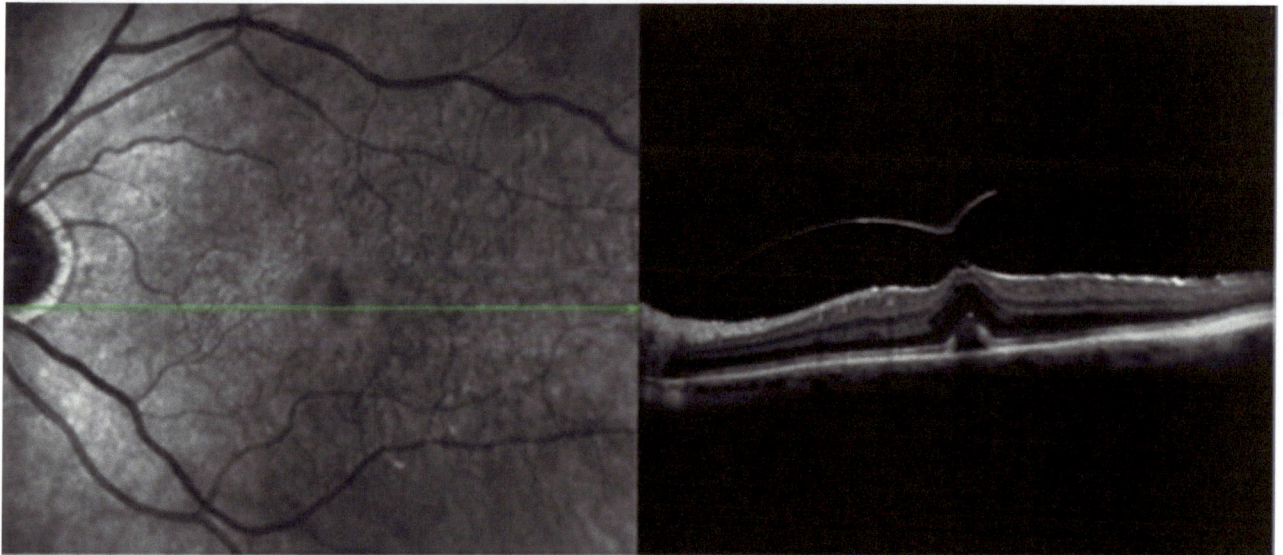

Depending on the orientation of the vitreous surface to the OCT beam, parts of the vitreous may be invisible on the image. However, the presence of retinal distortion and the contour of the overlying vitreous can be helpful. In this case the downward trajectory of the posterior vitreous surface and the elevation of the retina immediately below that region is consistent with VMT.

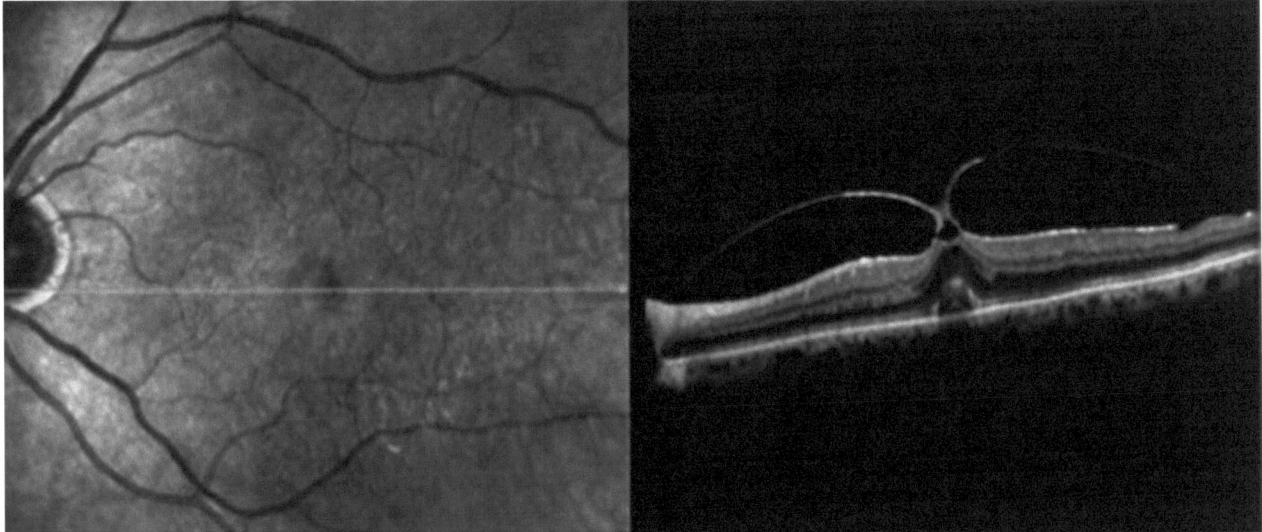

B-scan OCT on the same subject as above demonstrates the VMT much more clearly after moving the scan, with VMT now clearly revealed. Use of raster scan patterns may be helpful in identifying the full extent of vitreomacular changes.

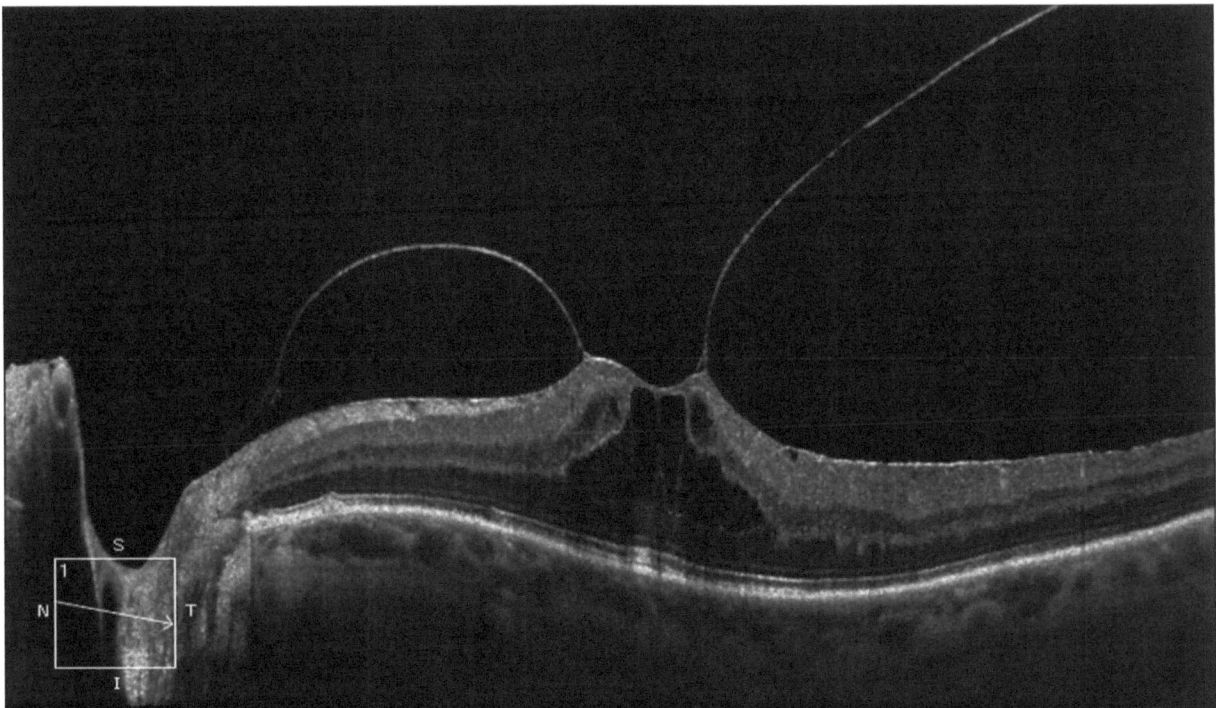

Vitreomacular traction causing retinal distortion. There is also an epiretinal membrane (ERM) extending along the entire retinal surface. Note that the vitreous is still adherent to the nerve.

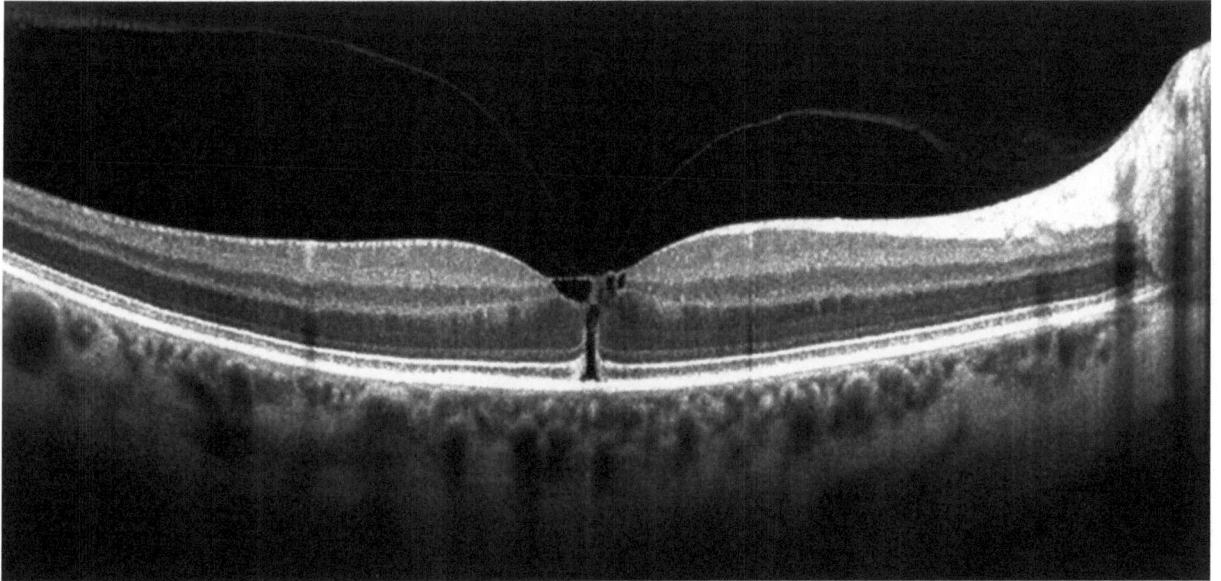

Vitreomacular traction with retinal distortion and likely full thickness macular hole (FTMH)

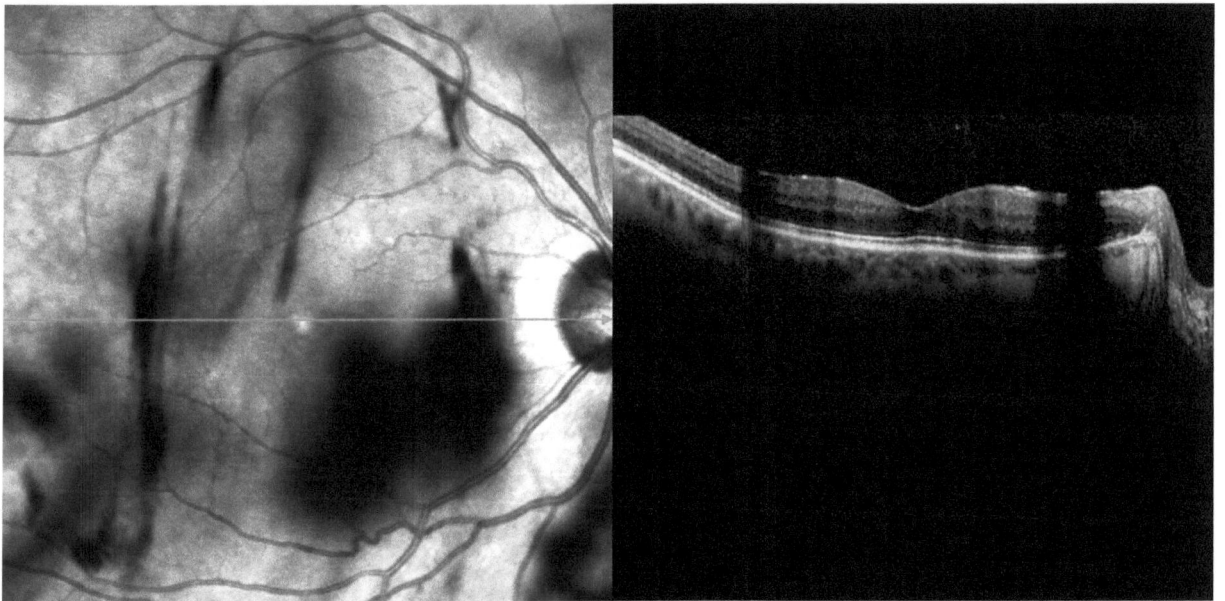

B-scan OCT and corresponding fundus image of a patient with a vitreous hemorrhage. As OCT uses light to image the retina, anything in the vitreous, lens or cornea that can block light will result in missing data. These lesions are collectively called media opacities and can cause "shadowing" defects on the OCT image. Note the areas of black shadowing on the OCT that represent missing data due to the light being blocked by the vitreous hemorrhage.

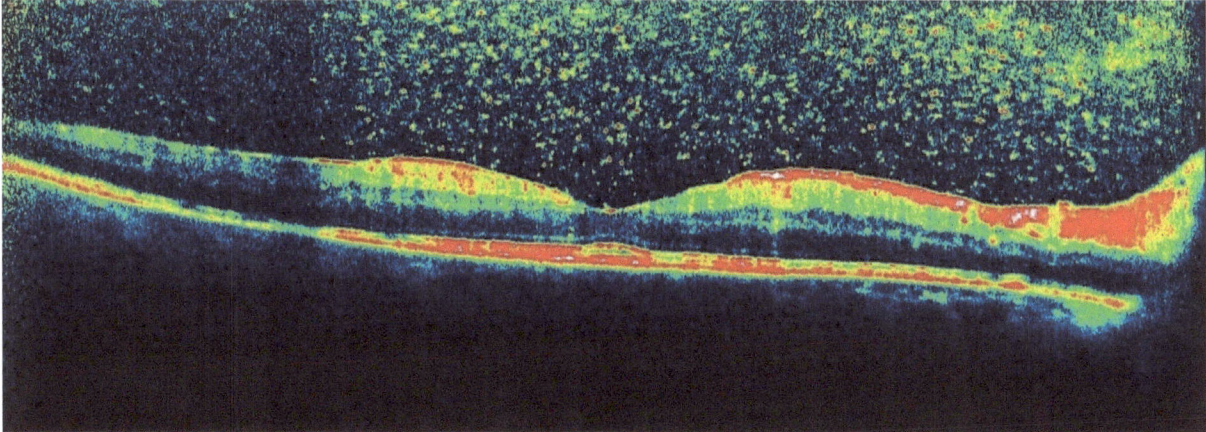

These vitreous opacities are consistent with vitreous debris, hemorrhage, cell or asteroid hyalosis

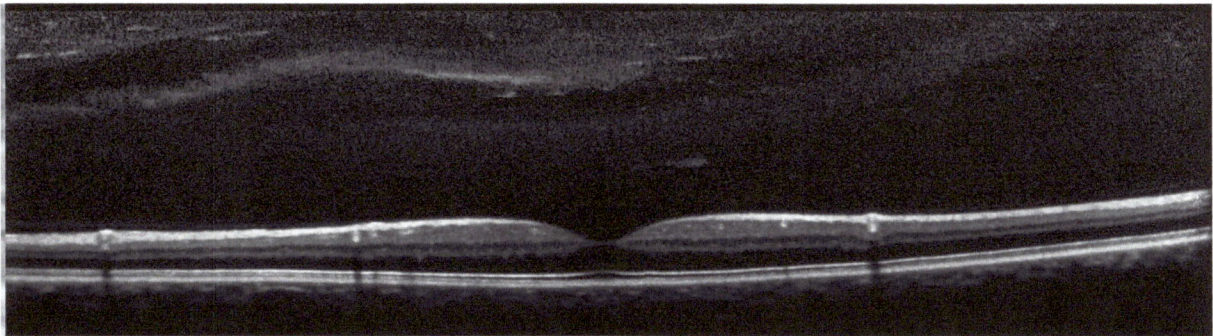

Note the variable appearance of the overlying vitreous on this B-scan OCT. The posterior hyaloid is still attached to the retina throughout the image.

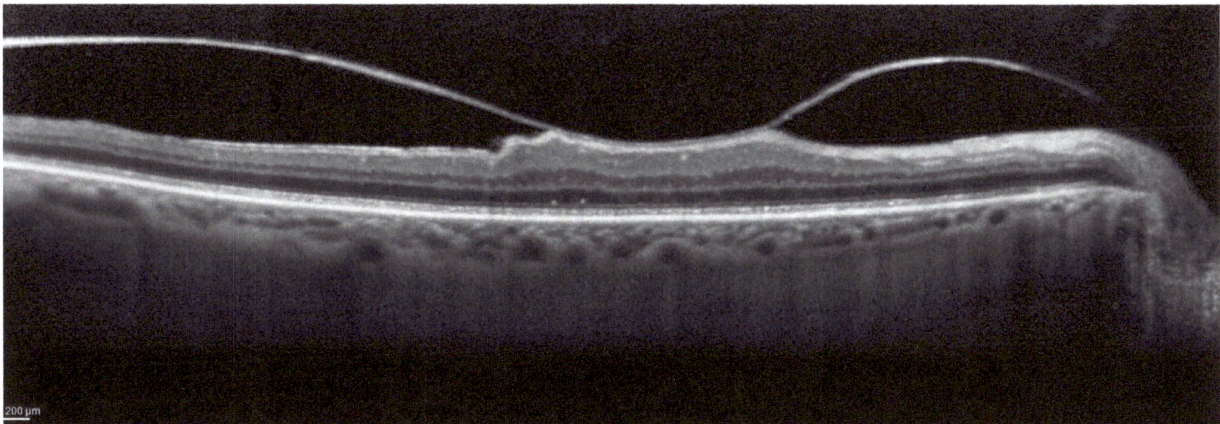

B- scan OCT demonstrates vitreoretinal traction, which is a more general form of traction that occurs outside the macula. In this case the vitreous is adherent to the central region of retina in the image and causing a mild distortion (elevation) of the retina.

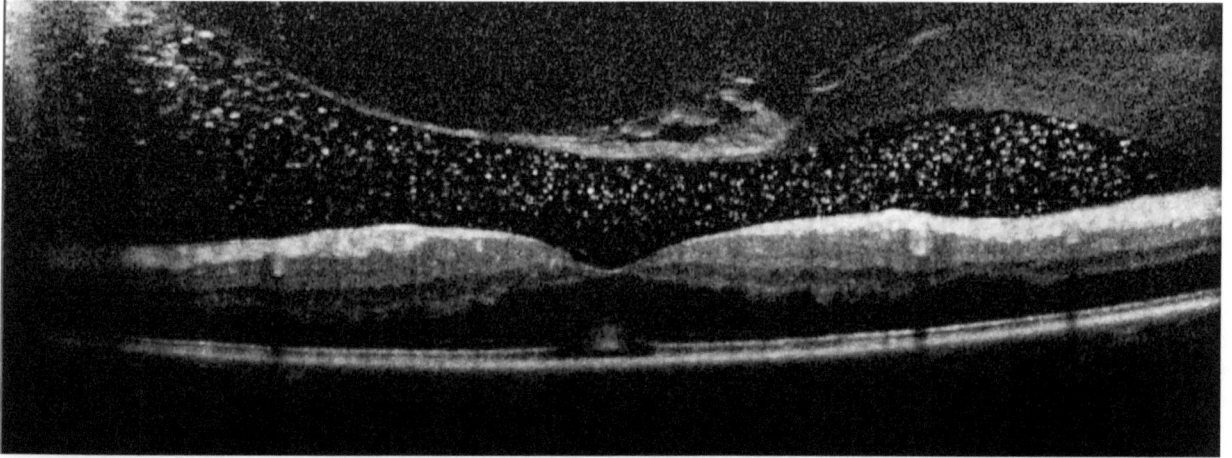

Vitreous hemorrhages, debris or cell can cause focal hyperreflectivity in the vitreous space overlying the retina that is consistent with the appearance on this B-scan OCT.

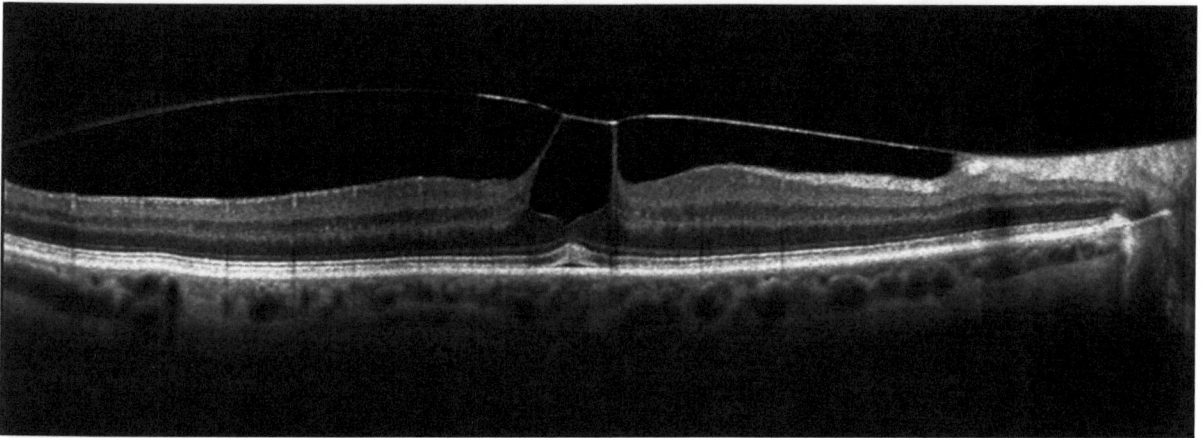

This B-scan OCT is consistent with classic vitreomacular traction, with attachments in the central macula causing a large macular cyst.

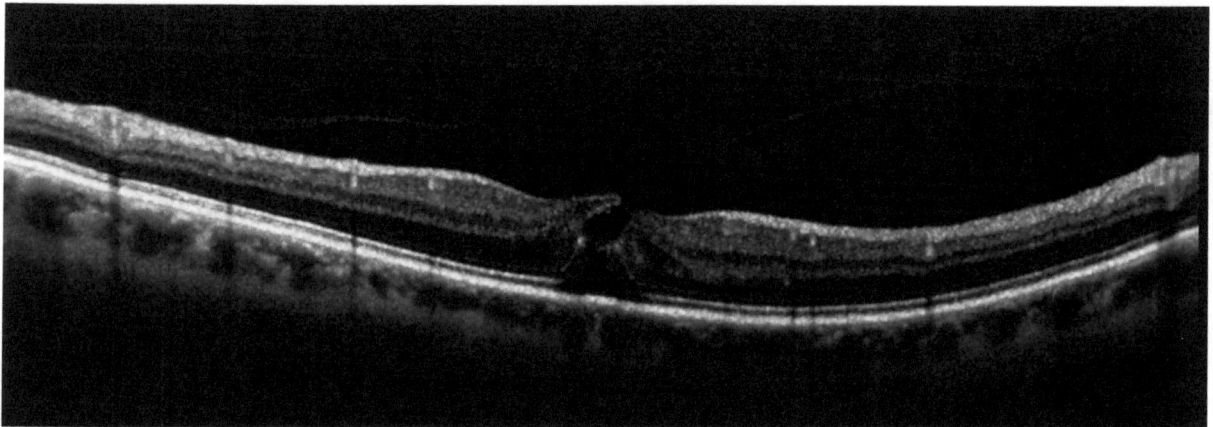

This B-scan OCT is consistent with vitreomacular traction with partial thickness macular hole.

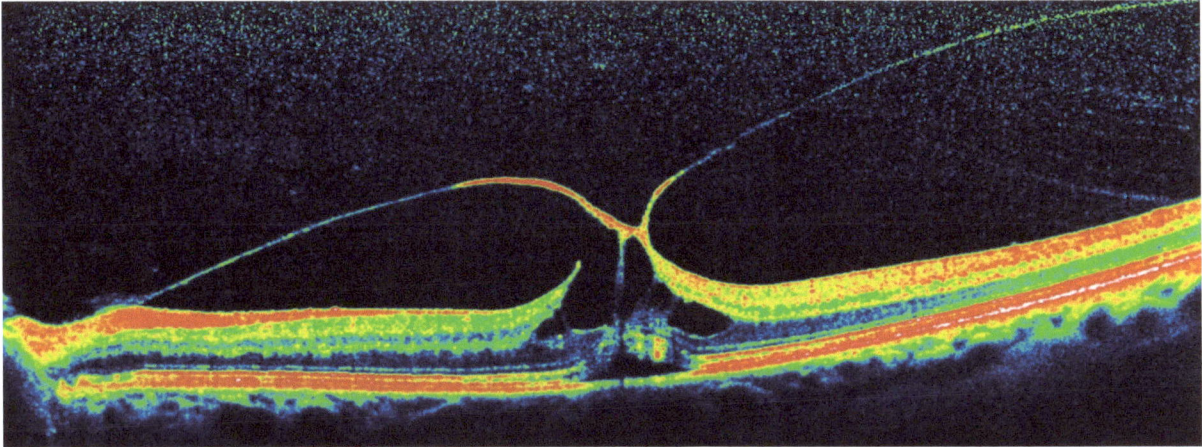

This pseudocolor B-scan OCT is consistent with vitreomacular traction and FTMH.

Epiretinal Membrane

Epiretinal membranes (ERM) are known by other names including macular puckering and cellophane retinopathy. ERM are very thin sheets of tissue that grow along the surface of the retina and are commonly found in the macular area. ERMs are easily identified on OCT scans but the effects of ERMs on retinal tissue can be visualized on other imaging modalities, including fluorescein angiograms and en face fundus images. ERMs appear as hyperreflective lines that are visible on top of the retina in OCT scans. ERMs can cause significant changes in the underlying retinal structure and marked tortuosity or distortion of surrounding retinal vessels in en face imaging methods such as fundus photographs. Visual symptoms from ERM range from asymptomatic to severe visual distortion that results from the underlying distortion of the retinal tissue. This distortion can be accompanied by focal accumulation of intraretinal fluid or diffuse retinal thickening, depending on the extent of the fluid. Sometimes epiretinal membranes can cause a loss of foveal depression, making it difficult to identify the location of the fovea.

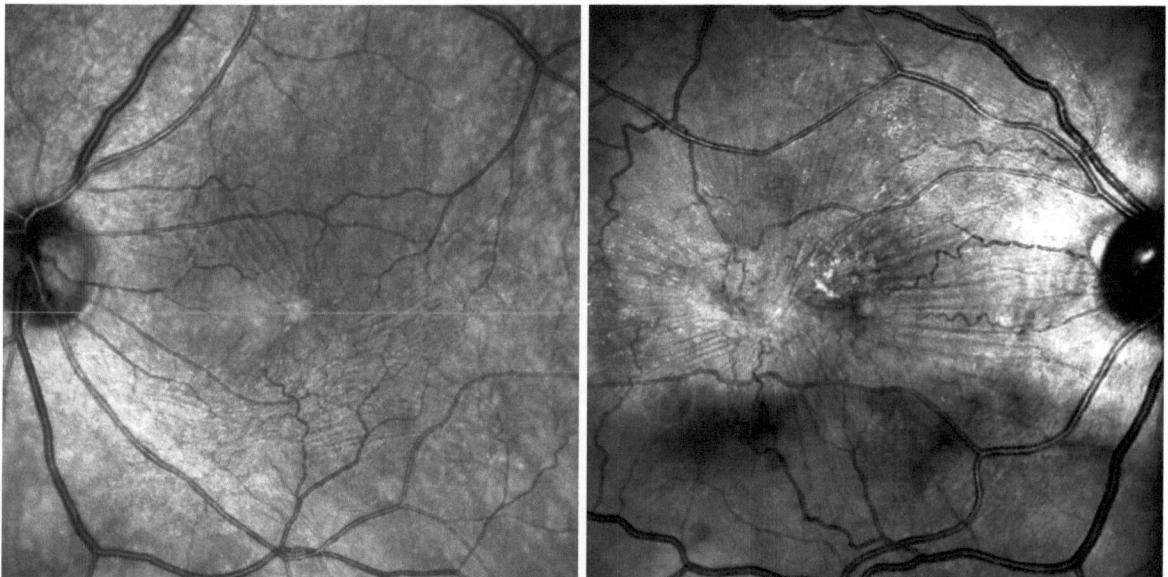

Fundus infrared images of epiretinal membranes. Note that the actual membranes are not visible in these en face images but the mechanical forces of the ERM on the retina cause lines or "wrinkles" in the retinal appearance that radiate in different directions. These lines or "wrinkles" are also known as retinal striae and indicate the presence of an ERM. The presence of an ERM is also indicated by the increased tortuosity of the retinal vessels in the central macula.

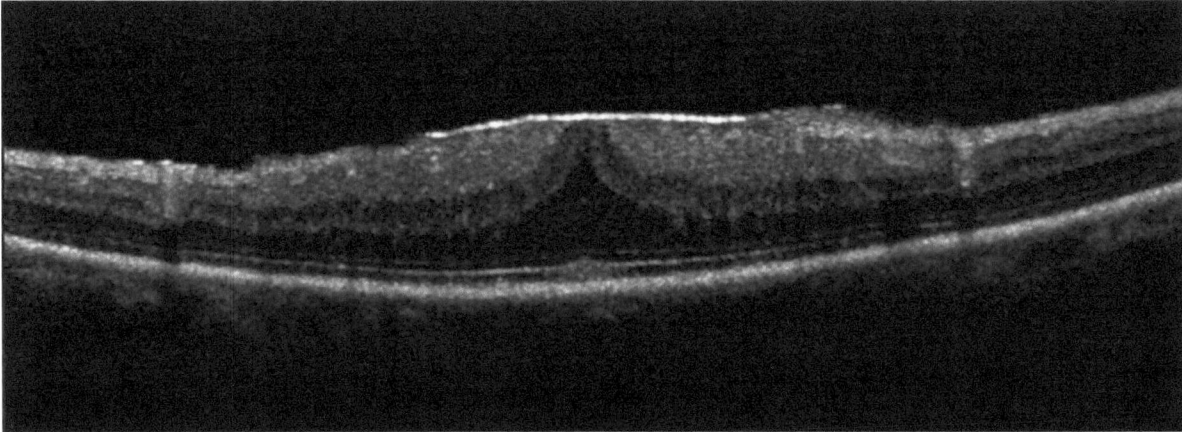

Epiretinal membranes appear as a hyperreflective line along the surface of the retina. In this case the ERM is most prominent over the fovea, the foveal depression has been blunted by the ERM and the surrounding retina is slightly thickened but no clear intraretinal edema is visible. The inverted funnel shape of the outer nuclear layer in the center of the image suggests the location of the fovea.

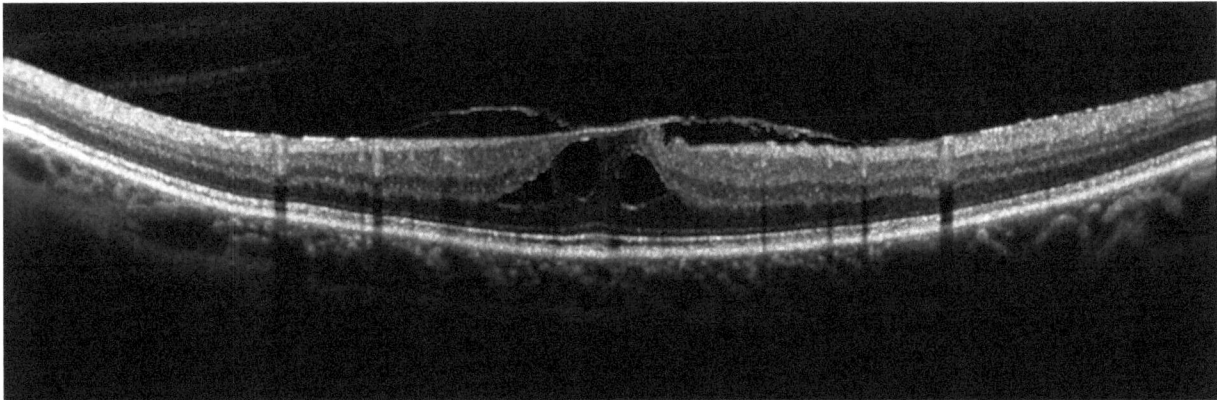

An epiretinal membrane is evident on several portions of this retina. The overlying vitreous is still adherent to the retina and the ERM in this case, thereby causing vitreomacular traction.

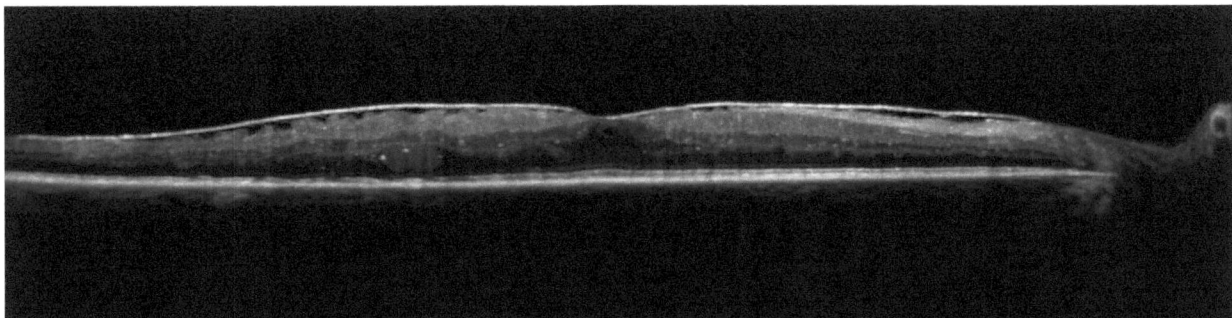

An example of an epiretinal membrane that is causing mild undulations in the underlying retinal surface most evident on the left side of the image. There are two large cystoid spaces to the left of the fovea (in the outer nuclear layer) that contain hyperreflective material and there are numerous foci of hyperreflectivity throughout the retina, which may be consistent with hard exudates.

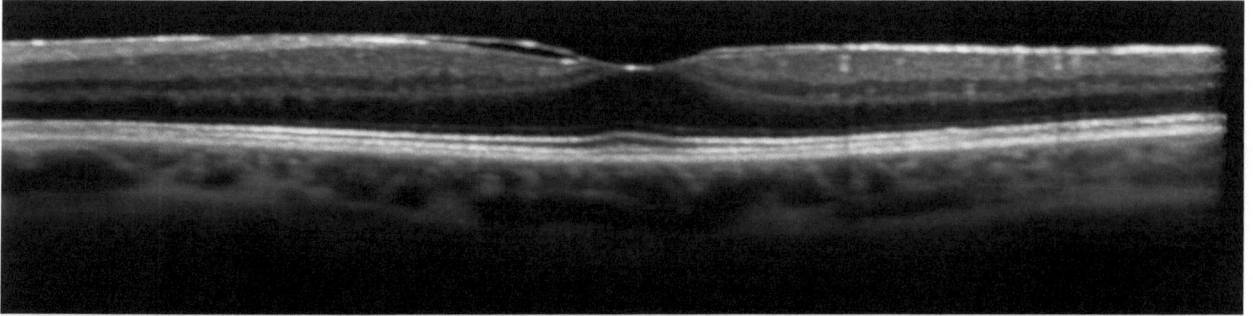

An ERM is notable along the entire surface of the retina in this case, but a slight separation just to the left of the fovea clearly defines the ERM as well.

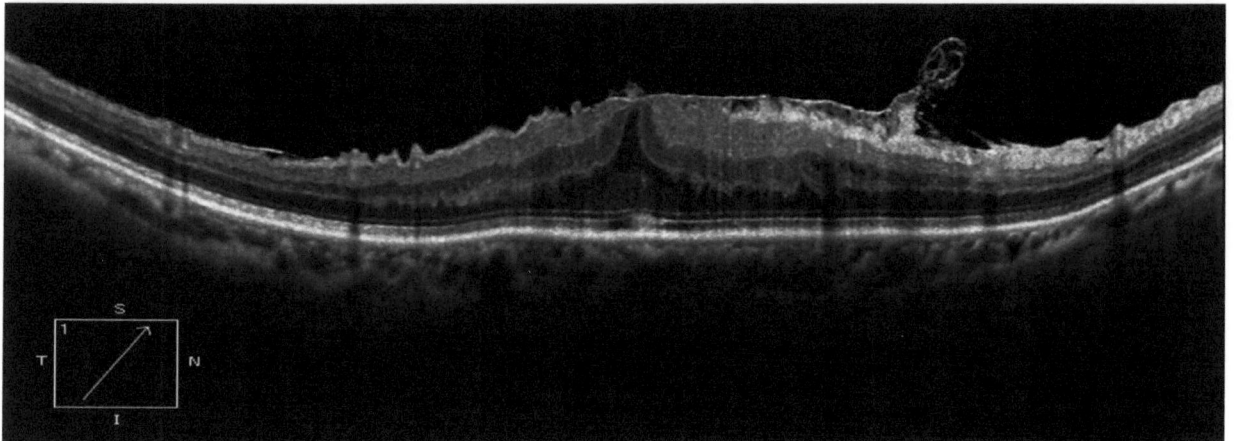

The ERM on the surface of this retina is causing severe distortion of the underlying retina. The foveal contour is completely blunted. The ERM edge on the right side of the image has a scrolled appearance and is elevated into the vitreous space. The inverted funnel or pyramid shape indicates the approximate location of the fovea in this case.

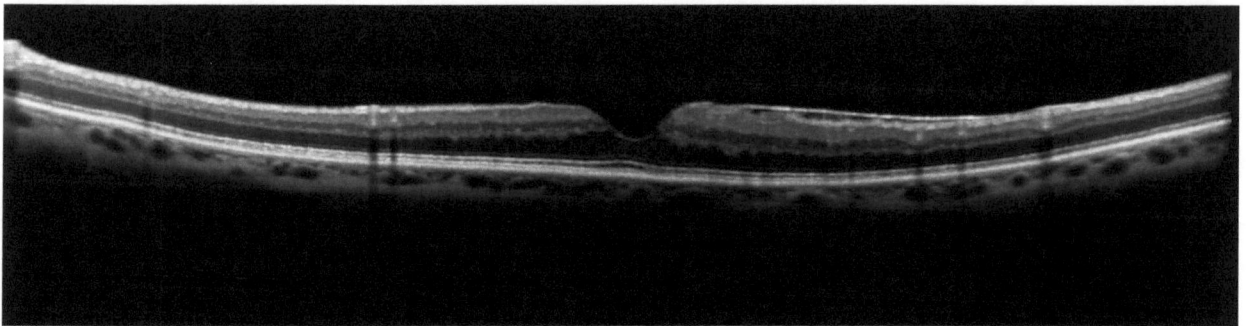

An ERM is visible along the right side of the fovea and is separated from the underlying retinal surface in some regions. In this case a clear ERM is not visible on the left side of the fovea.

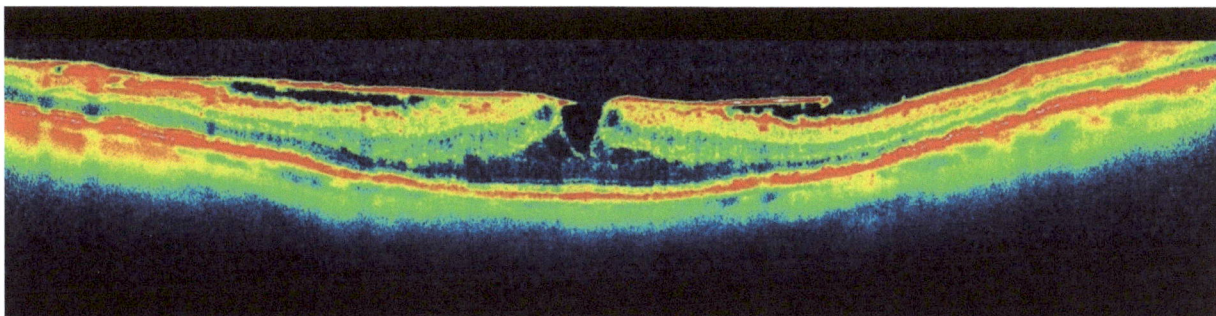

Epiretinal membranes can cause significant distortion of the underlying retina. In this case the ERM seems to extend on either side of the foveal depression for some distance (more on the left than the right side). The foveal contour is visible but clearly irregular and the surrounding retina has small cystoid spaces. This appearance is sometimes referred to as a lamellar hole.

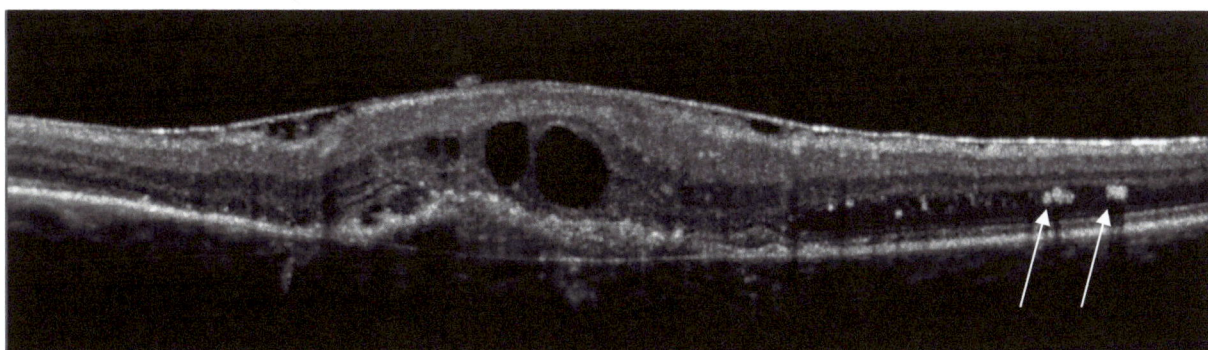

Epiretinal membrane extends over the entire retinal surface here. Note that there is also a pigment epithelial detachment with both serous and fibrous components consistent with a choroidal neovascularization. There are multiple retinal cysts overlying the pigment epithelial detachment consistent with the underlying choroidal neovascularization. The overlying ERM is most likely unrelated to the macular degeneration and intraretinal cystoid spaces in this case. Multiple hyperreflective foci are visible in the outer nuclear layer and consistent with lipid exudation or "hard exudates".

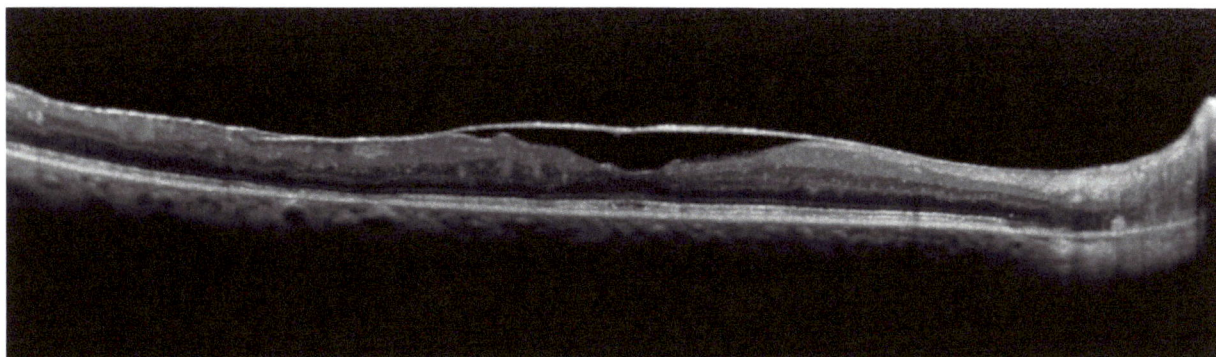

Epiretinal membrane that is not adhered to the fovea

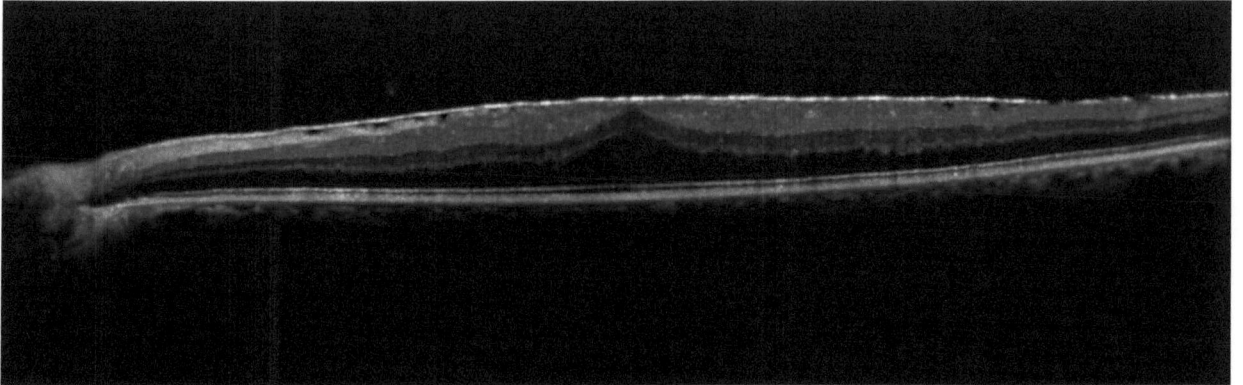

This ERM extends along the entire length of the retina and completely flattens (blunts) the foveal contour. The pyramid shape or inverted funnel appearance in the center of the image indicates the approximate location of the fovea.

The following pages are examples of ERM flattening the normal foveal contour, however, the imager was able to move the scan to find the apex of the fovea by looking for the pyramid shape of the outer nuclear layer:

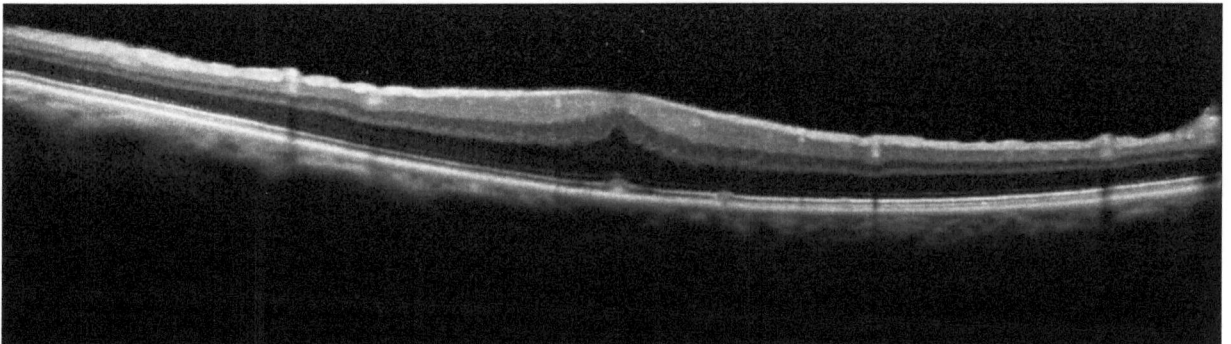

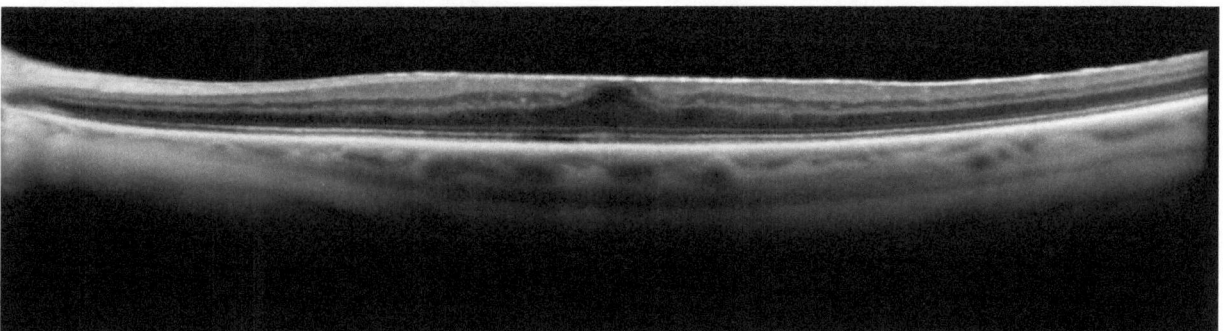

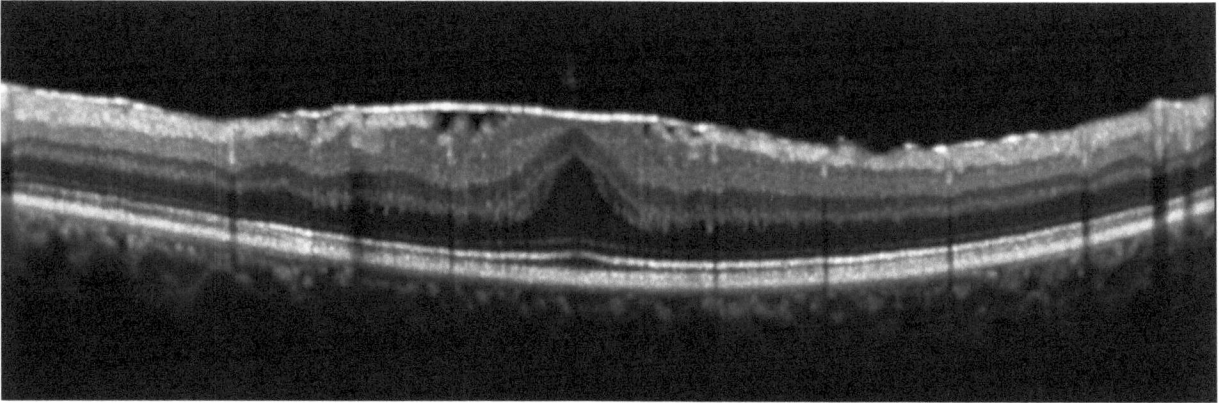

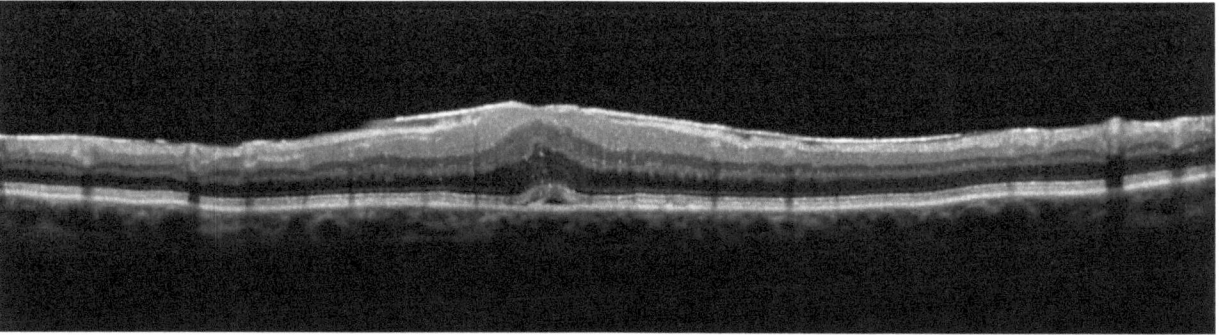

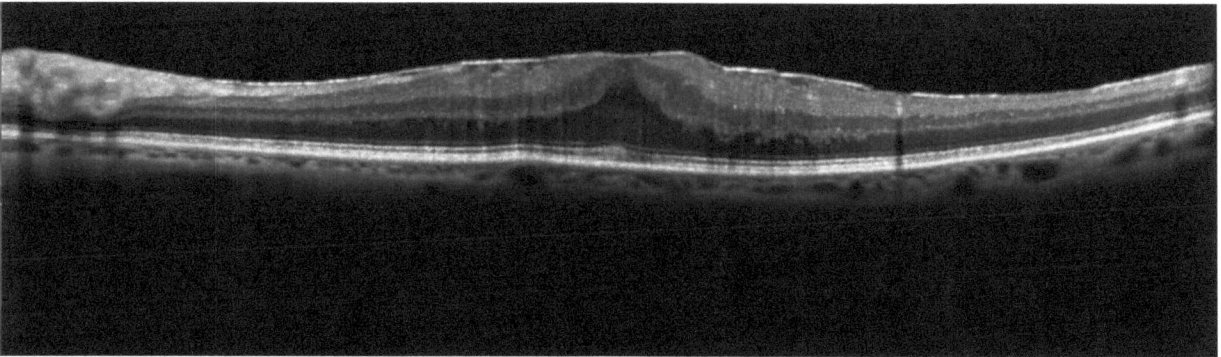

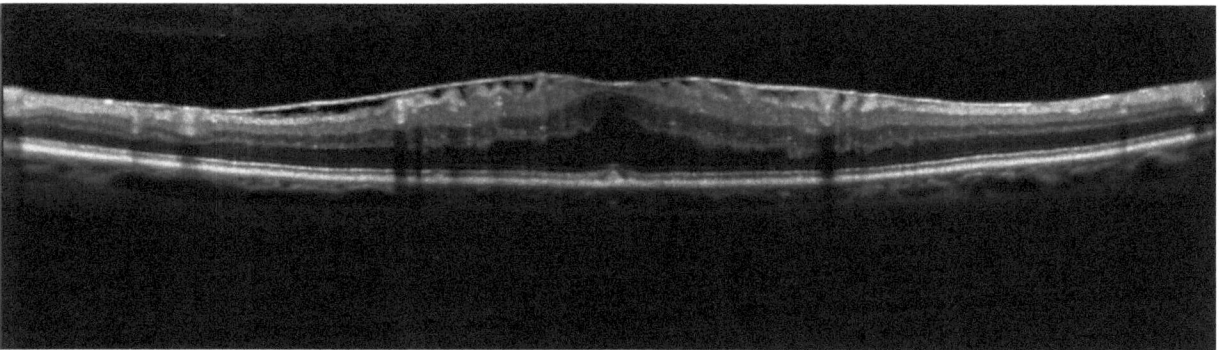

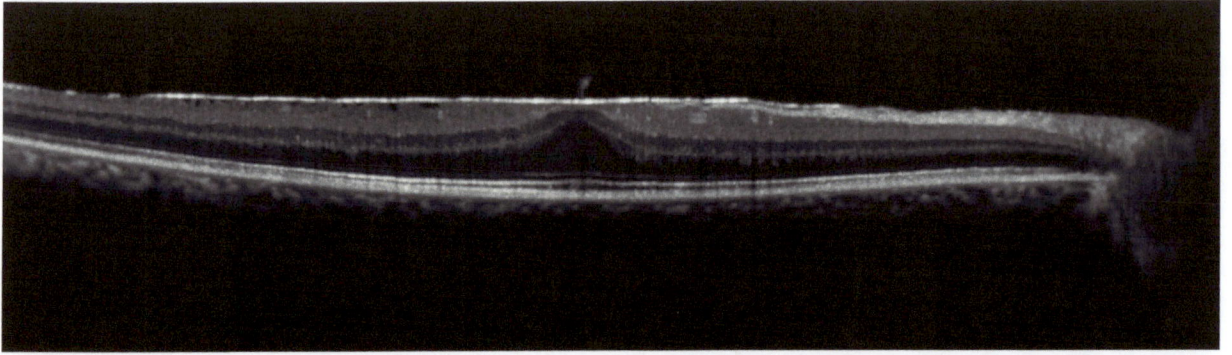

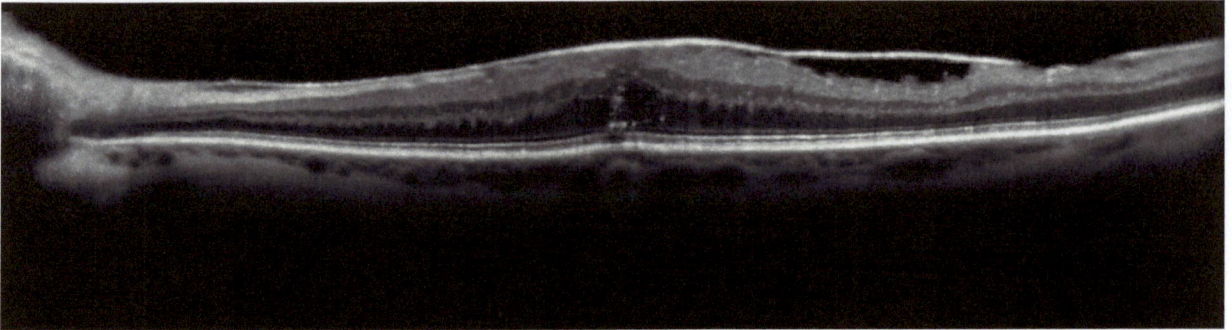

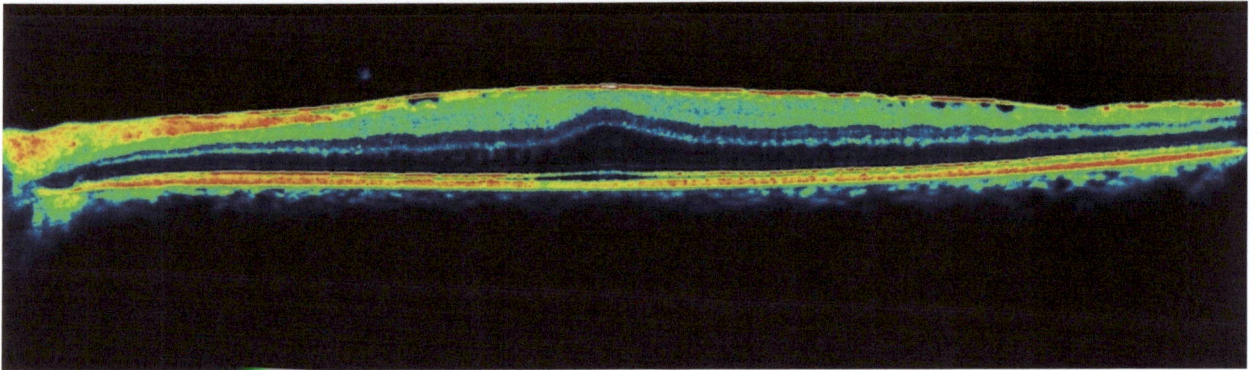

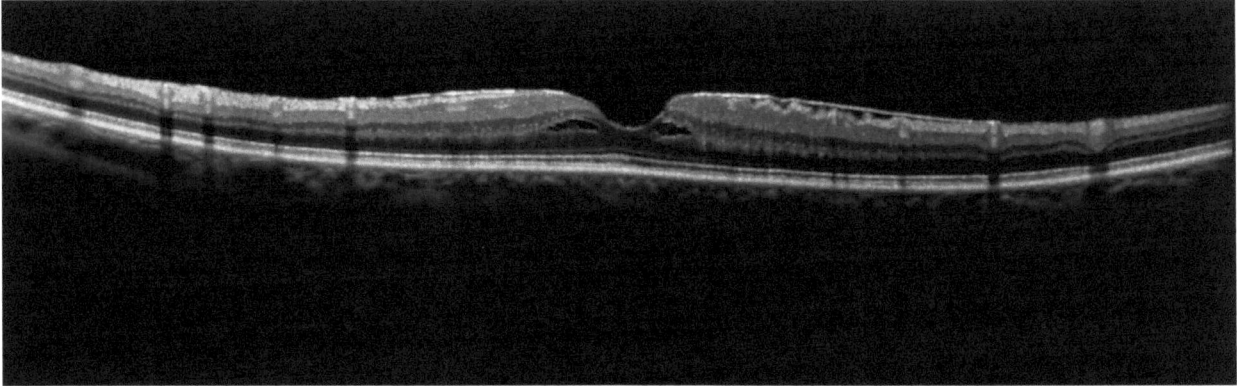

The epiretinal membrane in this example extends across the majority of the retina on either side of the fovea. There is mild wrinkling of the retinal surface on the right side of the fovea. There are some cystoid spaces on either side of the foveal depression but these are not likely to be macular edema in this case, as this pattern is most consistent with a lamellar hole associated with the ERM. Evaluation of the OCT B-scans on either side of this would help to further evaluate the extent of the lamellar hole.

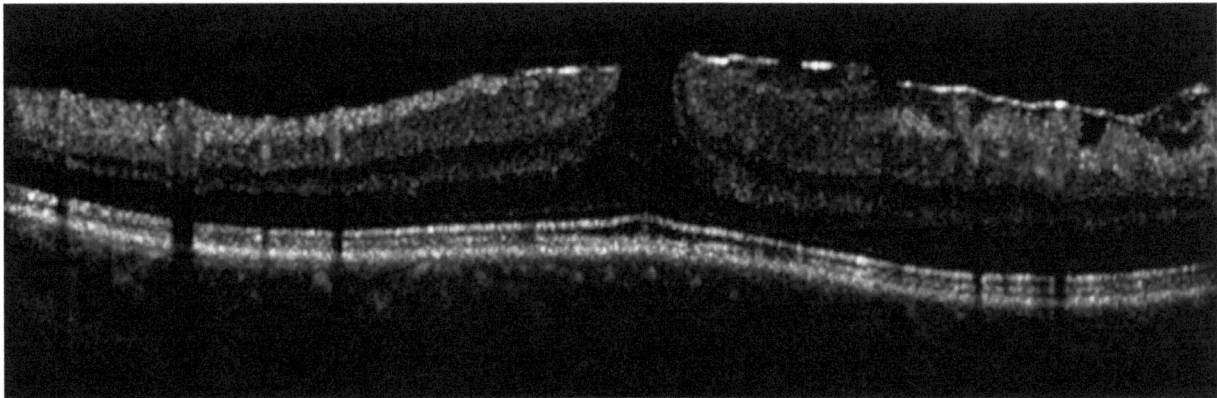

This epiretinal membrane extends along the right surface of the retina to just over the foveal depression. The foveal depression is irregularly shaped and consistent with a lamellar hole associated with the overlying ERM.

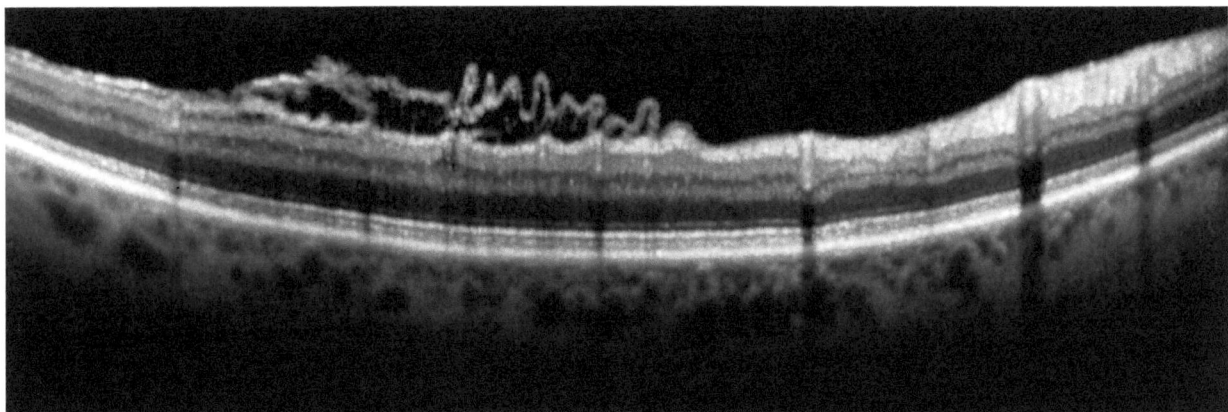

In some cases, the epiretinal membrane can break and coil above the retina. This scan was done outside the fovea, hence the absence of a foveal depression.

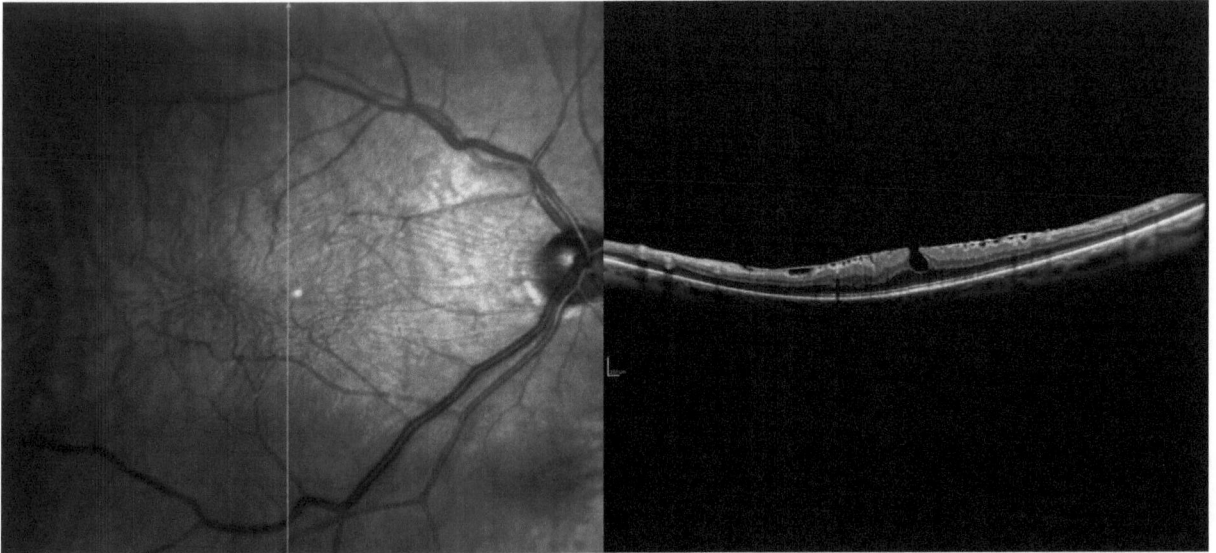

Epiretinal membrane is clearly visible on the surface of the retina (right). An irregularly shaped foveal depression suggests that the ERM is causing significant retinal distortion. The infrared image on the left shows fine horizontal lines corresponding to the retinal striae radiating between the fovea and disc. The retinal striae in this case correspond with the retinal wrinkles underneath the ERM on the OCT.

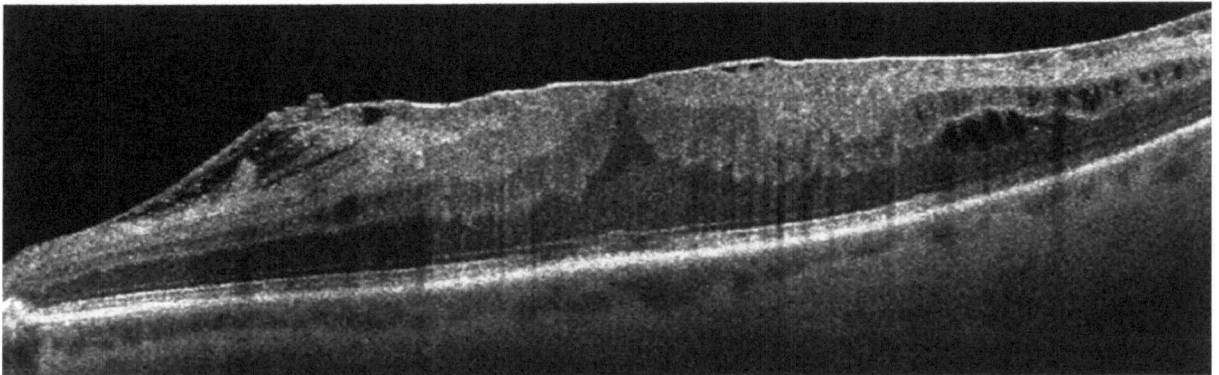

Another example of an ERM and flat fovea with the classic pyramid shape beneath it. The retinal distortion in this case is severe and associated with some retinal cysts most prominent on the right side of the image.

Lamellar and Macular Hole

The term "macular hole" is commonly used to refer to a Full Thickness Macular Hole (FTMH). This can be confusing as there are partial thickness macular holes, which are also known as "lamellar holes" or "pseudoholes." The advent of OCT advanced our understanding of the anatomic findings in FTMH and lamellar holes.

FTMH is a condition in which there is a full thickness defect through the retina extending to the RPE. In contrast, lamellar holes typically only have a partial thickness defect that extends to the outer nuclear layer. Both FTMH and lamellar holes are usually found at the fovea but can be extrafoveal as well. FTMH are often associated with vitreomacular traction and lamellar holes are generally associated with epiretinal membranes. In this section we will be discussing both lamellar holes and FTMHs.

Depending on the size of the FTMH, patients will complain of central visual defects and will not be able to fixate with their fovea. Therefore, they may fixate parafoveally, that is, outside of the fovea and imaging of the subject may be challenging. The resulting line scans will be centered on an area slightly outside of the fovea. There-

fore, the imager must take into account the patient's visual history and complaint, and adjust the fixation

target and scan pattern accordingly. It is also important for the clinician to review the entire OCT cube manually so that an off-centered scan does not misrepresent the severity of the pathology. In general, obtaining an OCT raster pattern throughout the central macula is a good idea so that small changes in fixation do not obscure relevant pathology and so that parafoveal changes can be regularly evaluated.

Lamellar macular holes are also known as partial thickness macular holes or pseudoholes. Lamellar holes can take many configurations but are characterized by the common feature that the outer nuclear layer is intact.

In the example on the following page, the first scan was done through the patient's subjective fixation. **(Figure 1)** The imager then directs the patient to maintain fixation, and then moves the scan manually to find the area of interest; in this case, the fovea. **(Figure 2)** The resulting images are drastically different, and may even alter the physician's diagnosis or the patient's treatment.

OCT images of a subject with FTMH. The image on the left is parafoveal while the image on the right is foveal and clearly demonstrates the FTMH. Moving the scan outside the patient's subjective fixation often reveals different pathology and may be necessary when doing a line B-scan OCT. Note the intraretinal cystoid spaces on either side of the FTMH, which are common findings in acute FTMH. Performing a raster pattern will often help identify extrafoveal pathology and its relationship to the fovea without the need to manually adjust the scan pattern. Higher resolution line B-scans can then be done in the region of interest based on the raster pattern.

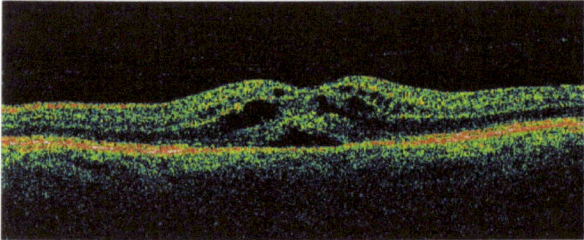 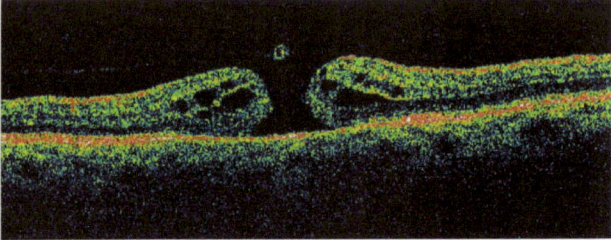

Figure 1   **Figure 2**

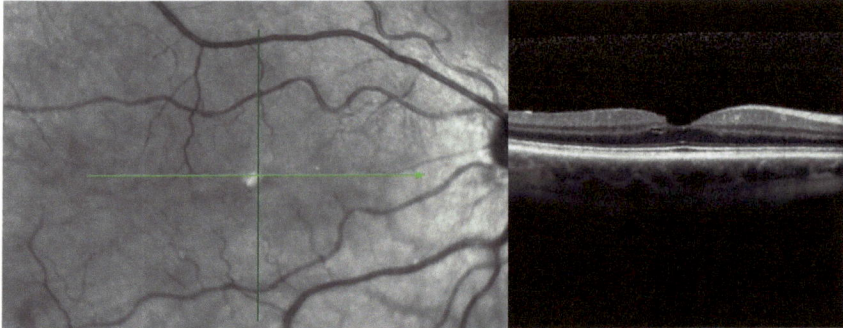

Subjective fixation in this patient shows a relatively normal foveal contour with trace cystoid spaces temporal to the fovea.

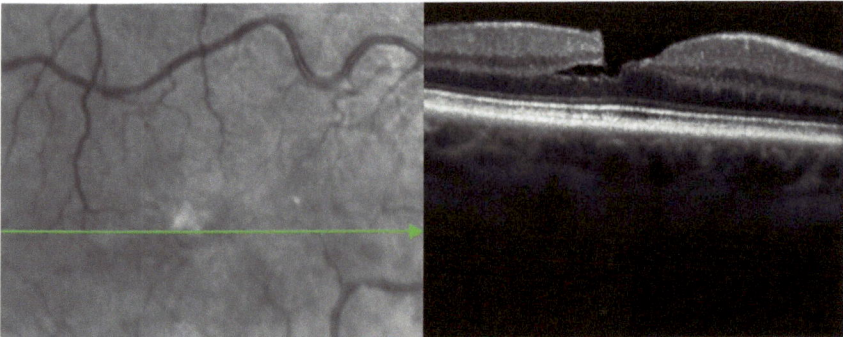

After moving the line scan, a lamellar hole is clearly visible.

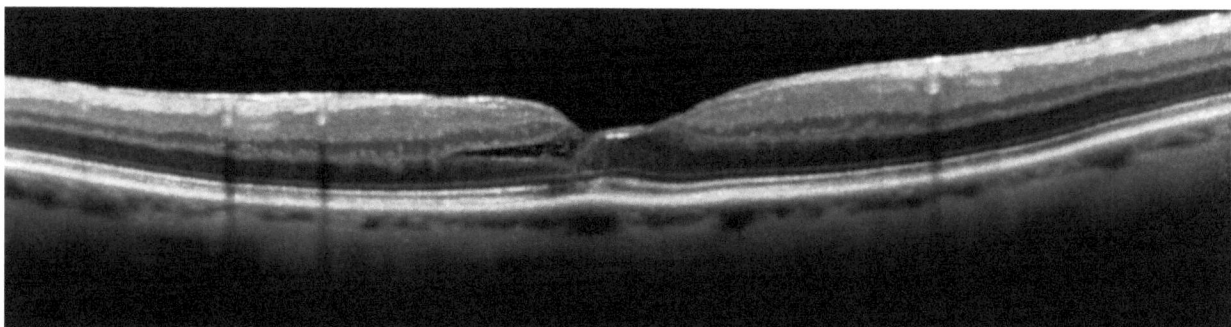

When there is suspicion of a macular hole, scanning the patient with subjective fixation may reveal some pathology.

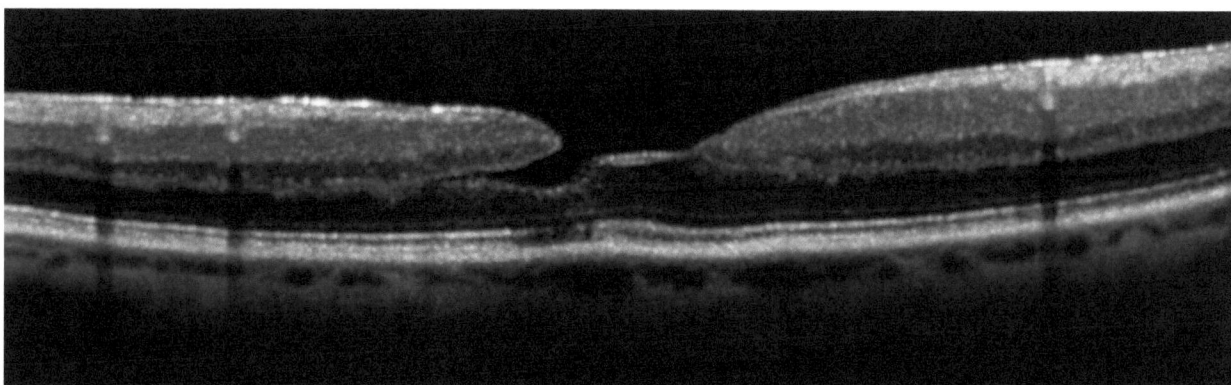

Evaluation of additional B-scans or moving the line scan and adjusting the magnification may reveal additional pathology.

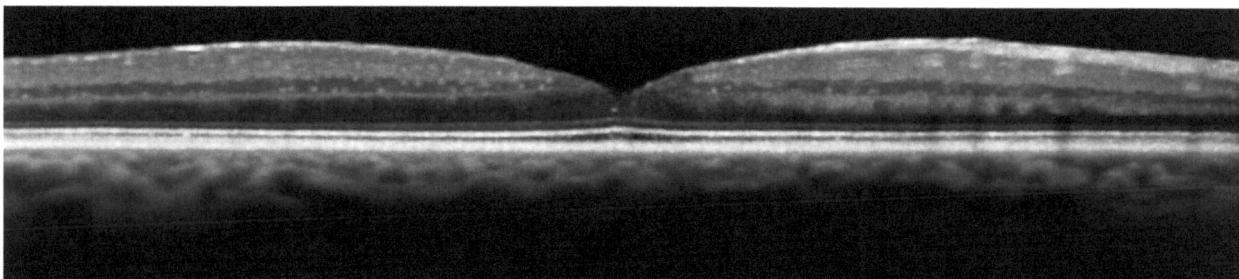

Another example of the appearance of the fovea with subjective fixation in a patient with central vision complaint. The foveal contour appears relatively normal.

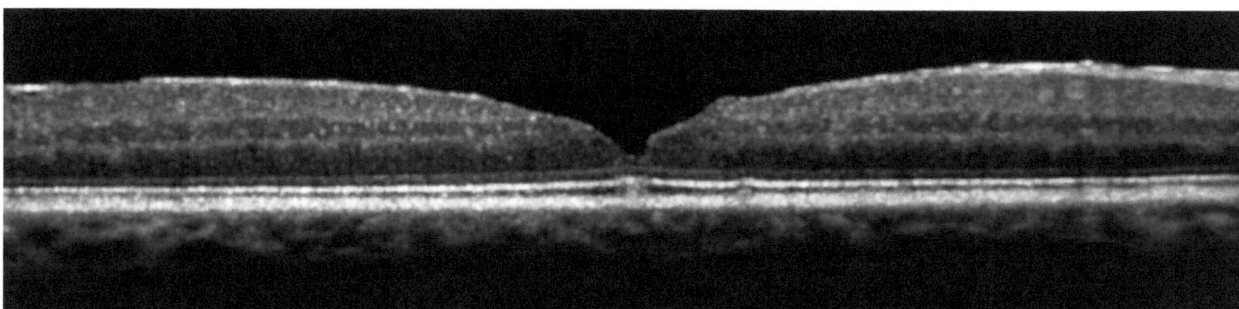

Increasing magnification and adjusting the scan location assists the imager in finding subtle changes.

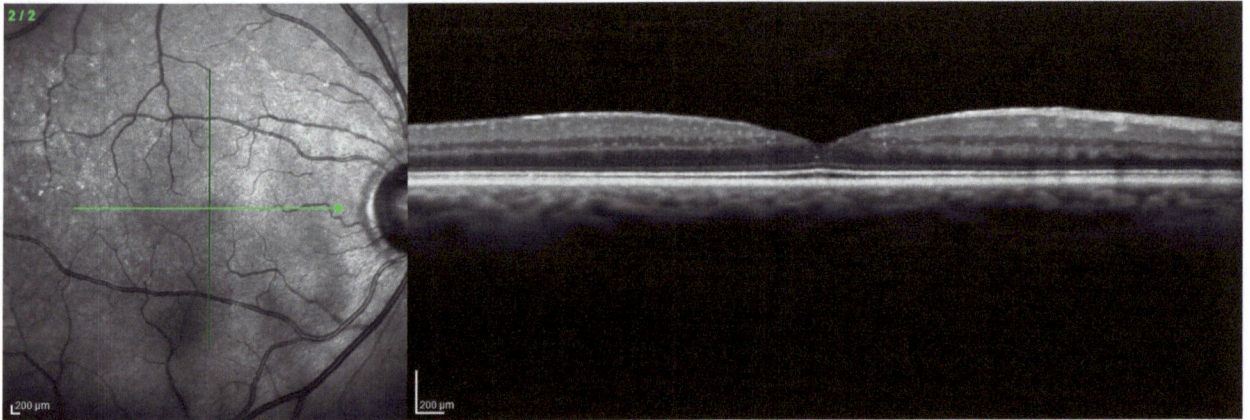

A scan through a patient's subjective fixation

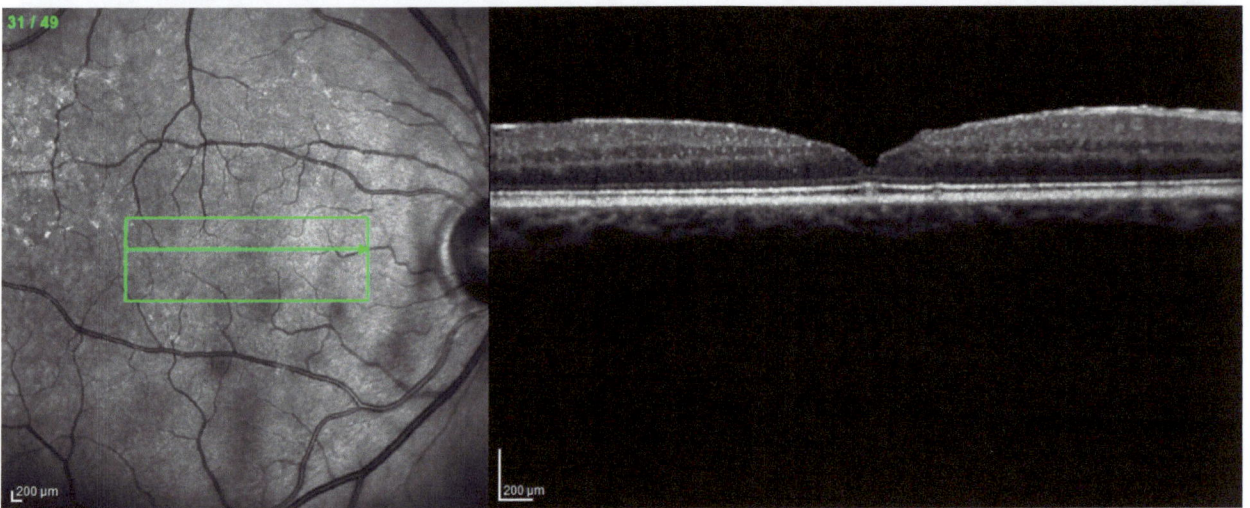

The same patient after the imager has moved the scan. Although there is a minimal excavation of the fovea, an enlarged view of the fovea shows IS/OS disruption.

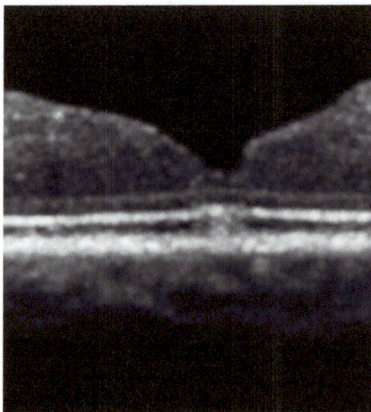

IS/OS disruption on post op

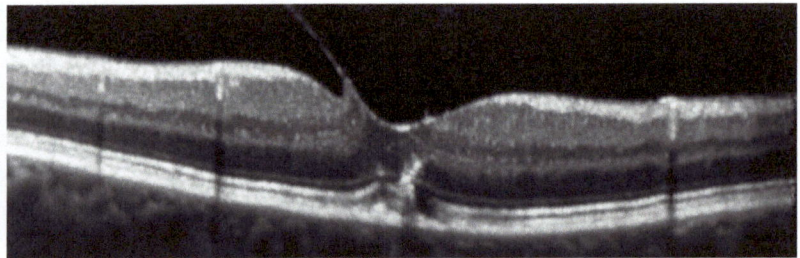

IS/OS disruption secondary to VMT

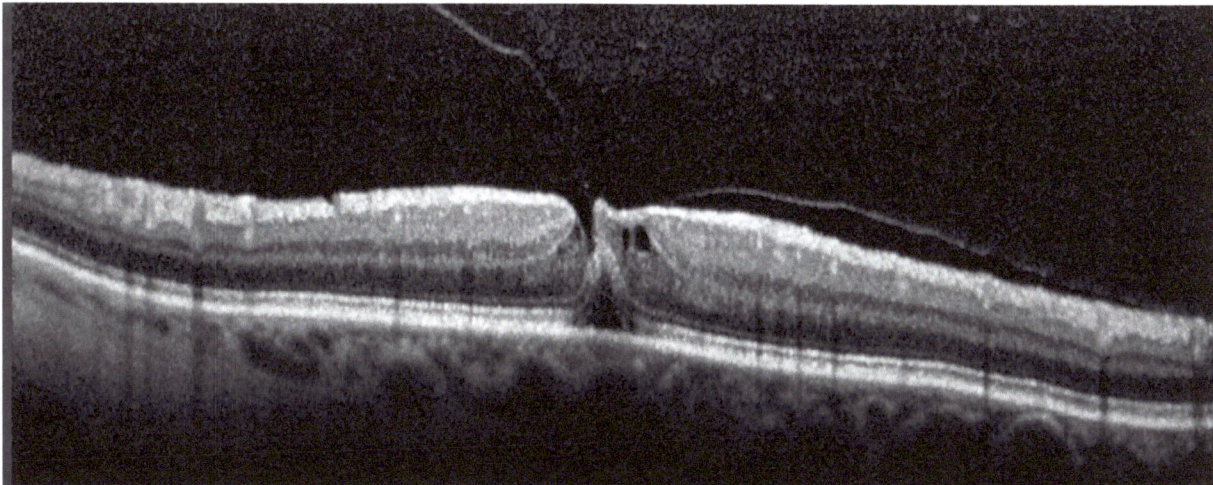

Another example of scanning through a patient's subjective fixation. Note the hyperreflective line that attaches to the tip of the retina in the center of the image. This is characteristic of VMT.

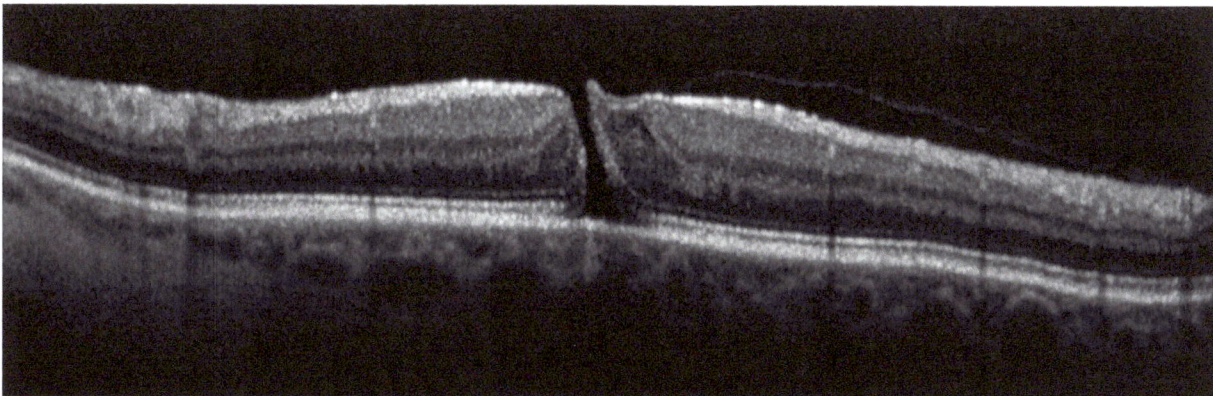

After moving the scan, a full thickness macular hole is revealed.

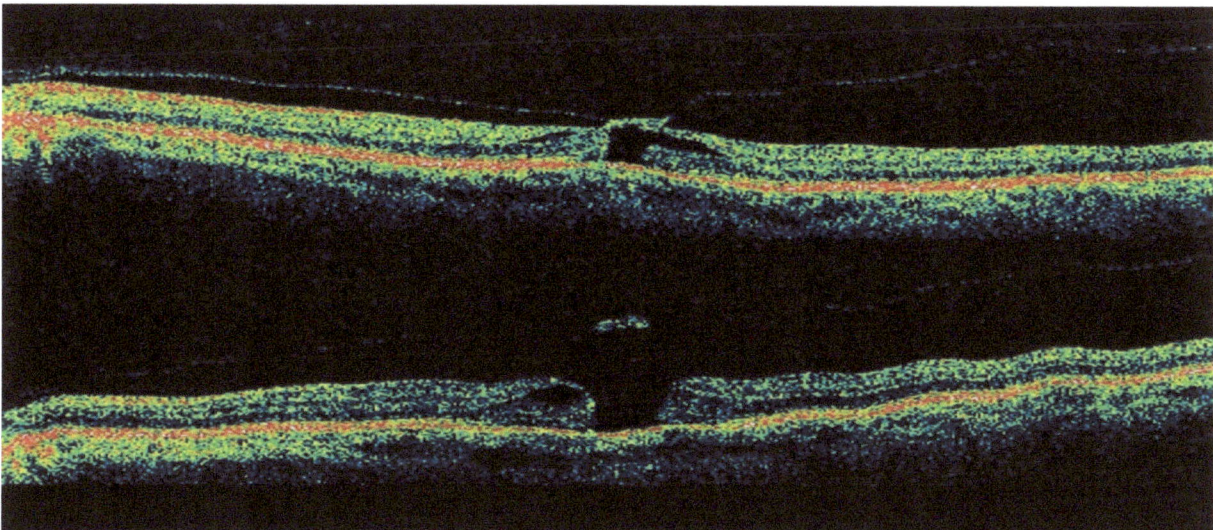

Macular traction (top) progressed to macular hole (bottom) on subsequent examination.

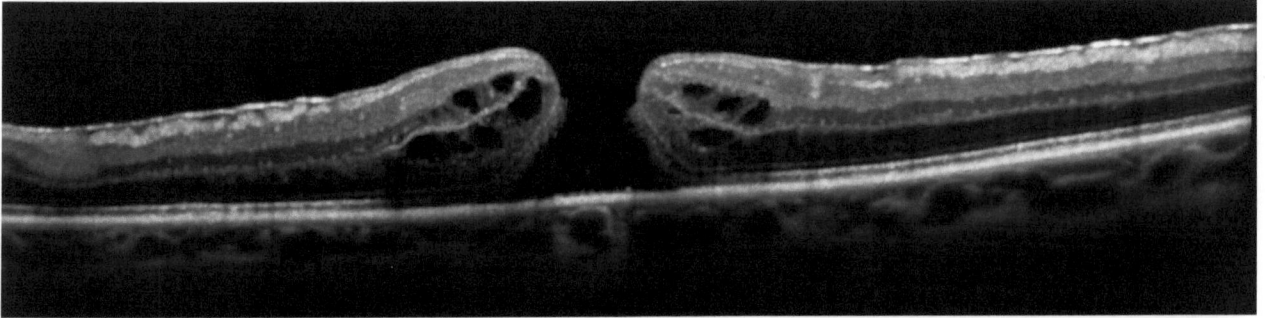

Preoperative full thickness macular hole. Note the epiretinal membrane that extends along the entire length of the retinal surface in either direction from the FTMH. There are cystoid spaces within the edges of the retina surrounding the FTMH. The choroid immediately under the FTMH is hyperreflective due to the decreased tissue attenuation and increased penetration of light in that region.

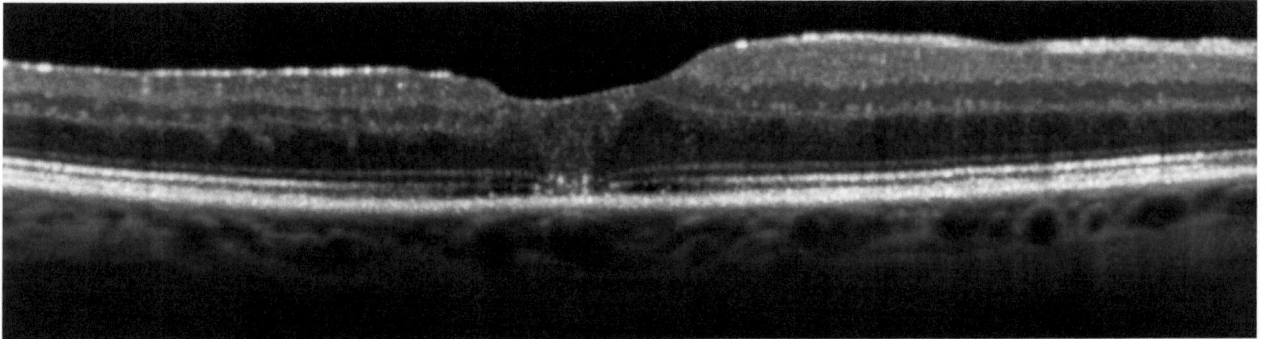

Post-operative OCT of FTMH shows that the hole is closed. The foveal depression appears abnormal and the outer retinal structures are abnormal. The external limiting membrane is not continuous and the ellipsoid band of the photoreceptors (also known as the inner segment-outer segment junction or IS/OS junction) is also broken.

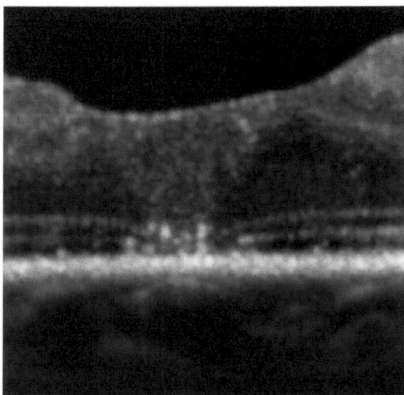

Magnified view of IS/OS junction

OCT can be used to follow patients with FTMH throughout the recovery period:

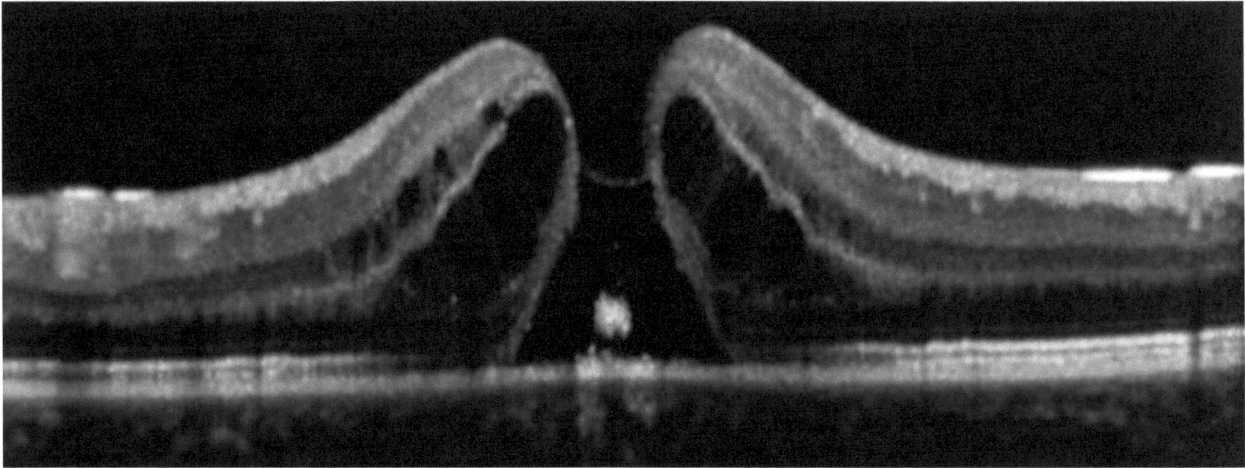

Pre-operative full thickness macular hole shows intraretinal cystoid spaces, hyperreflective retinal debris in the hole, and hyperreflective choroid in the center of the FTMH. There is a partial ERM that is evident in the peripheral regions of the retinal surface.

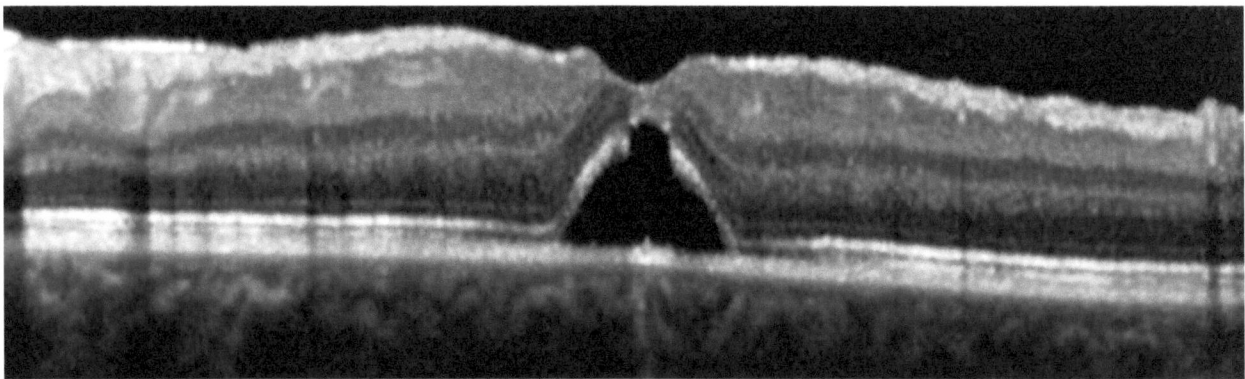

Post-operative 1 month OCT shows closure of the FTMH with persistent subretinal fluid. This is a not an uncommon post-operative finding in FTMH.

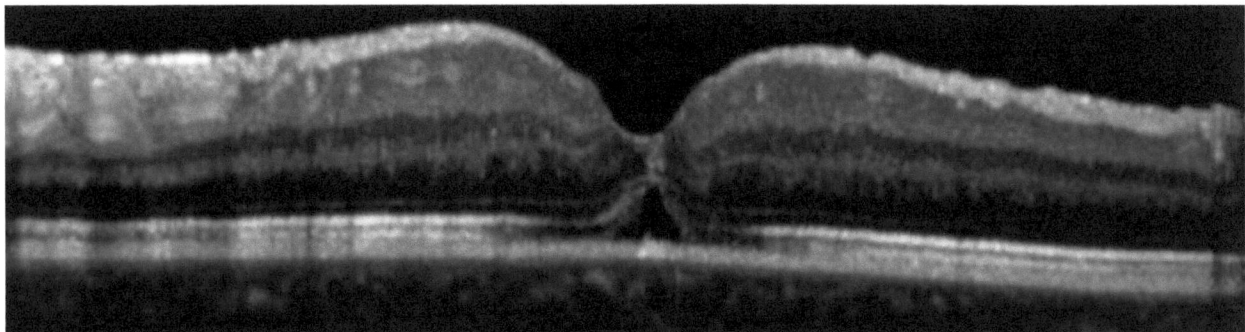

Post-operative 3 month OCT shows closure of the FTMH with significantly improved sub-retinal fluid.

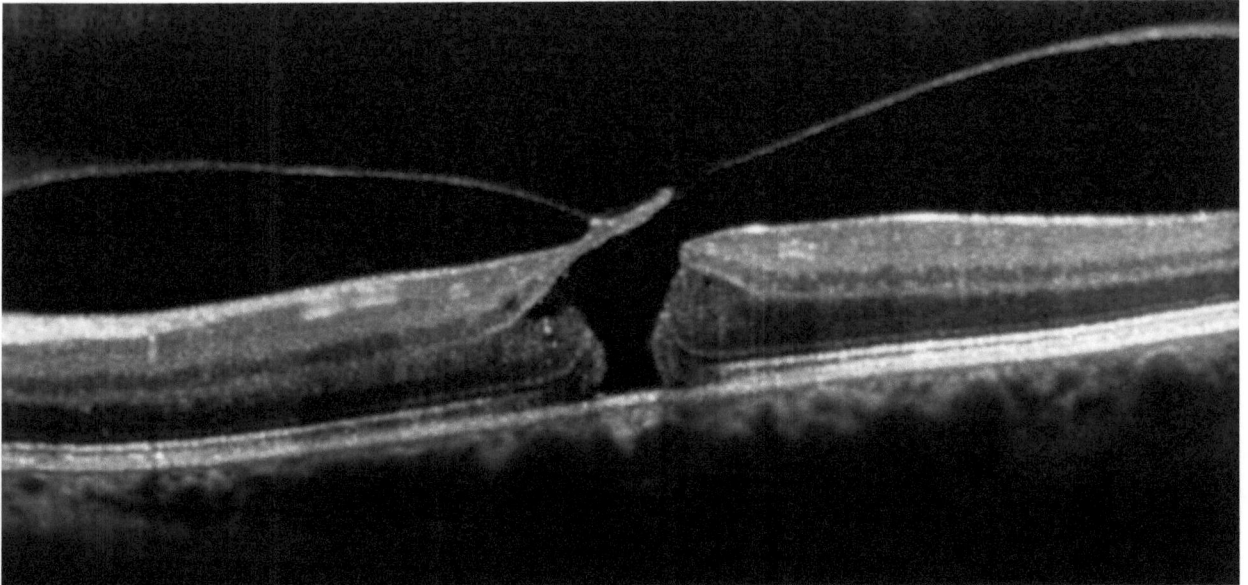

Pre-operative full thickness macular hole secondary to vitreomacular traction

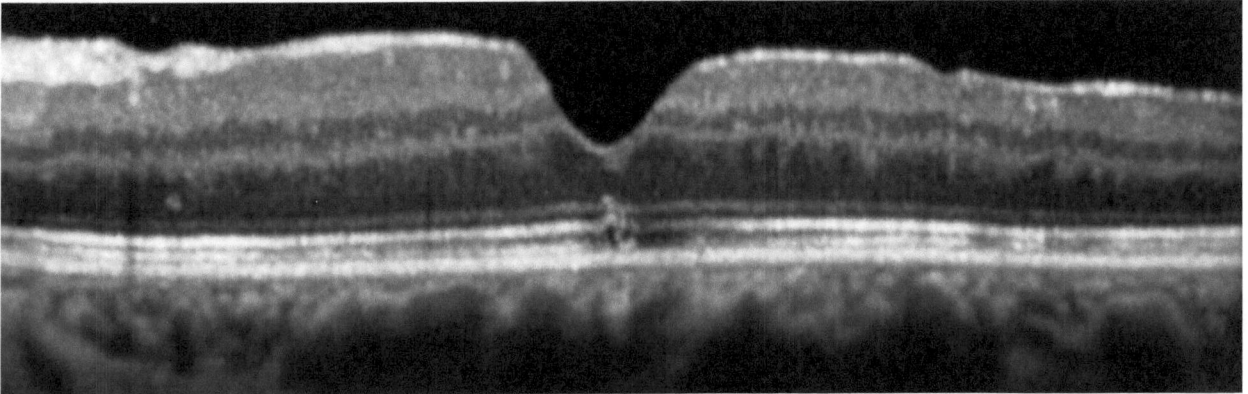

Postoperative macular hole is closed with persistent disruption of the external limiting membrane and ellipsoid band (also known as the inner segment-outer segment junction or IS/OS junction). Another example of a similar case is below:

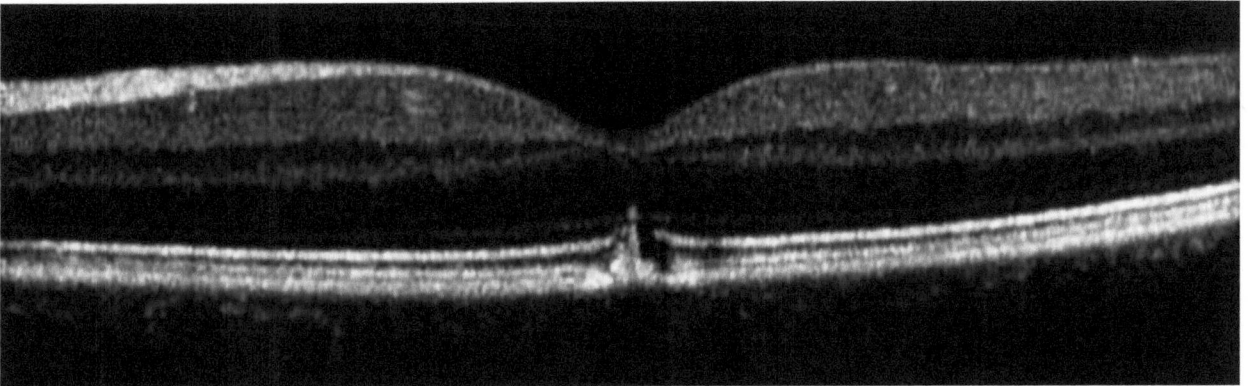

IS/OS disruption

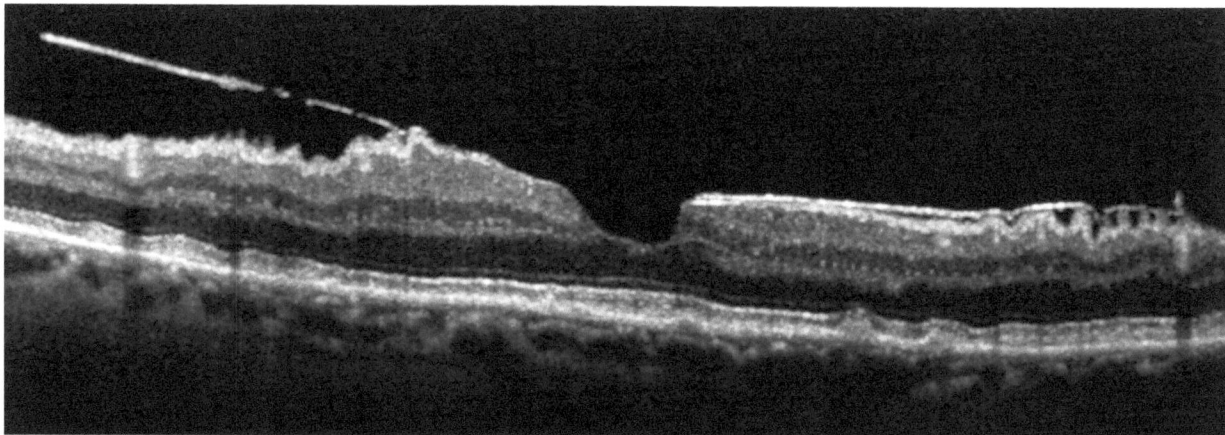

Partial thickness macular hole and epiretinal membrane

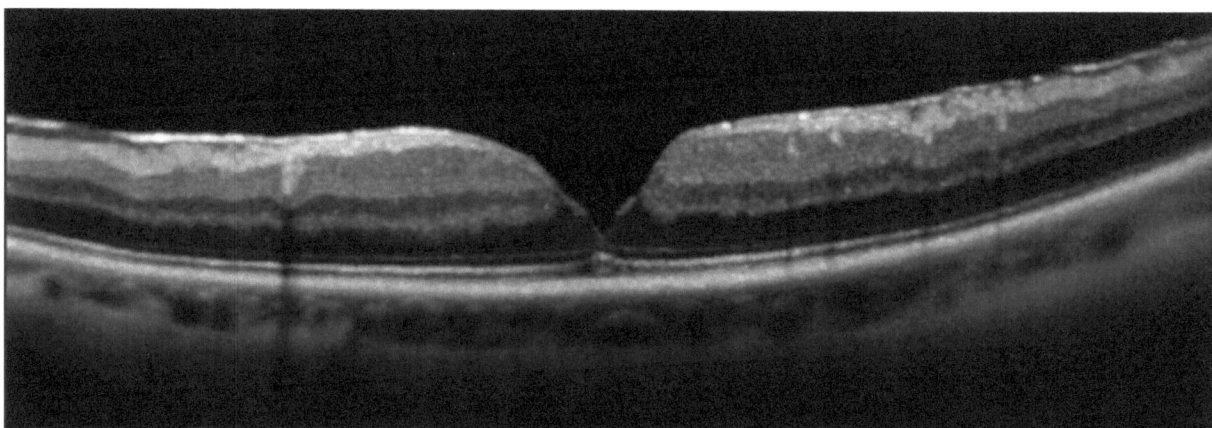

Lamellar macular hole with epiretinal membrane. Note that the outer nuclear layer is still intact.

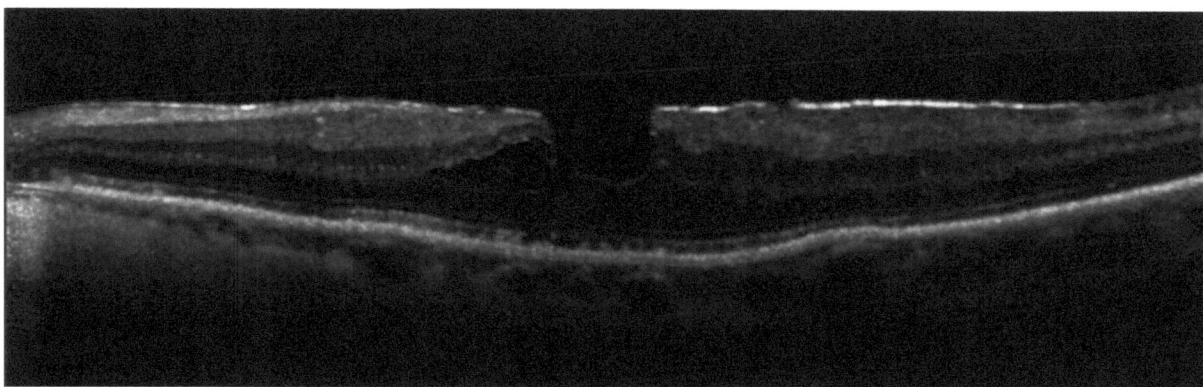

Lamellar macular hole with an ERM extending over the entire retinal surface but most evident on the right side of the fovea. The foveal depression is abnormal and the defect extends to the level of the outer nuclear layer.

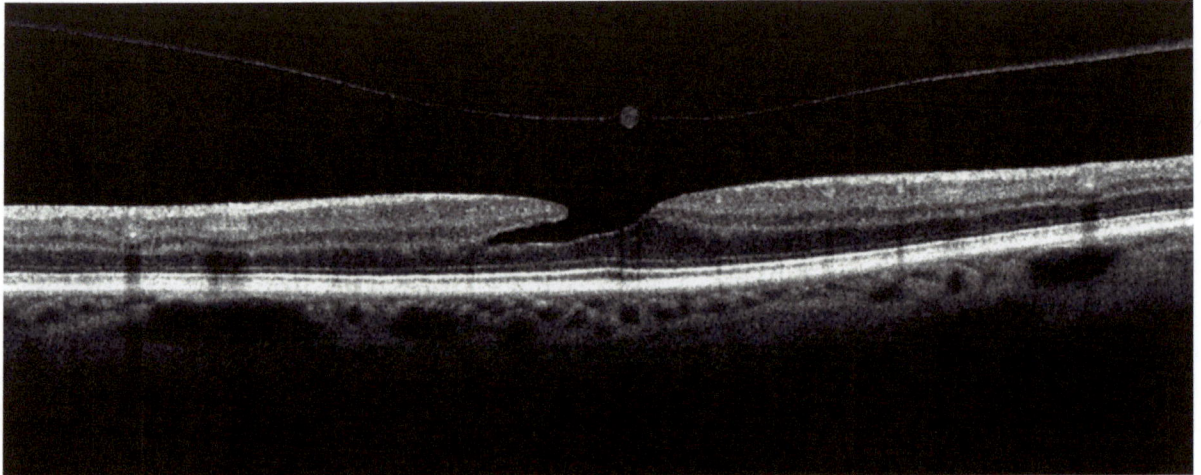

Lamellar macular hole with operculum in vitreous interface

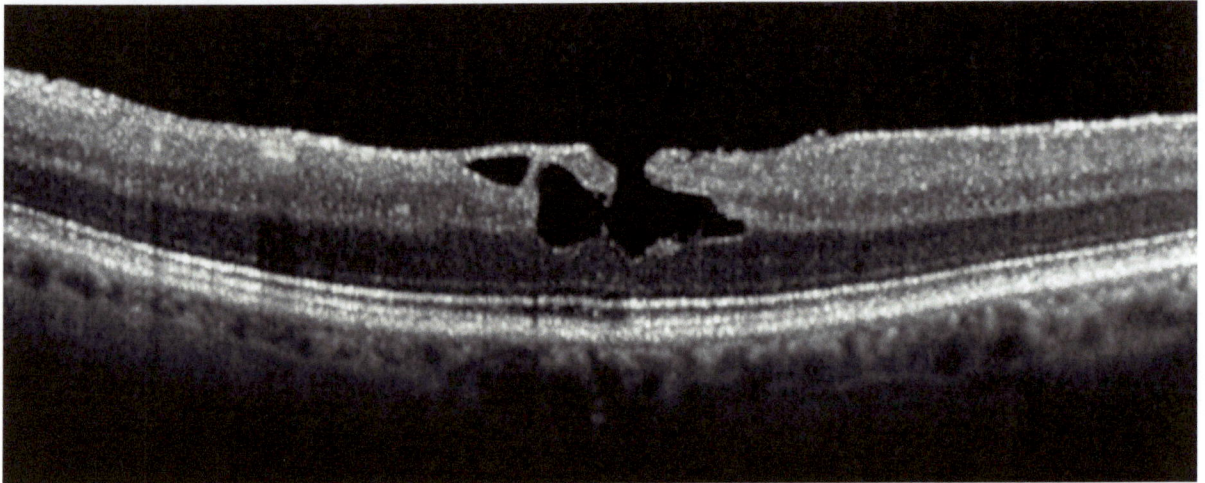

Lamellar hole- note that the outer nuclear layer is intact

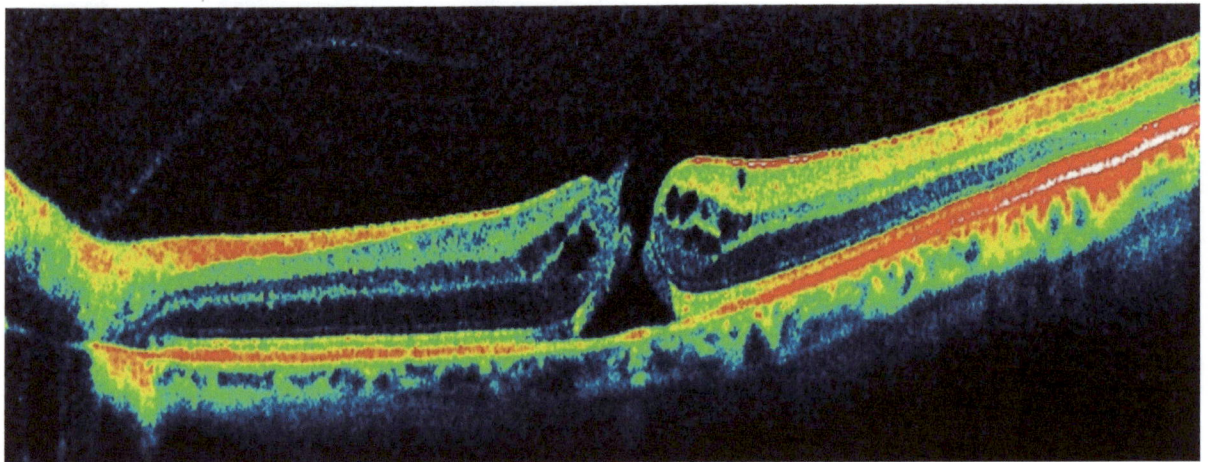

Pseudo-color full thickness macular hole with overlying vitreomacular traction on the nasal side of the FTMH. Intraretinal cystoid spaces are also evident on both sides of the FTMH.

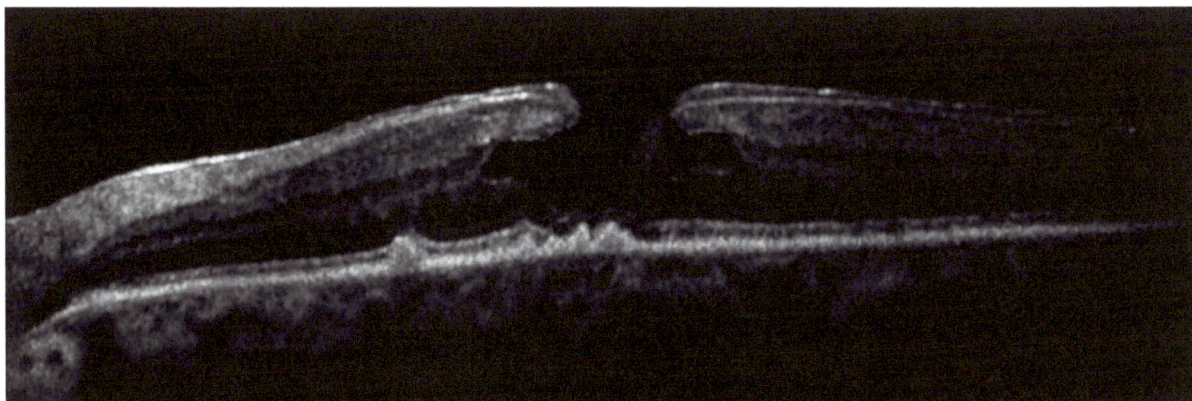

Pre-operative lamellar macular hole with overlying ERM and epiretinal proliferation

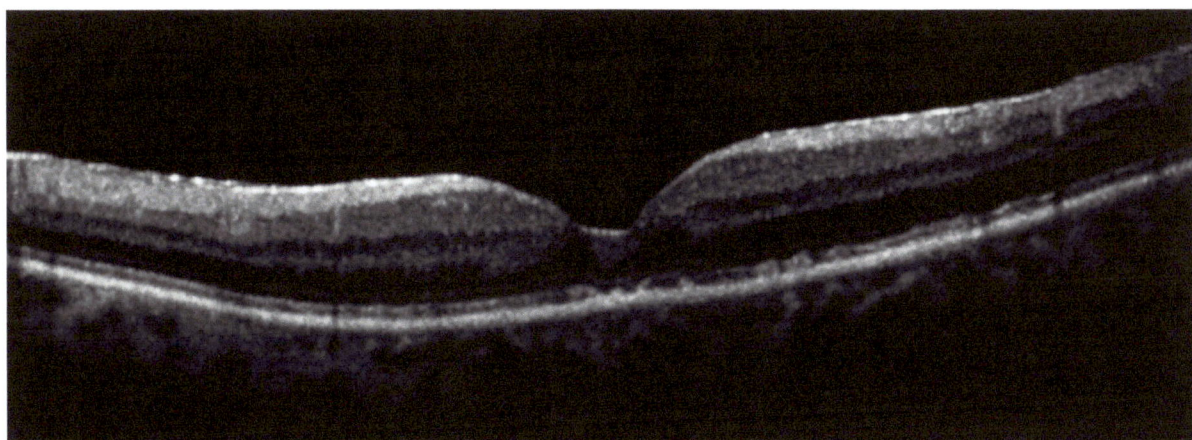

Post-operative lamellar macular hole is resolved

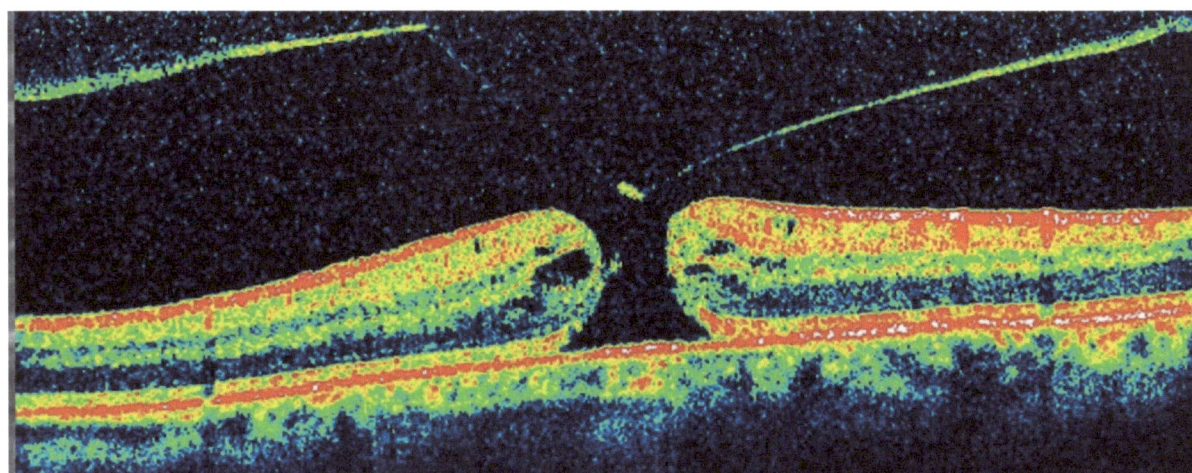

Full thickness macular hole with operculum

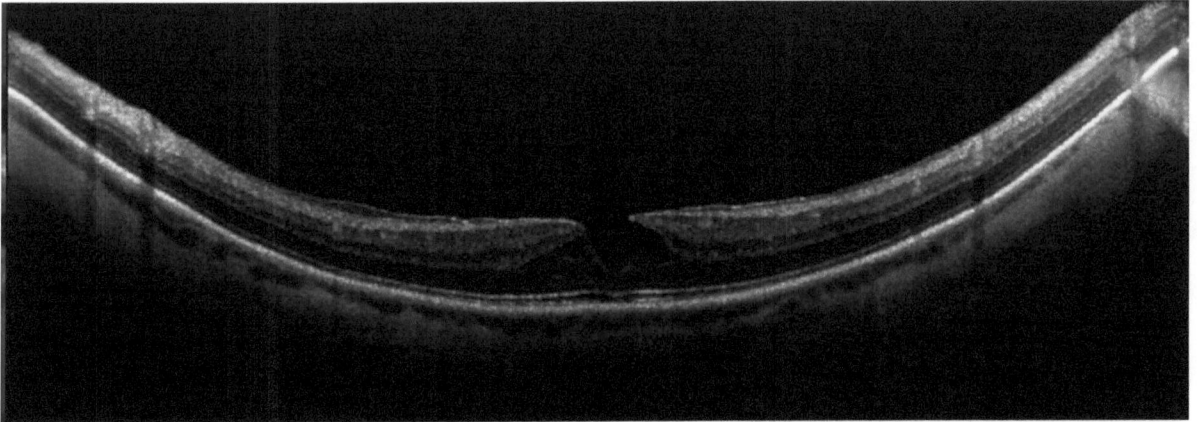

Partial thickness (lamellar) macular hole in high myope. Note the prominent curvature of the retina, which is indicative of the myopic eye. There is an ERM along the central portion of the macula and a prominent lamellar macular hole. Note that the outer nuclear layer is intact.

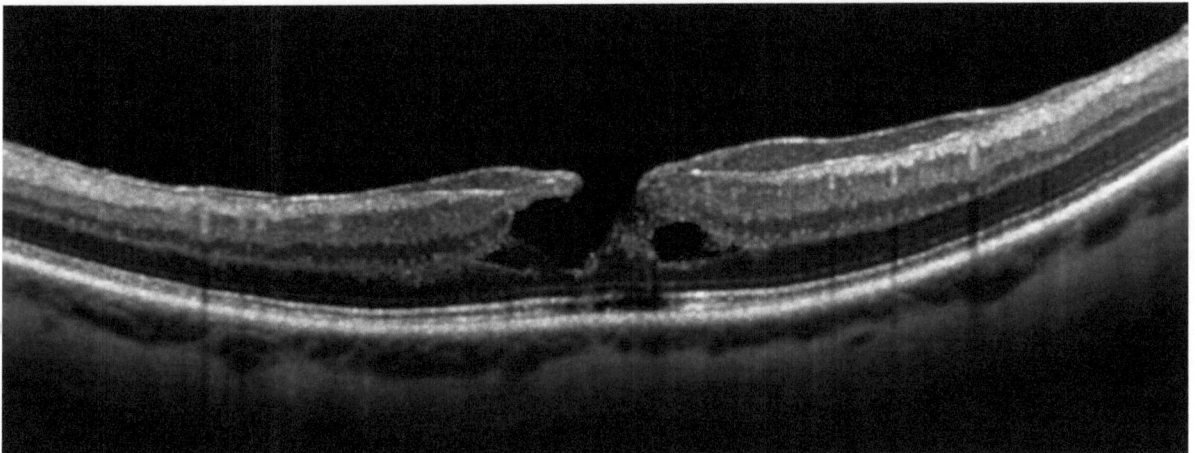

Partial thickness (lamellar) macular hole

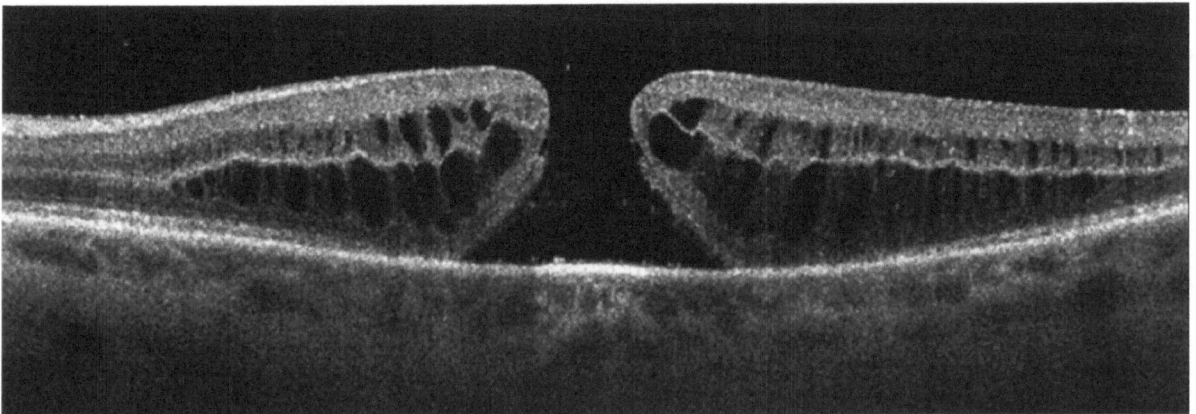

Full thickness macular hole on OCT B-scan

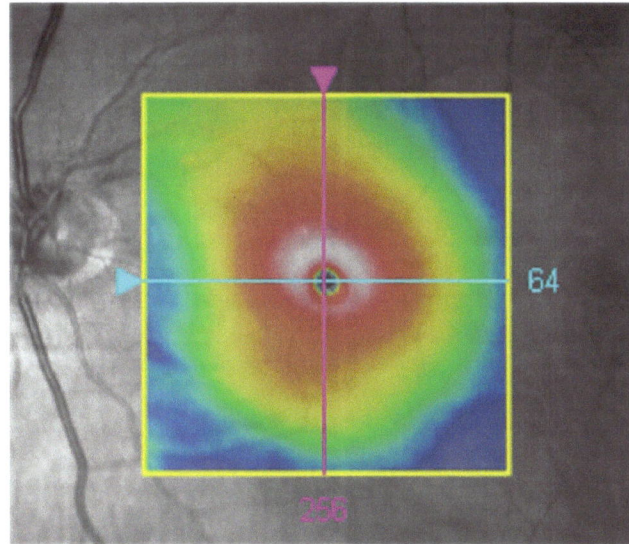

Volumetric display of macular hole on Spectral Domain. Note the excavation centrally, with elevated surrounding macula, represented by the red area.

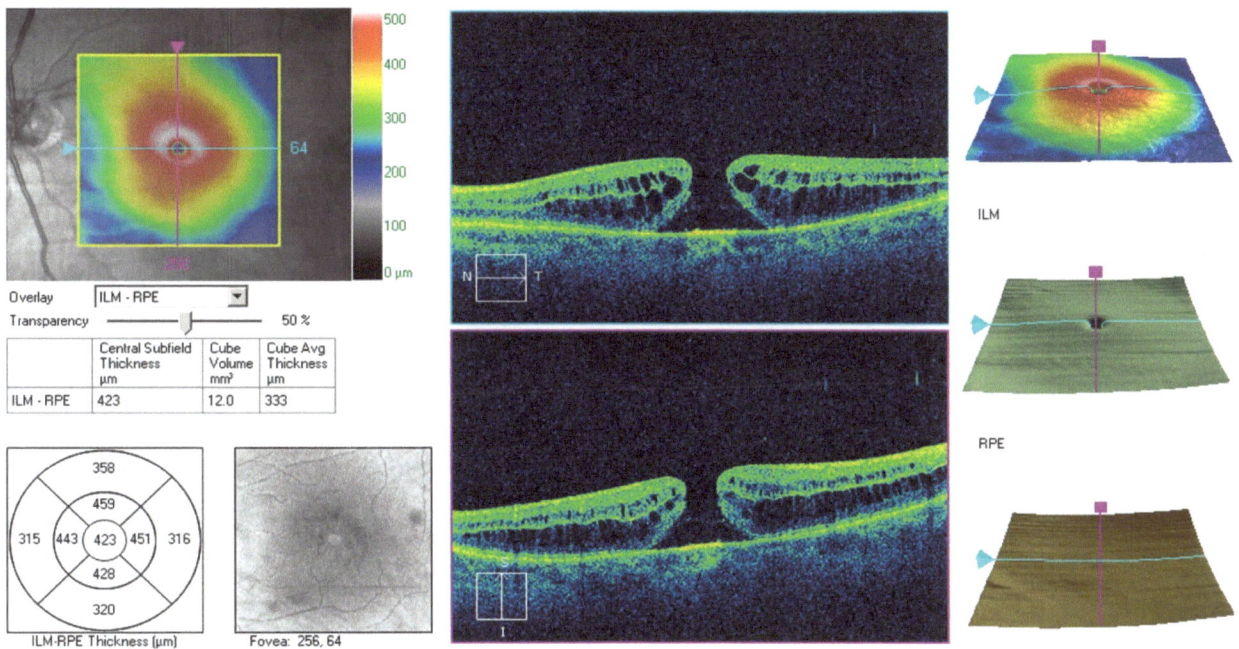

OCT display of full thickness macular hole with volumetric and individual layers

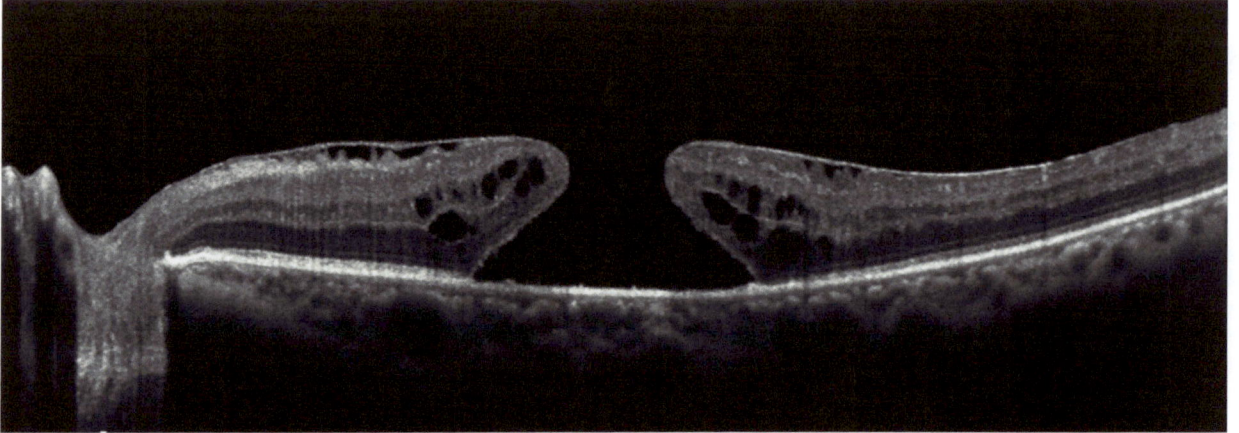

Full thickness macular hole with epiretinal membrane. Note the areas of intraretinal cystoid spaces on either side of the FTMH.

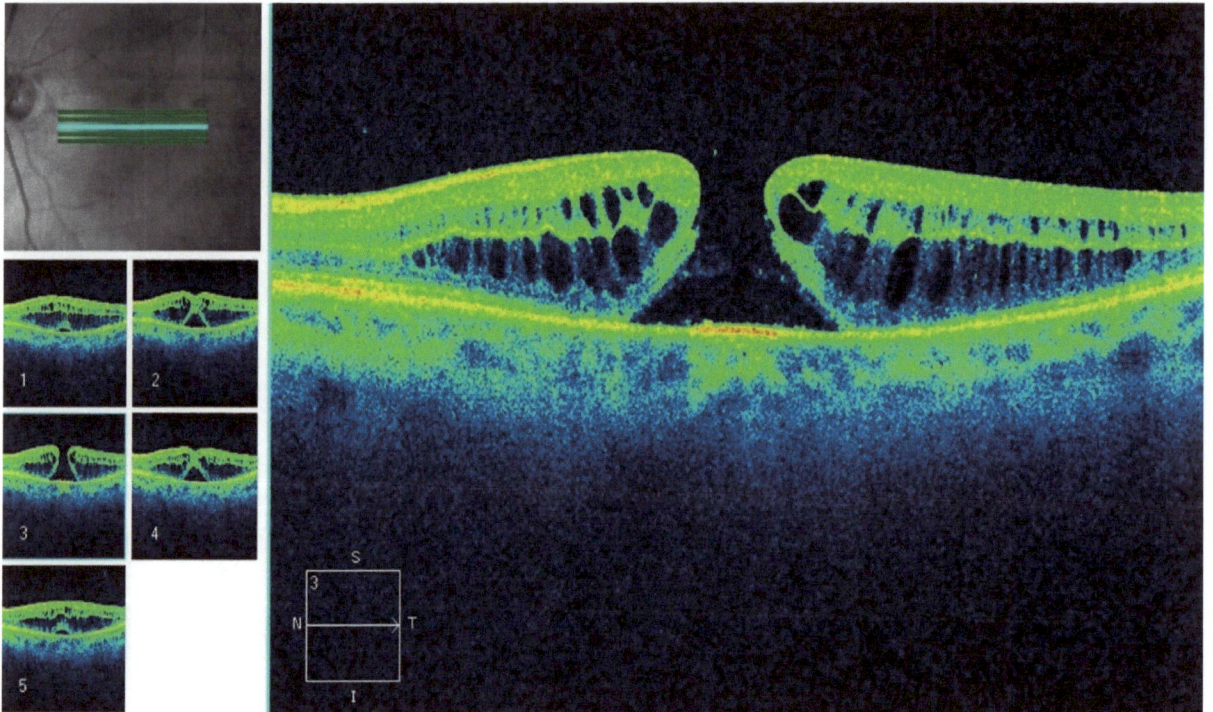

Full thickness macular hole. The top fundus image shows raster type scan, which uses multiple horizontal scans across a designated area.

A majority of OCT systems offer a preset crosshair or radial scan pattern that the imager can center on the fovea. In some instances, alternatively angled scans may better reveal pathology. In the example below, only presenting the horizontal scan does not offer the physician the entire story.

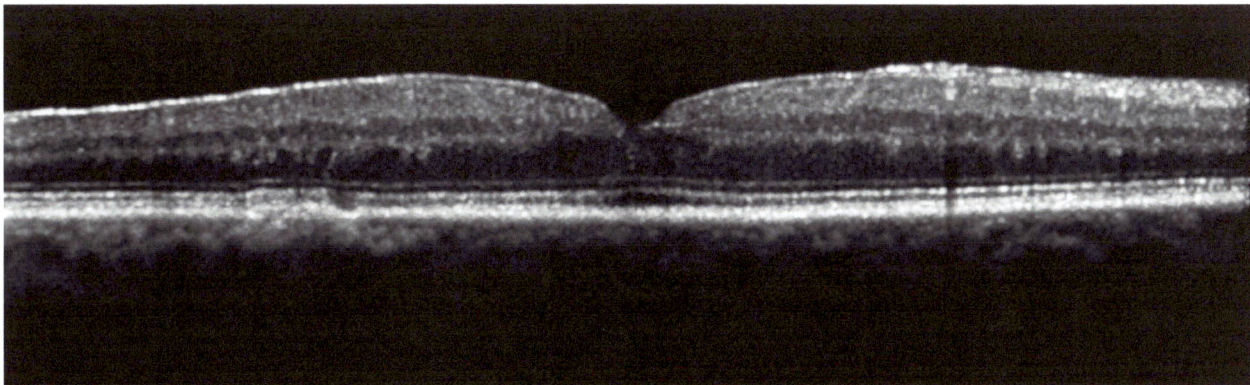

Horizontal scan

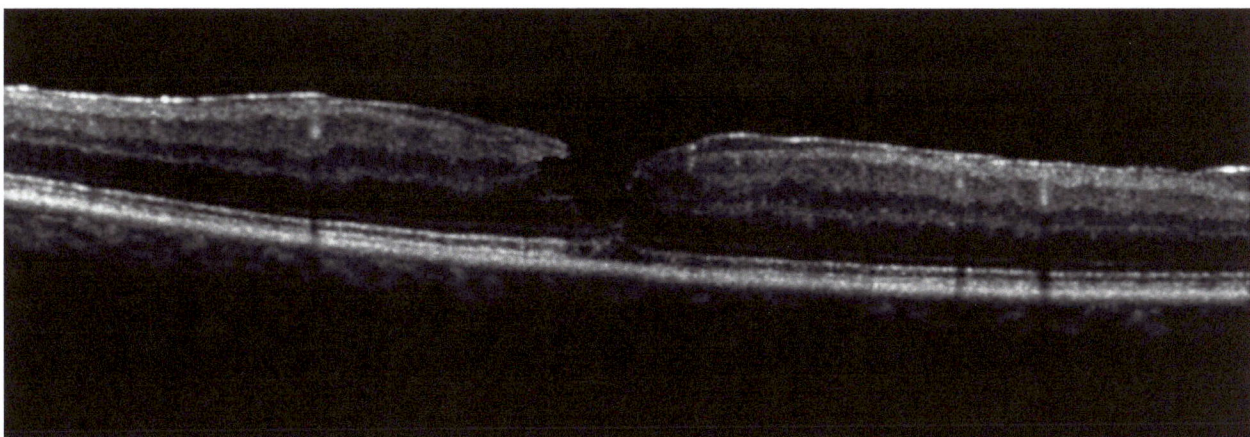

Vertical scan, revealing a partial thickness macular hole with an epiretinal membrane

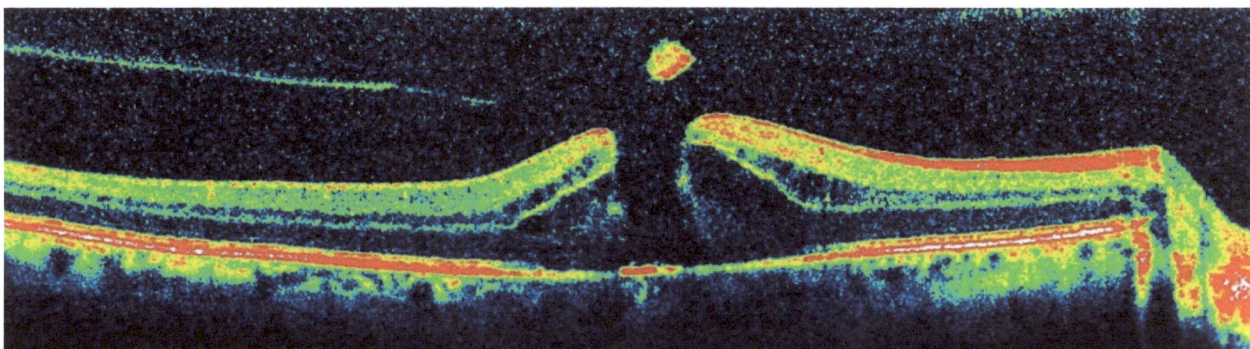

Full thickness macular hole with large operculum. Note that the false color display in this image renders some separation of layers indistinguishable.

Cystoid Macular Edema (CME)

There are several terms that are used interchangeably when referring to intraretinal fluid. These terms are largely interchangeable but some are used more commonly to refer to specific pathologies. In general, "intraretinal fluid" and "macular edema" are very general terms that refer to the presence of hyporeflective cystoid spaces within the neurosensory retina on OCT. Cystoid Macular Edema (CME) is a specific type of macular edema that is usually associated with retinal vein occlusions, post-operative retinal edema ("Irvine-Gass"), and uveitis. In the setting of Diabetic Retinopathy, macular edema is generally referred to as Diabetic Macular Edema (DME). Therefore, DME and CME refer to specific types of macular edema. Intraretinal fluid associated with choroidal neovascularization is commonly referred to as just "intraretinal fluid" or "macular edema." The discussion below will be largely limited to CME. Macular edema associated with DR and AMD will be discussed in the chapters specific to those diseases.

CME typically appears in and around the foveal avascular zone. The etiology of CME is unclear, but it is thought to be related to incompetent retinal capillaries and consequent leakage of serous fluid into the intraretinal space. CME is best visualized with fluorescein angiography and OCT. Fluorescein angiography may demonstrate a classic late petaloid leakage pattern centered on the fovea or a more nonspecific diffuse leakage pattern (see image on next page). The advent of OCT has provided much more information regarding the extent and location of CME. Today, OCT is the mainstay of CME diagnosis and management, although fluorescein angiography may still be necessary for a complete evaluation. Both B-scan line and volumetric OCT scans of macular edema can be used to visualize and quantify the volume of fluid in the intraretinal space. With most OCT systems, the software can show differences in the volume of edema between scans. However, when evaluating OCT for presence or absence of CME, it is critical to manually inspect each OCT B-scan, since small pockets of fluid can occur in a few B-scans without impacting the volume measurements.

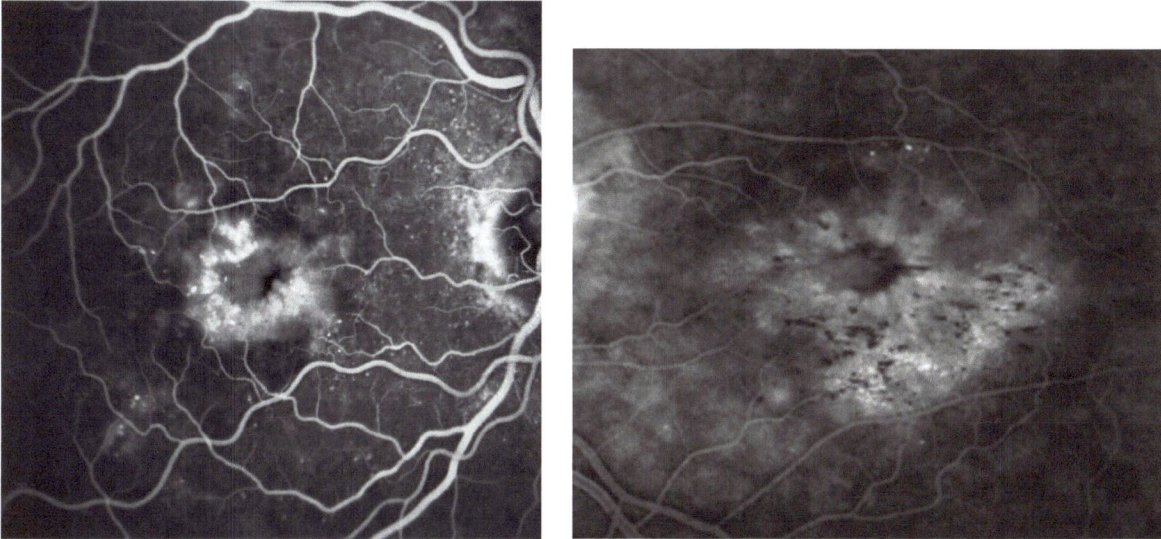

Fluorescein angiogram of subjects with CME. Note the somewhat symmetric petaloid appearance of the hyperfluorescent areas around the fovea in both examples. CME is typically best illustrated on late phase fluorescein images.

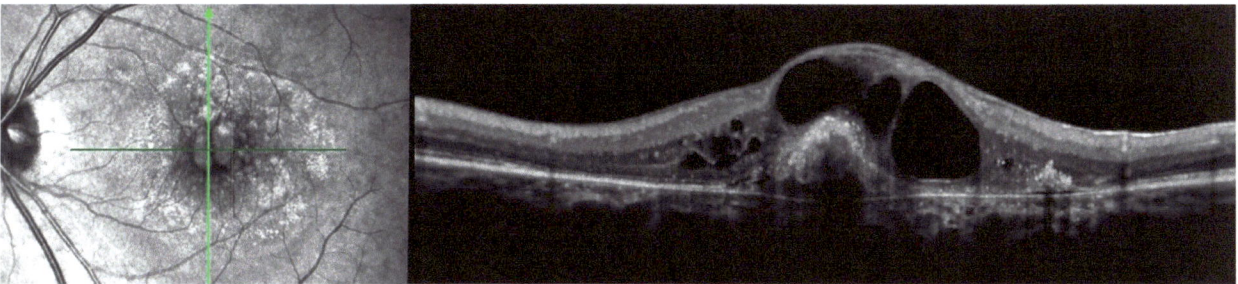

Macular edema can be seen on the infrared image (left) and on the OCT (right). Underlying the area of intraretinal fluid is a pigment epithelial detachment and likely a choroidal neovascular membrane.

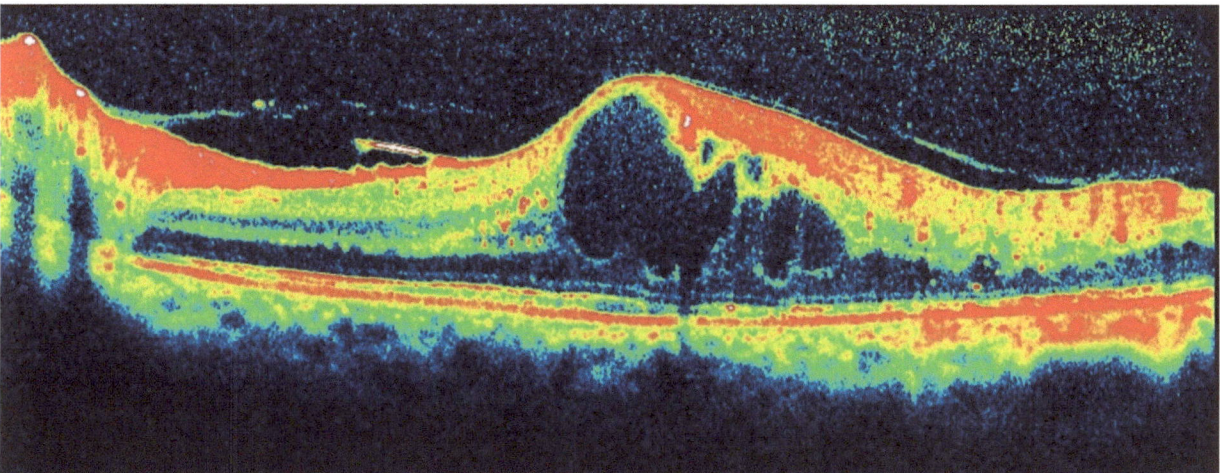

Typical cystoid macular edema with oblong, cystic spaces in the fovea

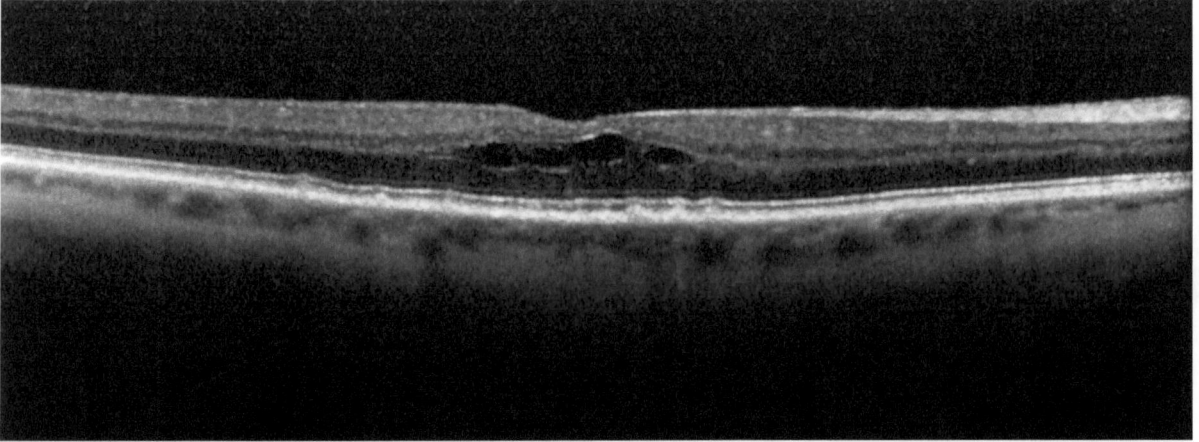

Even mild CME can blunt the foveal contour. It is important to manually scan through the individual OCT B-scans to identify cystoid spaces that may be too small to cause retinal thickening on the volume maps.

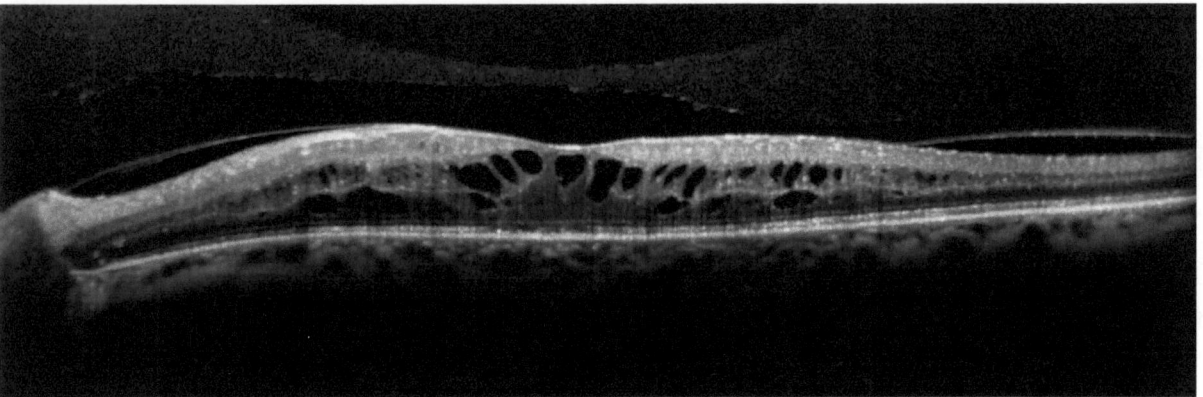

CME with overlying vitreous attachment. In this case, it is difficult to determine whether the CME is caused by the vitreomacular traction, by some other process or by a combination of the two.

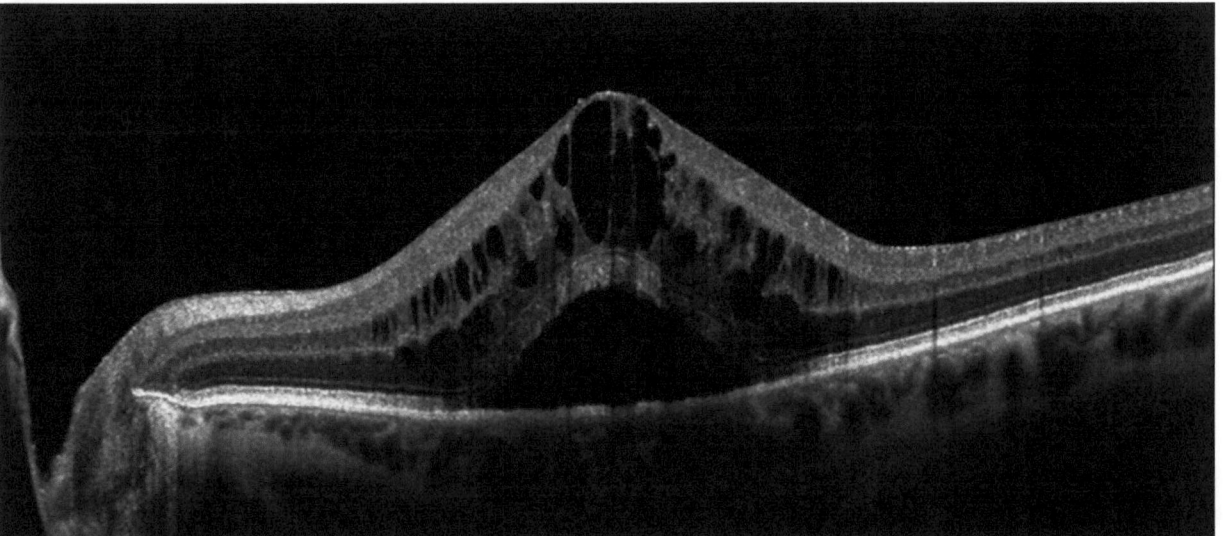

Severe CME with associated sub retinal fluid. Note that there is no overlying vitreous that is detectable on the OCT. This patient likely has a complete PVD, unlike the previous case.

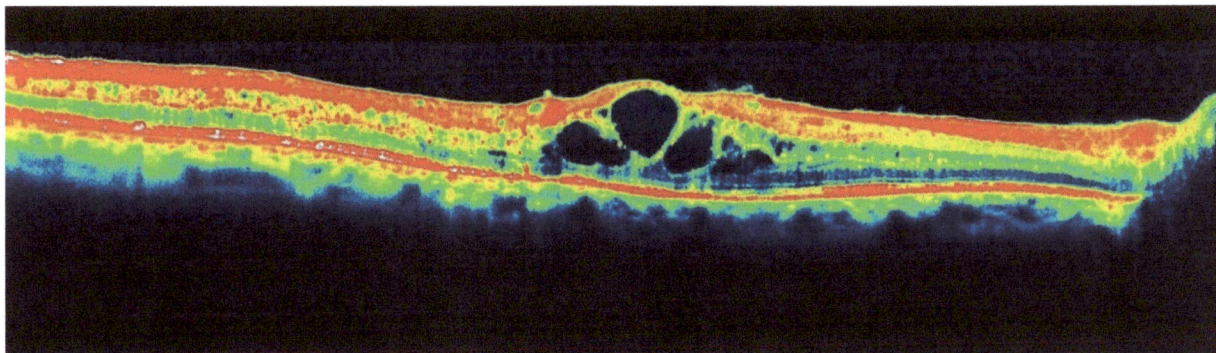

Pseudo-color OCT of CME with typical petaloid pattern of cystoid spaces

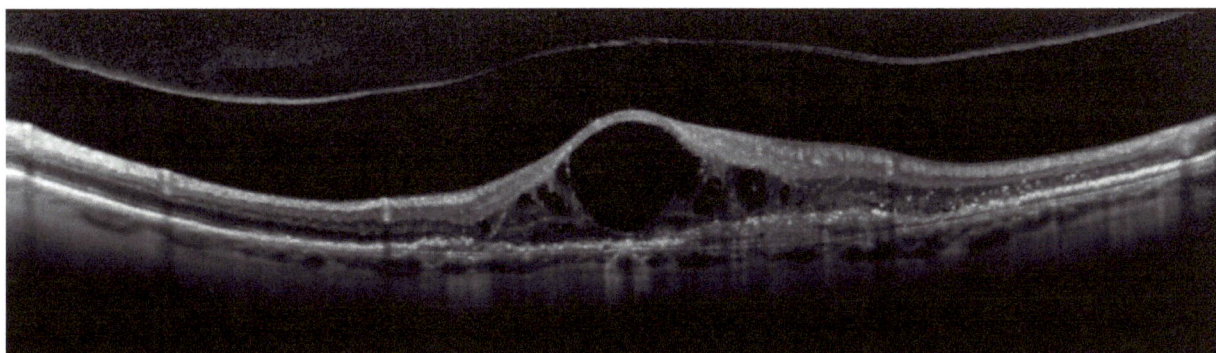

Subject with neovascular age related macular degeneration and overlying macular edema. Note the partial posterior vitreous separation indicated by the hyperreflective line above the retina.

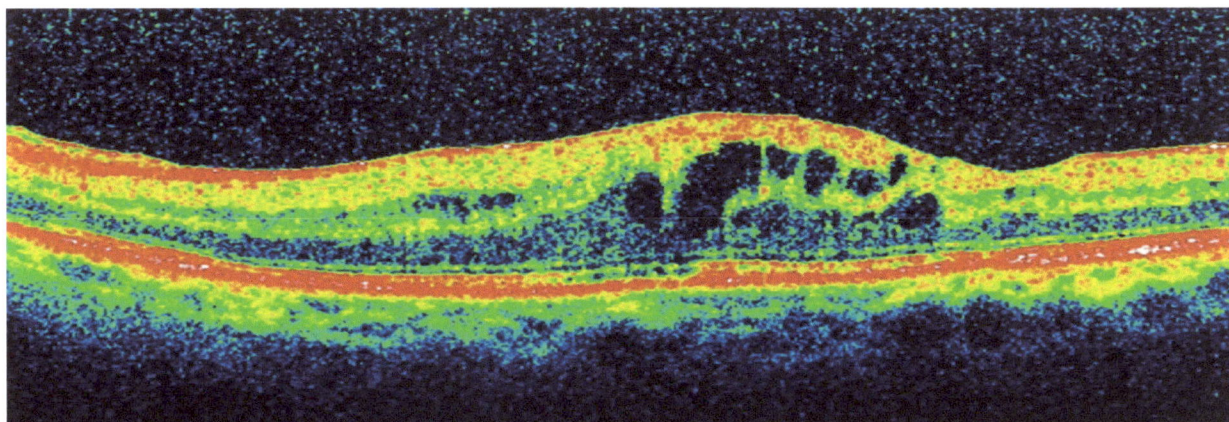

CME may distort the macula and make it difficult to locate a foveal depression.

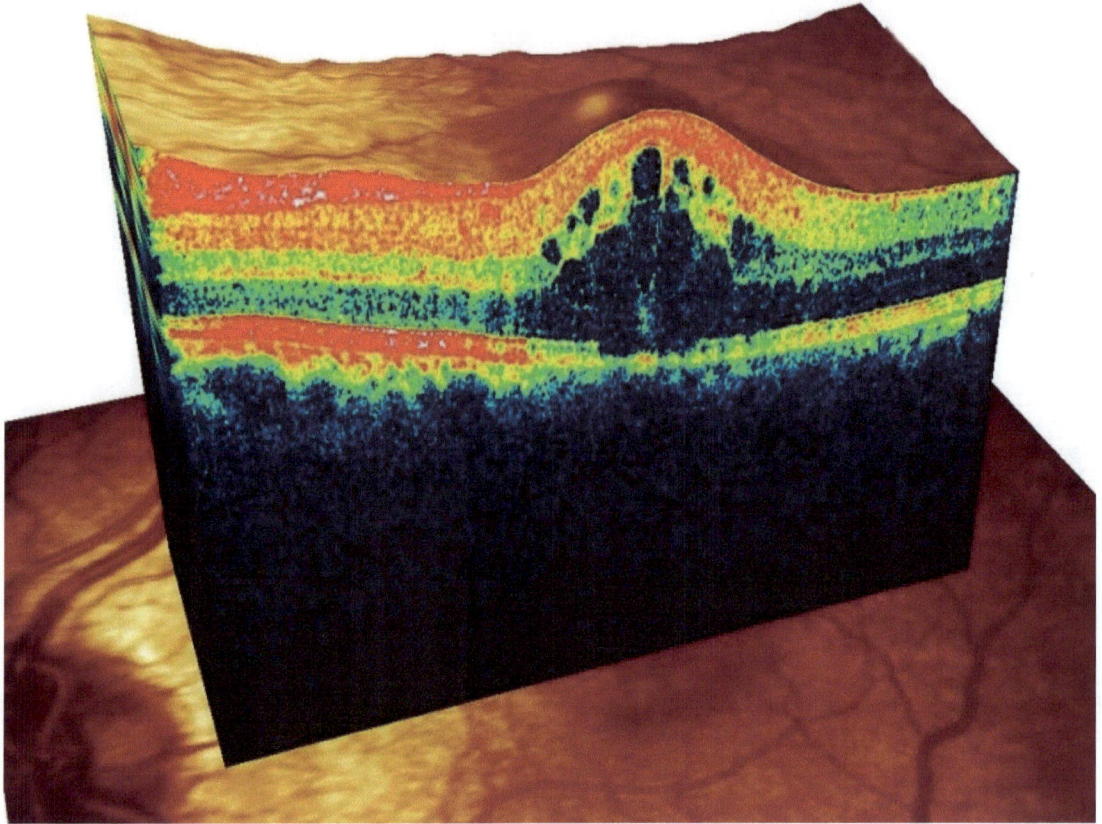

Three-dimensional cube showing CME and retinal thickening

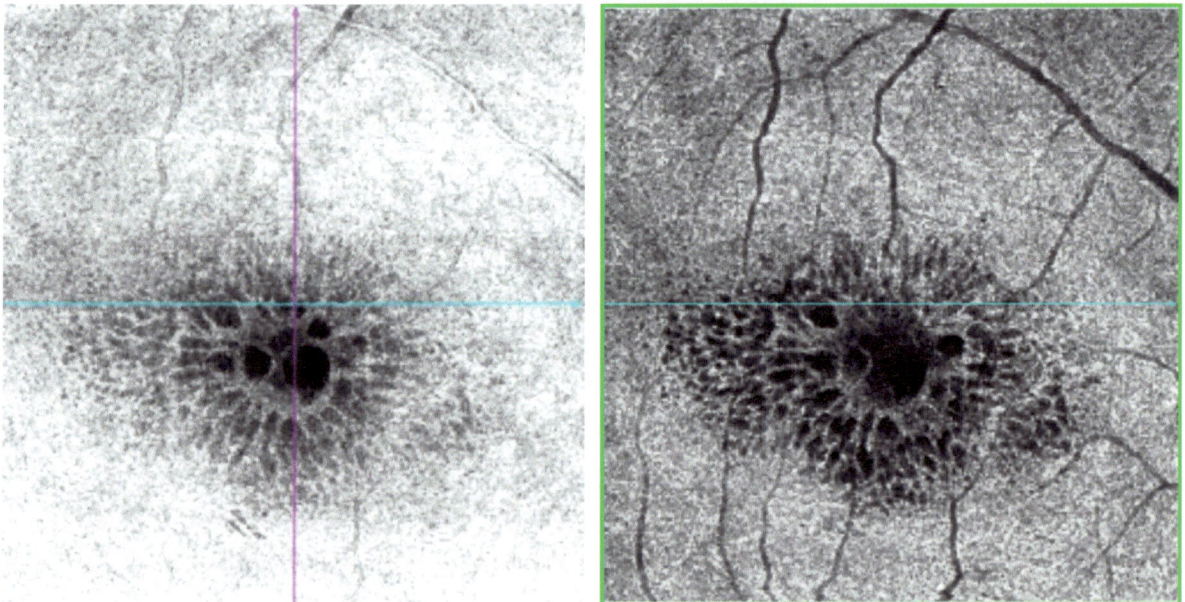

En face IR images of CME, clearly showing cystic patterns. These patterns are visible on the OCT en face intensity image, which is essentially an IR image. Note that these are not OCTA images but just raw intensity images. The cystoid spaces attenuate the OCT signal and appear as relative hyporeflective spaces.

Diabetic Macular Edema (DME)

Macular edema that occurs in the setting of diabetic retinopathy (DR) is called DME. DME may present like CME, with intraretinal cystoid spaces, but DME is commonly not symmetrically oriented around the fovea. DME can be very focal, and can occur anywhere in the macula, or it can occur diffusely throughout the large regions of the macula. DME can occur at any stage of DR, and depending on the severity may cause severe symptoms or no symptoms at all. When DME is severe enough to be detected on clinical examination it is sometimes referred to as Clinically Significant Macular Edema (CSME), although this terminology is infrequently used in the era of OCT and anti-VEGF therapy. It is important to note that mild DME can frequently occur within only a few B-scans and may not be detected on the volume measurements that are generated by commercial software. Careful manual inspection of individual B-scans is necessary to provide a definitive evaluation of DME.

DME may also be associated with hard exudates. These exudates are visible on clinical examination as yellow deposits and are visible on OCT as very focal hyper-reflective spots within the retina.

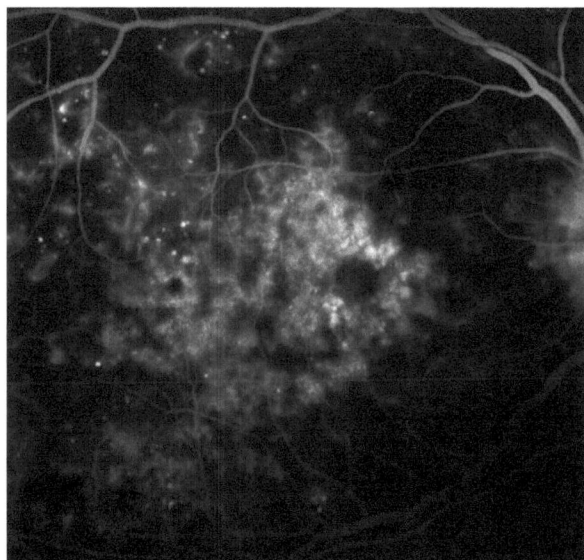

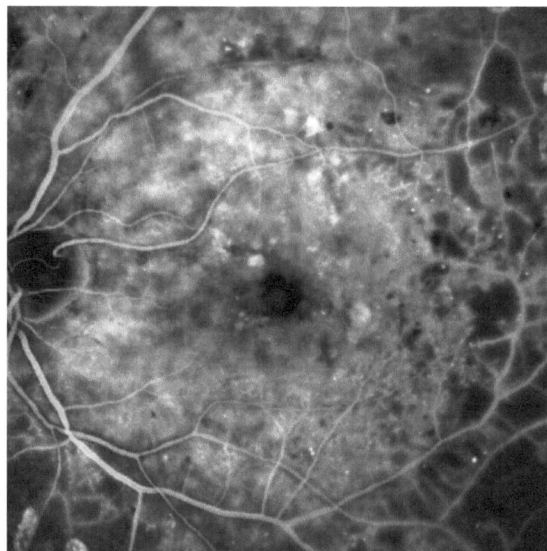

Late phase fluorescein angiogram of two diabetic patients with diffuse diabetic macular edema. Note the areas of hyperfluorescence throughout the majority of the macula in both cases. Numerous microaneurysms are visible in the image on the right as bright pinpoints of hyperfluorescence. Several areas of impaired capillary perfusion ("nonperfusion") are noted on the far right portion of the image on the right.

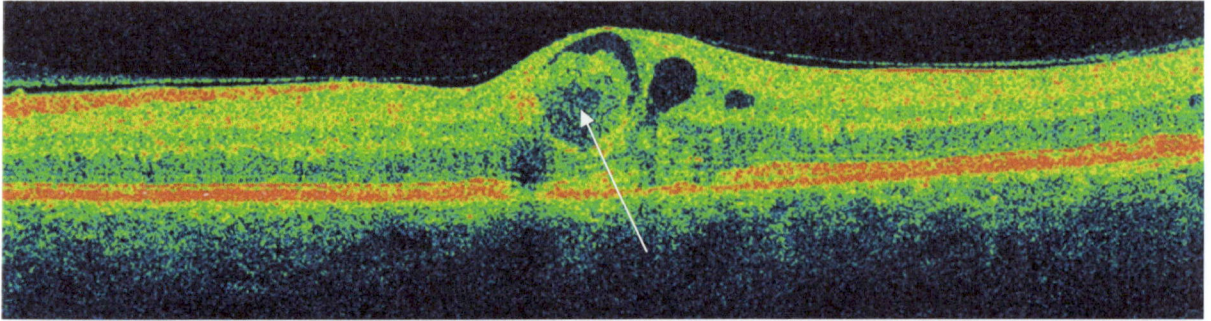

DME with hyperreflective material. In most cases, DME is associated with intraretinal cystoid spaces that are hyporeflective compared to the surrounding retina. In some cases, hyperreflective material may be noted within these cystoid spaces, as in the case illustrated above (white arrow). The etiology of this hyperreflectivity is unclear but is thought to be associated with the resorption of intraretinal fluid and the residual lipoproteinaceous material that remains in the retina and is observed clinically as hard exudate.

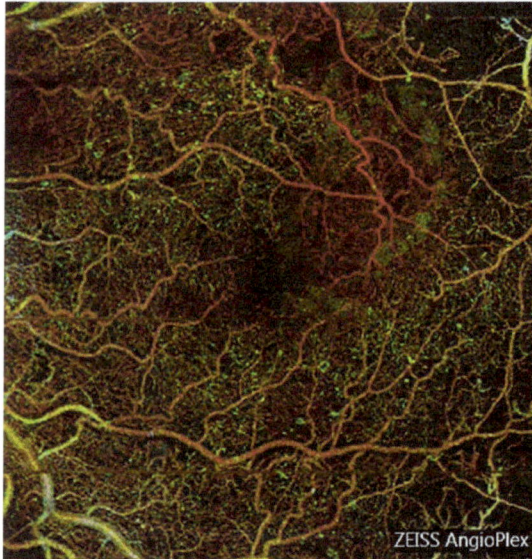

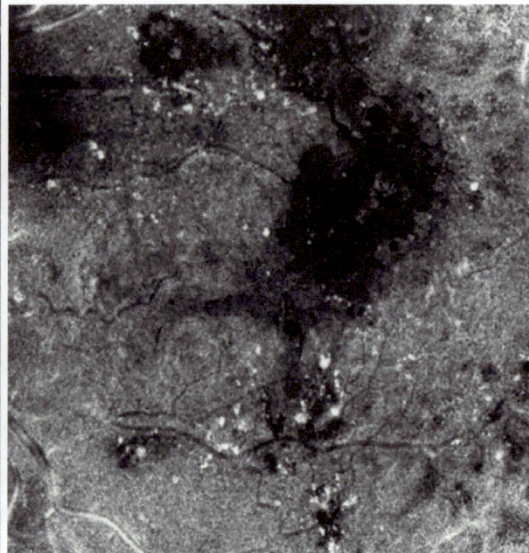

Depth encoded OCTA of DME. Note the superior superficial vessels in red, denoting intraretinal edema in that area, raising the normal vessels into a higher scan plane. The corresponding en face image on the right illustrates the areas of edema in high contrast of black on gray.

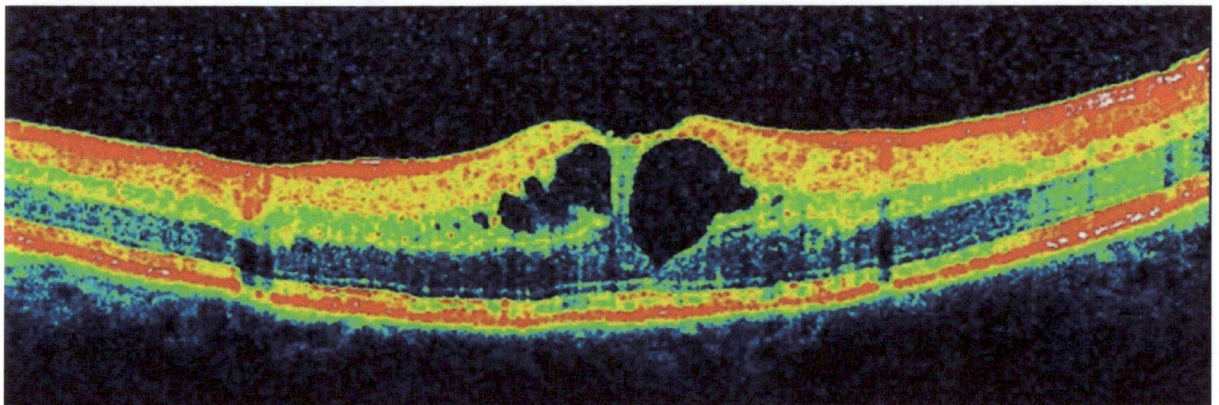

Diabetic macular edema presented as cystic spaces around the fovea

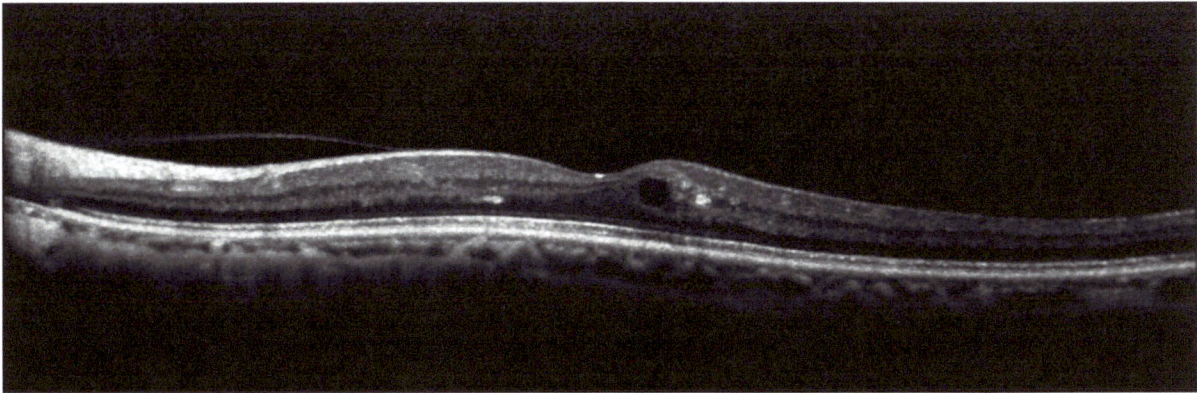

DME with associated foci of hyperreflectivity that are consistent with hard exudates

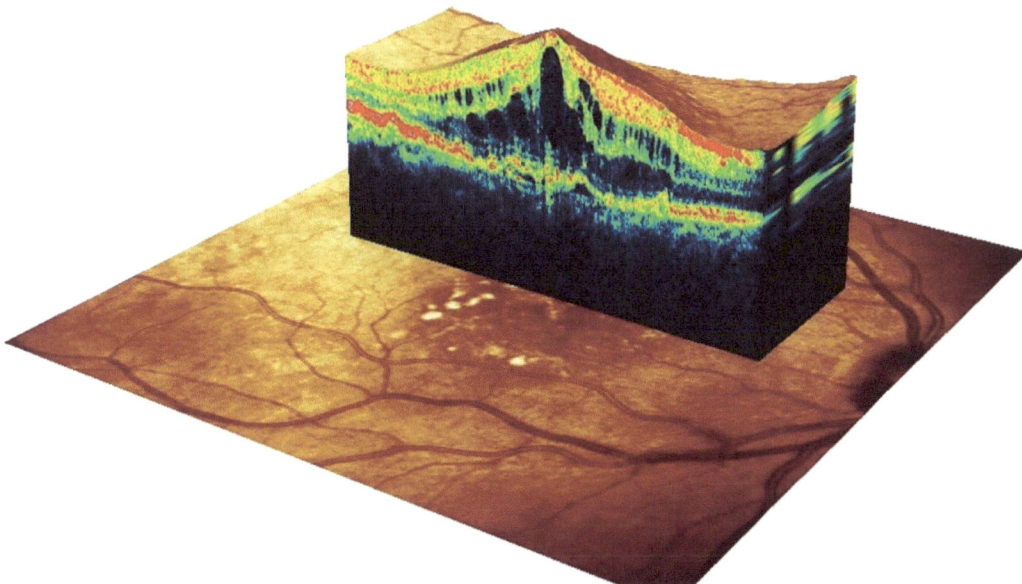

3D Volume Rendered OCT of DME

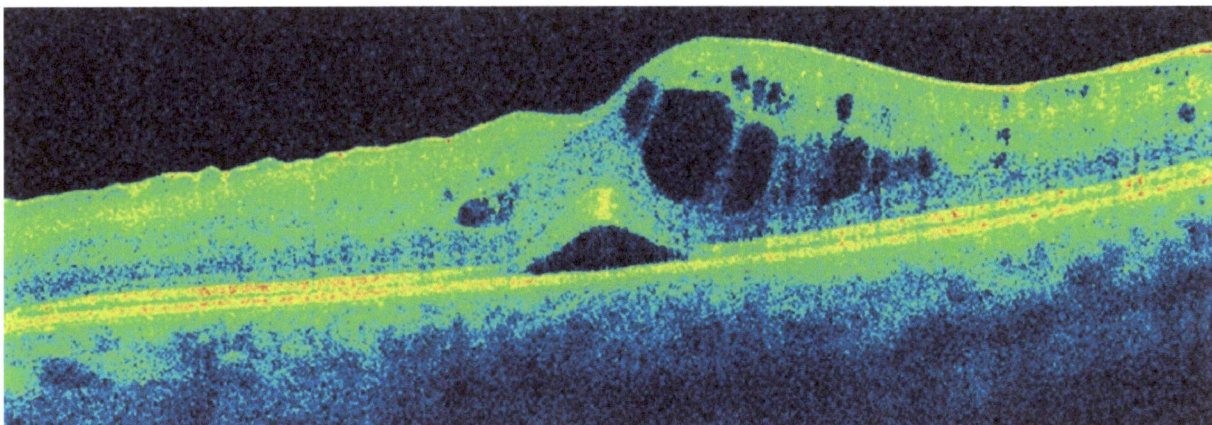

DME can be severe enough to cause or be associated with subretinal fluid, as in the case above.

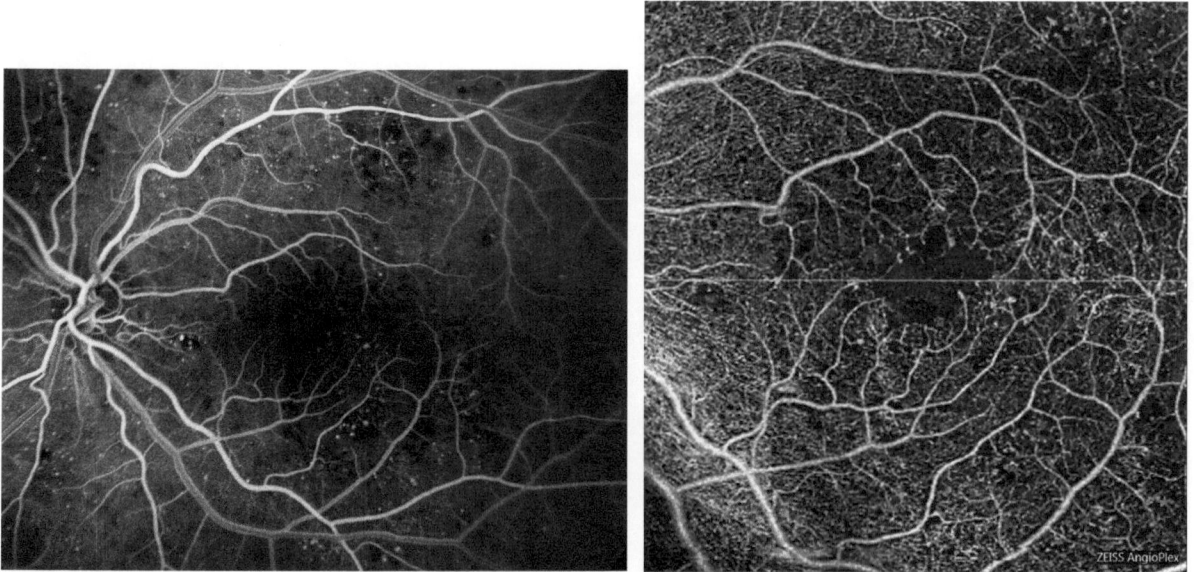

Fluorescein angiogram of DME with numerous microaneurysms (left). OCTA illustrates some microaneurysms but not all microaneurysms that appear on FA will appear on OCTA (right). OCTA demonstrates areas of impaired perfusion much more readily than FA since there is no late leakage on the OCTA.

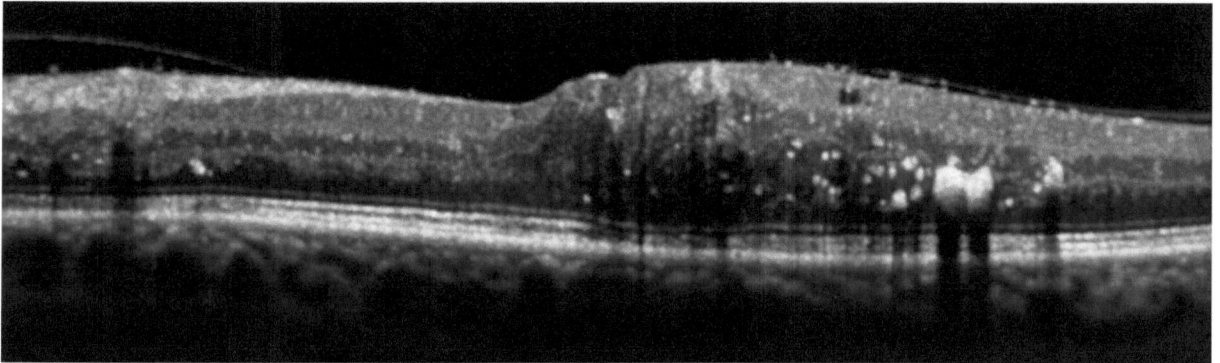

Corresponding horizontal OCT line B-scan of the above DME case

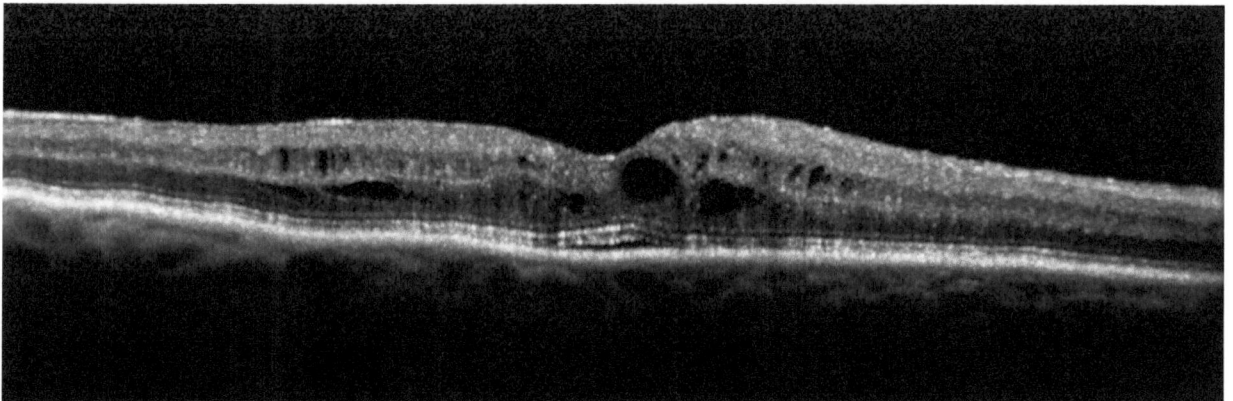

Multiple areas of cystoid spaces, both in the fovea and extrafoveally in DME

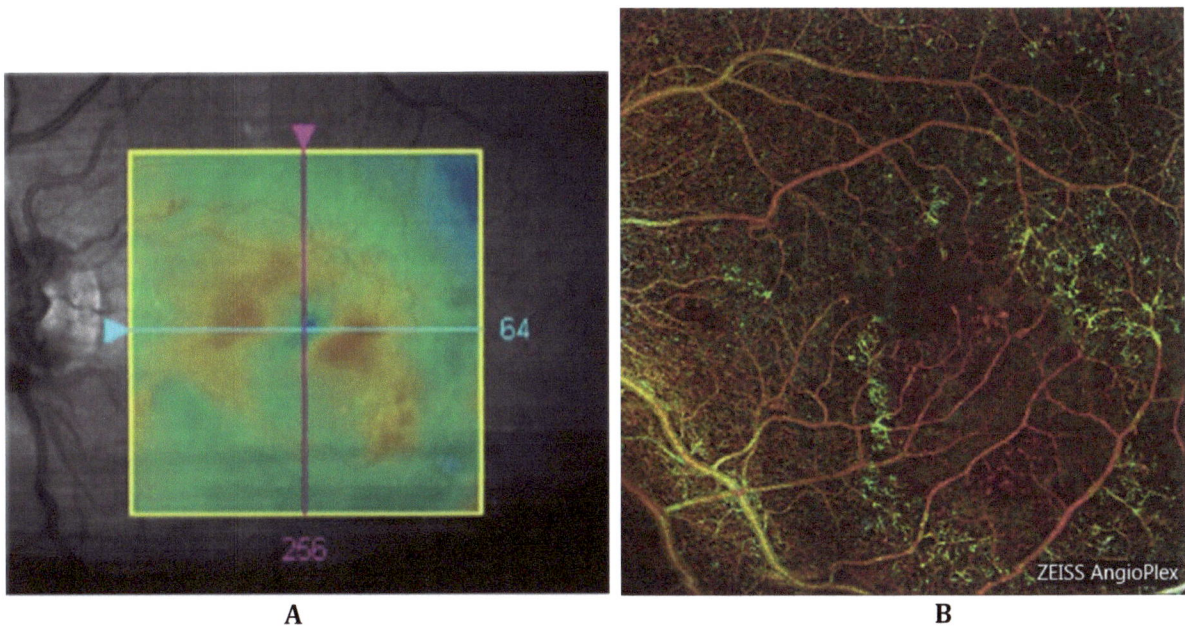

A

B

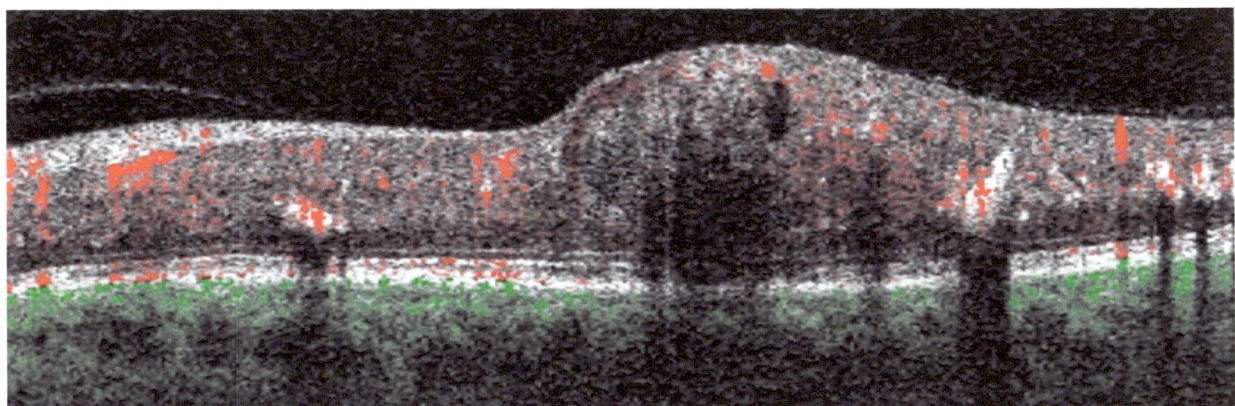

C

(A) Volume map OCT of DME. Note the areas of edema, marked by red in this image

(B) Depth encoded OCTA of subject with DME. Note the predominance of red vessels in the inferotemporal macula. This suggests that there is reduced perfusion in the deeper retinal layers (lack of green) or that the retina has been distorted enough to artifactually shift the deeper vessels into the superficial retinal plane. Interpretation of SD-OCTA images requires concurrent evaluation of the OCT of the area of interest.

(C) B-scan OCT illustrating vascular flow through the scan indicated in panel A and B. This image shows that the perfusion in the center of the B-scan is significantly attenuated compared to the surrounding region and is likely ischemic.

In areas of chronic edema, the deposits that are left after resorption of intraretinal fluid are visible as hard, or lipid exudates. On fundus exam, the lipid is white or yellow in appearance. Lipid exudates are highly reflective, and therefore appear bright white (hyperreflective) on OCT, usually associated with an area of present or former retinal edema (DME).

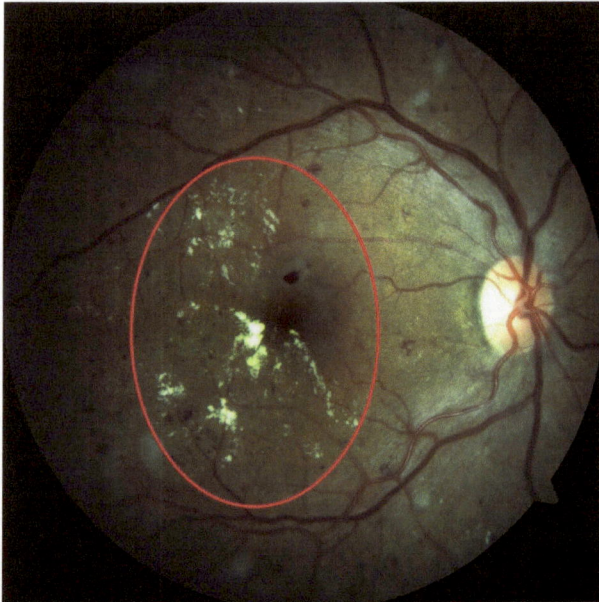

Color fundus image with lipid exudates and corresponding OCT line B-scan below

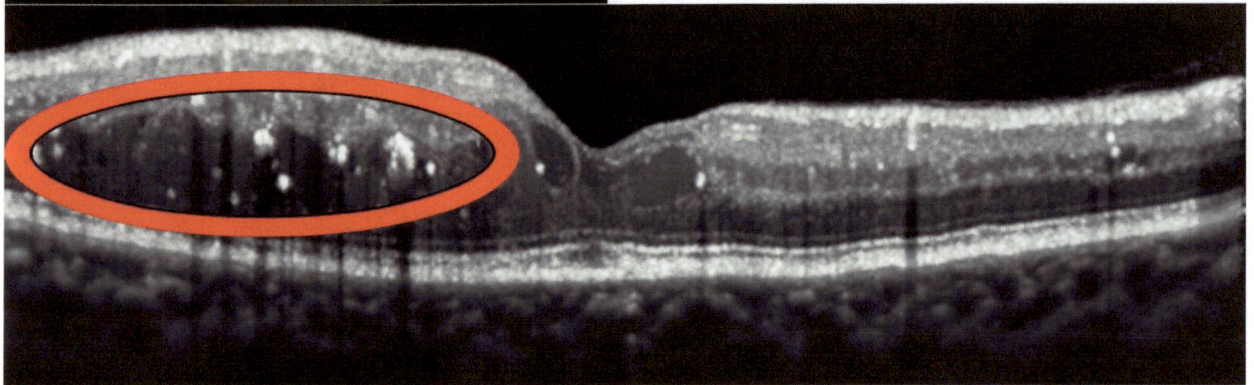

Once the edema has resolved, the lipid exudates may remain for some time until they break down and are absorbed.

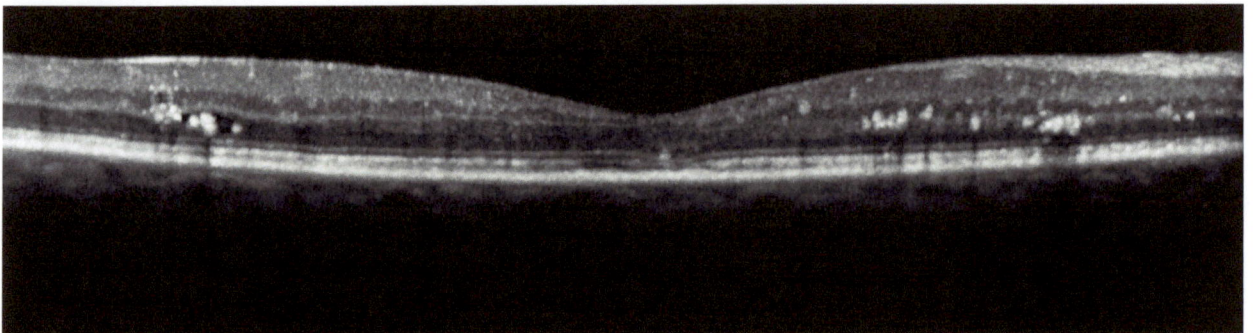

Diabetic with resolved macular edema, but residual lipid exudates visible as hyperreflective white foci throughout the retina in this case, but mostly around the outer plexiform layer.

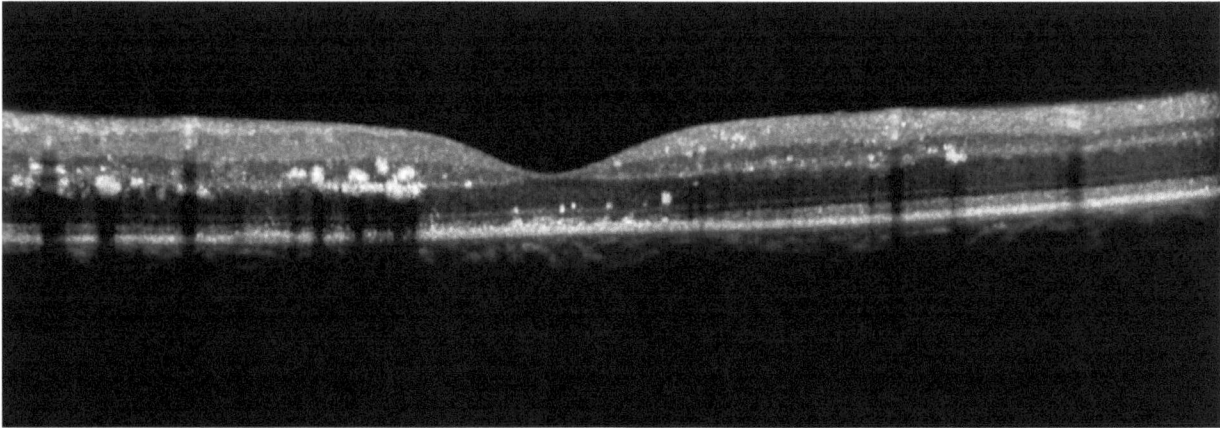

Hyperreflective foci are notable throughout the inner and outer retina in this case of a subject with resolved DME.

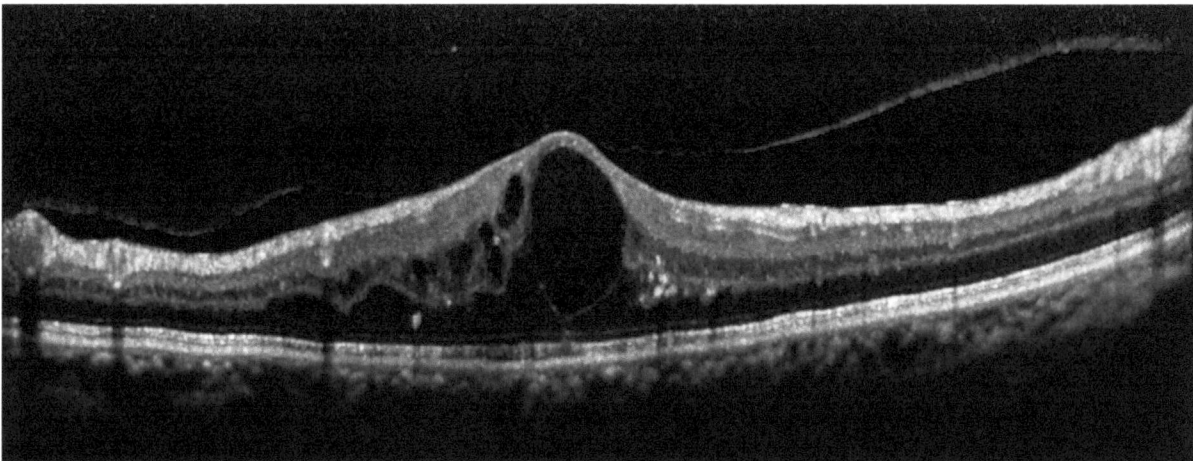

DME with large macular cyst that is blunting the foveal contour. There is vitreous attachment to the top of the retina. In cases where the overlying vitreous is adherent, it is sometimes not possible to determine if there is any contribution to the macular edema from vitreomacular traction, as in this case.

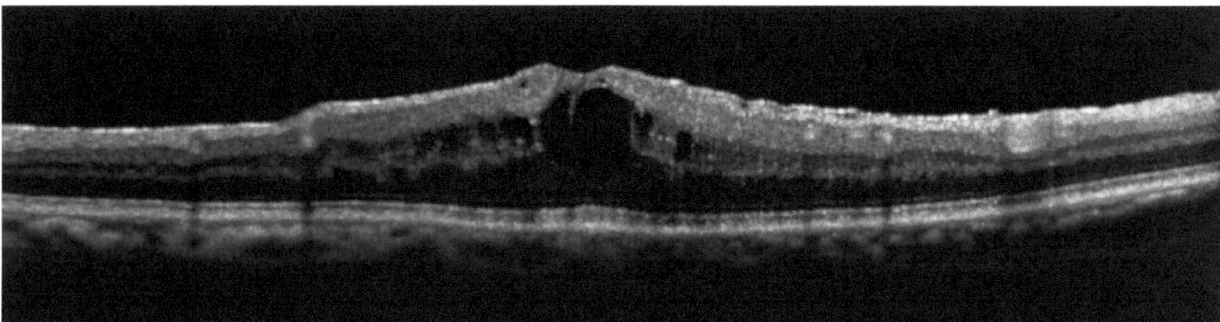

DME with intraretinal cystoid spaces and blunting of the foveal contour

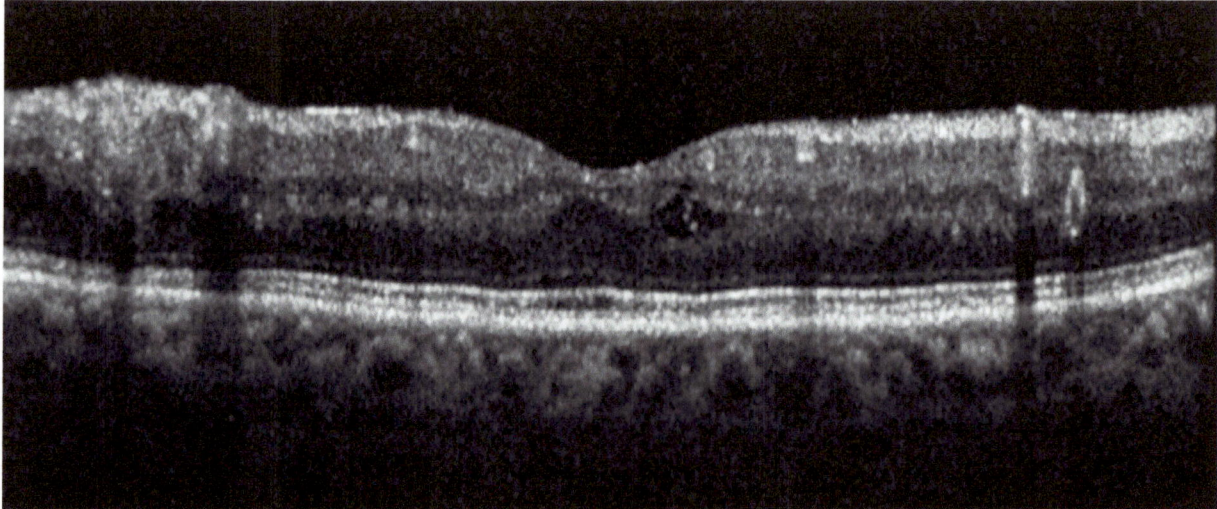

DME and hard exudates. Also note that there is a hyperreflective circular lesion in the far right of the image that is centered on the outer plexiform layer. This lesion is most consistent with a microaneurysm. Microaneurysms are not always visible on OCT sections.

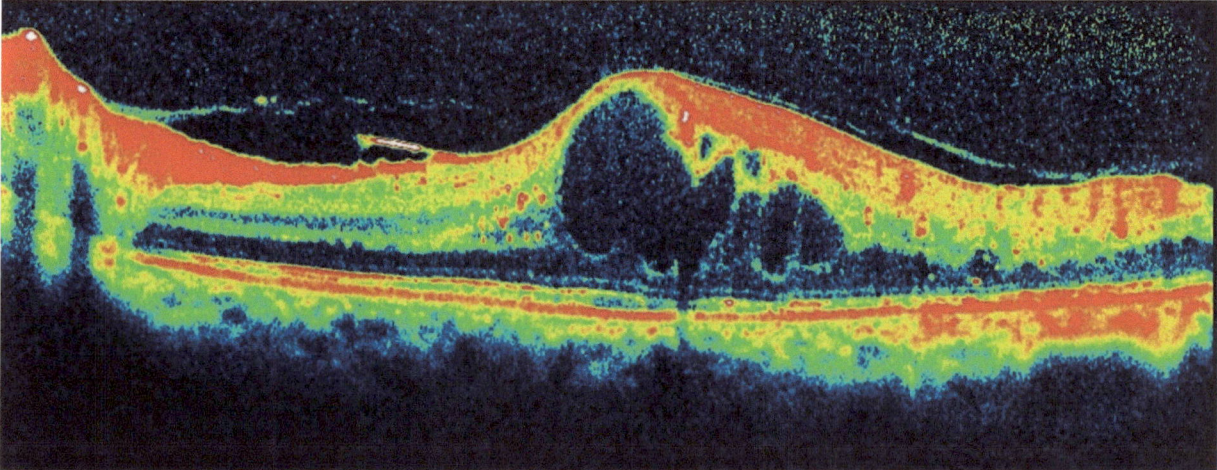

Multiple cystic pockets of fluid in a subject with DME

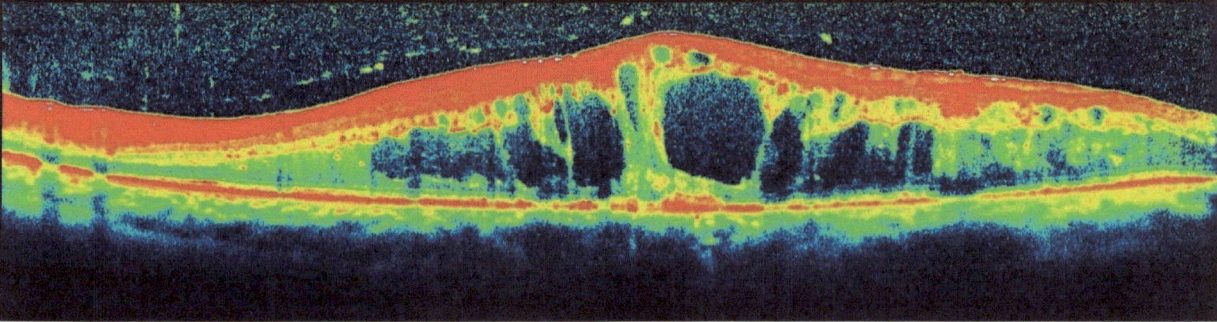

Multiple cystic pockets of fluid in a subject with DME

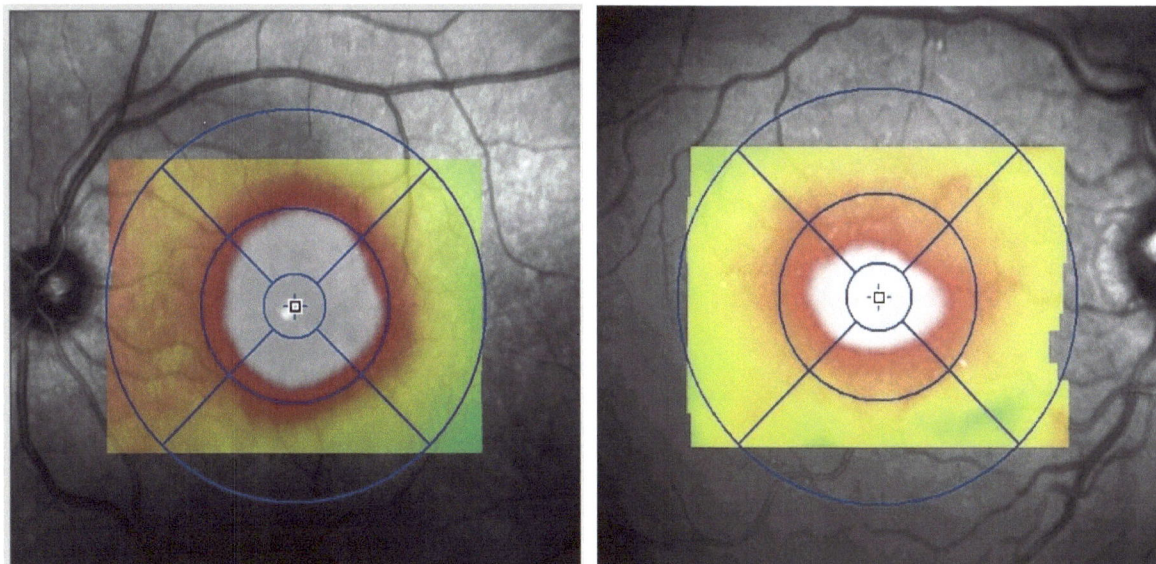

Volumetric OCT of two patients with DME shows severe thickening in the center of the macula.

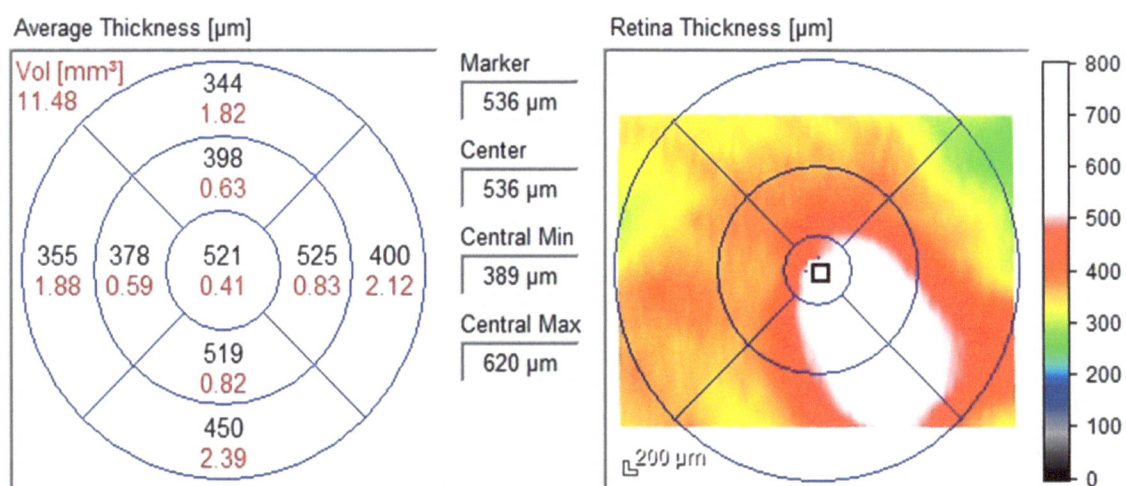

Quantified volumetric OCT (left) and false color designation (right). The color bar on the right provides a key for the retinal thickness display. Normal retinal thickness measurements appear in the green range.

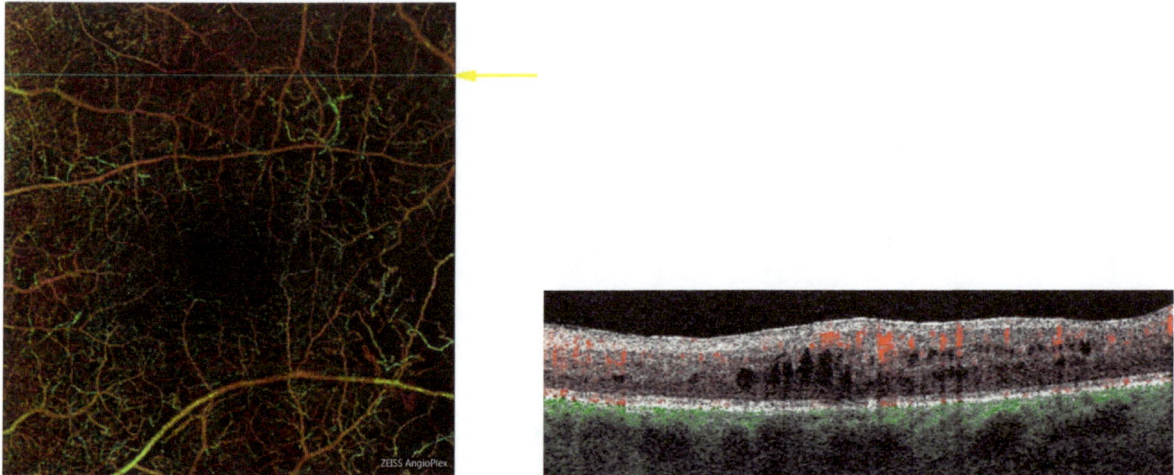

Depth encoded OCTA illustrating areas of impaired capillary perfusion most prominent on the right side of the image. There appears to be decreased OCTA signal from the deep retinal layers, which is indicated by the prominence of the red in the upper third of the image. The corresponding OCT line B-scan through the upper third of the image (scan line indicated by yellow arrow in depth encoded image) shows intraretinal edema and relative decrease in perfusion of the deep retinal layer. Note that some of the vessels in the superficial retinal layer appear enlarged in the region of the edema compared to the surrounding region. This may represent increased perfusion or displacement of deeper vessels into the superficial layer.

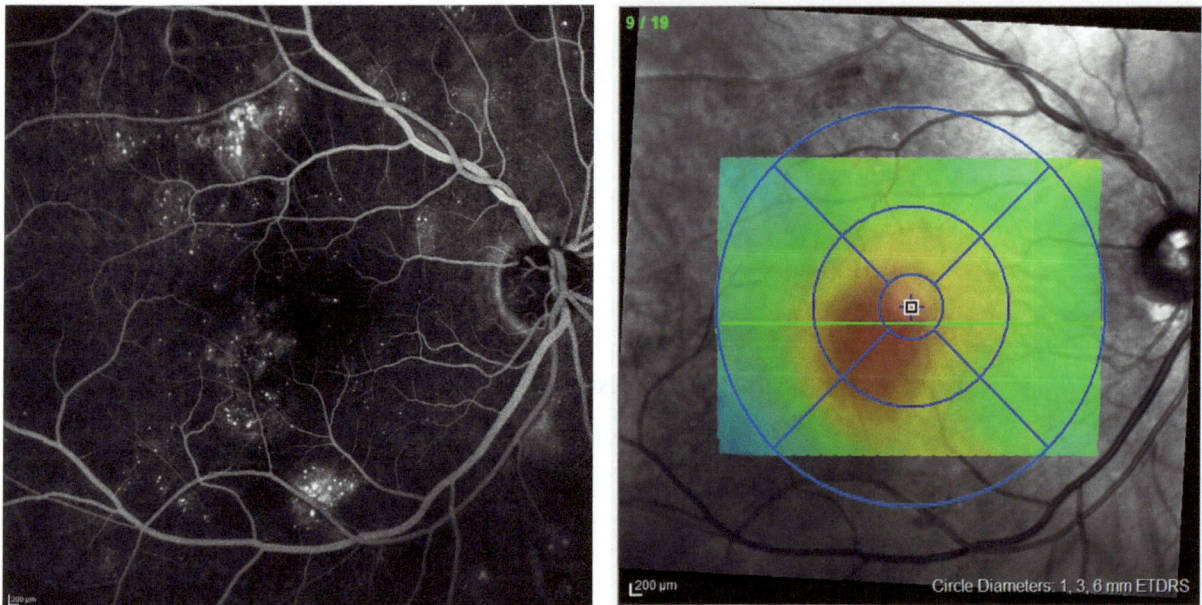

Late phase fluorescein angiogram (left) of subject with DME and numerous microaneurysms. Corresponding volumetric OCT (right) shows retinal thickening in the inferotemporal quadrant of the macula.

Diabetic Retinopathy

As with other small vessels in the body, diabetes can cause microvascular disease in the retina. The ocular manifestations of diabetes are numerous and include macular edema, microaneurysms, vessel dilation, cotton-wool spots, intraretinal hemorrhages, impaired capillary perfusion (also called "nonperfusion"), intraretinal microvascular abnormalities and neovascularization. Many of the macular findings in DR are captured on OCTA as effectively as FA. However, the peripheral changes in DR must still be identified with careful clinical examination, OCT and FA. Below we will outline the clinical findings and the ideal methods for imaging them.

Diabetic Macular Edema (DME): DME is best visualized with OCT as well as the cross-section of OCTA. In many cases, DME is subclinical and not detectable by clinical examination so OCT is essential in the management of any subject with DR. In cases where the edema is severe enough to be observed on clinical examination it is called clinically significant macular edema (CSME).

Microaneurysms (MA): MA range in size from 20-100 microns and are intraretinal. Large MA can be seen on clinical examination but all MA will be easily visualized on FA, and MA may be accompanied by intraretinal edema. MA are sometimes visible on OCTA, but their appearance can vary dramatically from that seen on FA.

Cotton Wool Spot (CWS): CWS are focal infarctions of the nerve fiber layer. On clinical examination and they appear as white feathery lesions. On fluorescein angiography they block the underlying fluorescence. OCTA of CWS demonstrates impairment mostly in the superficial retinal layer.

Intraretinal Hemorrhages: These appear as focal hemorrhages within the retina and are often called "dot and blot hemorrhages." Like all types of intraretinal hemorrhage they block the underlying fluorescence on FA. Hemorrhages generally appear hyperreflective on OCT and are not visualized on OCTA.

Impaired Capillary Perfusion: Areas of impaired capillary perfusion refer to regions that do not demonstrate clear filling on fluorescein angiography. It is generally assumed that these areas have no perfusion but this assumption may not be correct. These areas are often referred to as areas of "capillary non-perfusion" or "drop-out." Unfortunately, this term is a misleading descriptor of this finding and the term "impaired" perfusion is more accurate. OCTA can demonstrate macular areas of impaired capillary perfusion with excellent resolution. Unlike FA, OCTA can provide layer specific information in regions of impaired capillary perfusion. These areas are not typically observed on color images, clinical exam or OCT.

Intraretinal Microvascular Abnormalities (IRMA): These are areas of anomalous capillaries that are contained within the boundaries of the retina and are generally considered to be precursors to neovascularization, which extends outside of the retinal boundaries. These areas are most evident on fluorescein angiography and OCTA but also visible on careful clinical examination.

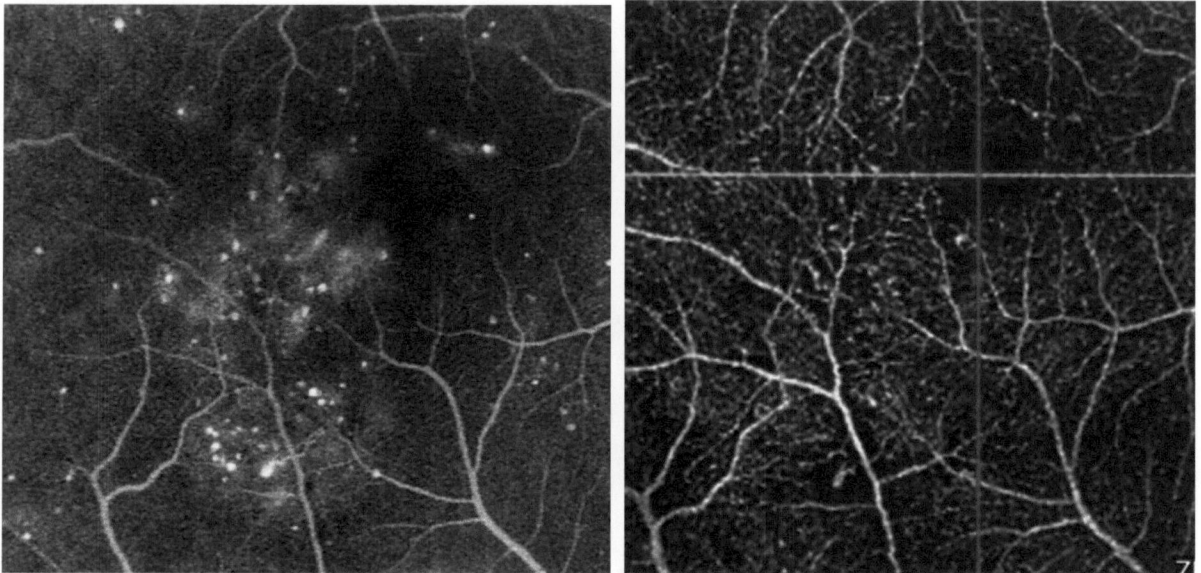

Fluorescein angiogram (L) and OCTA (R) of a subject with DR. Note the numerous pinpoint areas of hyperfluorescence in the FA, which represent microaneurysms. Also note the irregular foveal avascular zone, which implies impairment of capillary perfusion. Careful examination of the OCTA on the right demonstrates some of the MA seen on the corresponding FA. There are also multiple areas of impaired capillary perfusion on the OCTA that are not visible on FA. The FAZ is poorly outlined on OCTA, suggesting impairment in flow.

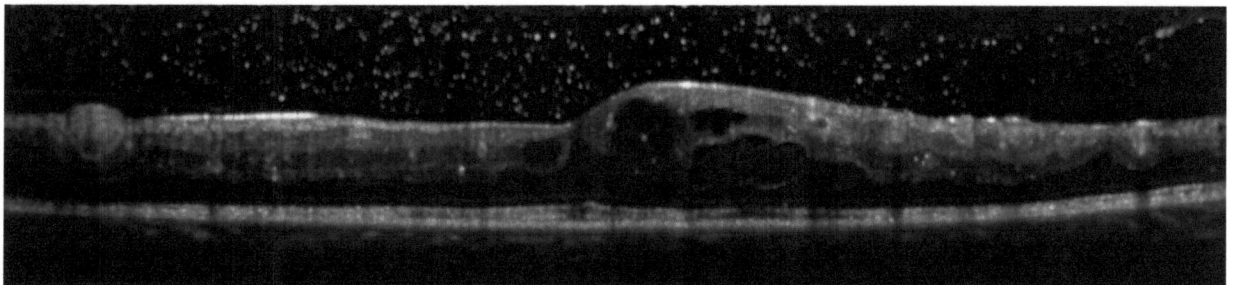

B-scan OCT of patient with diabetic retinopathy. The numerous hyperreflective spots in the vitreous are likely red blood cells from vitreous hemorrhage.

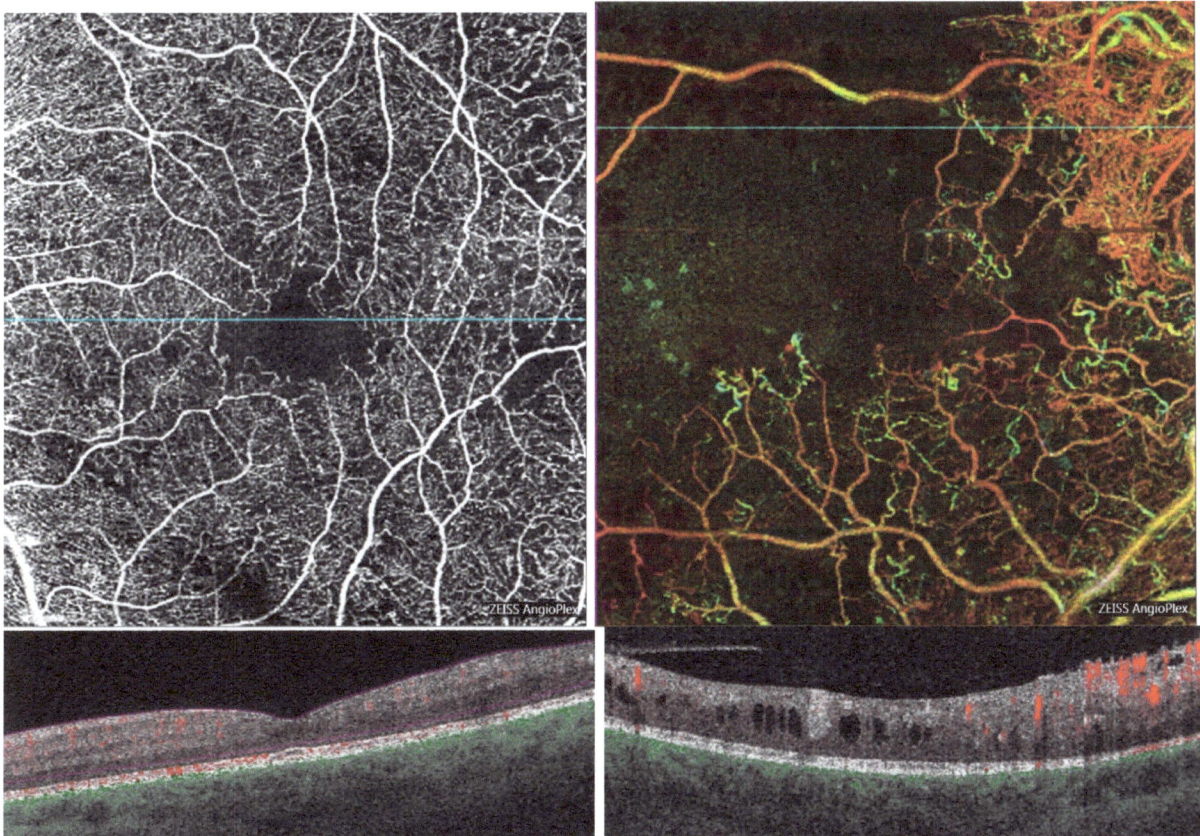

(Left) OCTA of the superficial retina layer demonstrates numerous small areas of impaired capillary perfusion, both adjacent to the foveal avascular zone as well as throughout the macula. Several large microaneurysms are also visible. (Right) depth encoded composite OCTA is of another subject with proliferative diabetic retinopathy, as evidenced by the neo-vascularization that appears in red in the top right corner image. Also note the diffuse area of impaired capillary perfusion involving almost all of the superior half of the macula, as well as extensive amounts of the inferior macula. The corresponding B-scans with retinal perfusion overlay in red show the distribution of perfusion throughout the retinal layers. The area of NVD appears as an area with intense red perfusion signal overlying the retina in the right of the image.

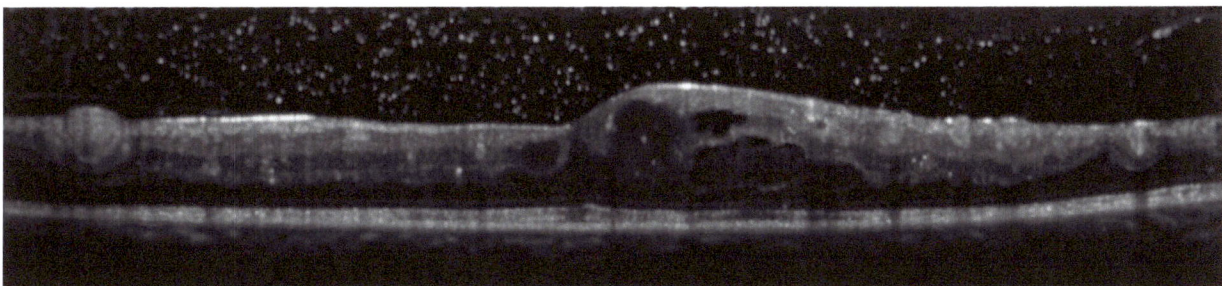

B-scan OCT of patient with diabetic retinopathy. The numerous hyperreflective spots in the vitreous are likely red blood cells from vitreous hemorrhage.

A

B

C

D

E

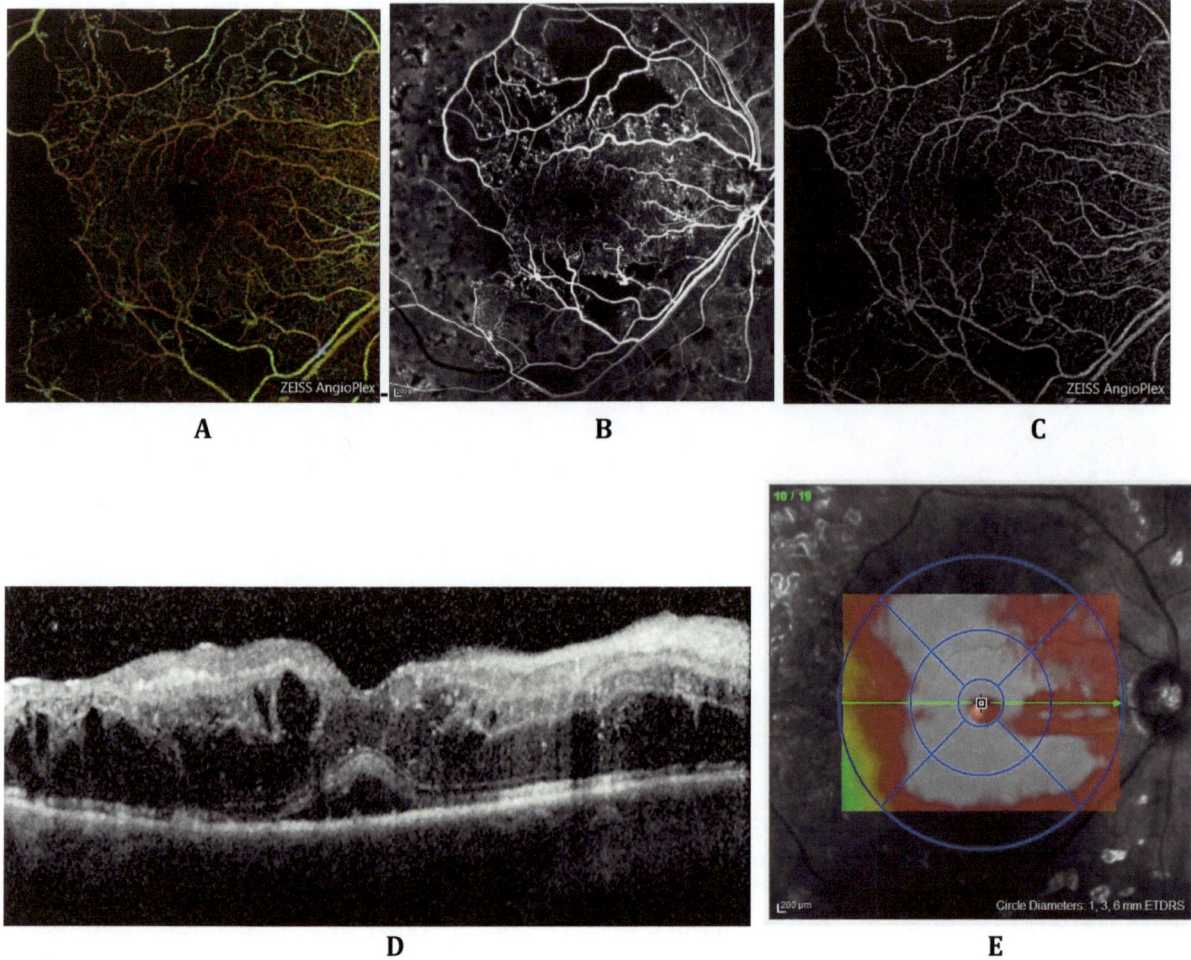

Several regions of impaired capillary perfusion seen on depth encoded OCTA (A), fluorescein angiogram demonstrates peripheral laser scars, multiple regions of impaired capillary perfusion (B), full thickness OCTA (C), line B-scan OCT demonstrates intraretinal edema and subretinal fluid. Also note the multiple fine hyperreflective dots that may be suggestive of hard exudates (D), and volumetric OCT demonstrates the severe retinal thickening throughout the macula (E).

Retinal Neovascularization

Impaired capillary perfusion (e.g. "capillary non perfusion") inherently leaves retinal tissue ischemic or hypoxic. Both of these conditions cause an overexpression of vascular endothelial growth factor (VEGF). When overexpressed, VEGF contributes to angiogenesis, which is the growth of new blood vessels, or neovascularization (NV), from existing vasculature. When these new blood vessels form in the retina, they are fragile and leak serous fluid, plasma and even bleed. In advanced cases, these new blood vessels may become fibrous and cause traction on the retina, leading to tears or detachments. NV can come in multiple forms including neovascularization of the disc (NVD) and neovascularization elsewhere (NVE). These findings are most evident on clinical exam and fluorescein angiography. In cases where the NV is located within the macula, OCTA can verify the extraretinal location of the vessels. Extramacular NV will definitely require clinical examination or FA, along with OCT, for evaluation.

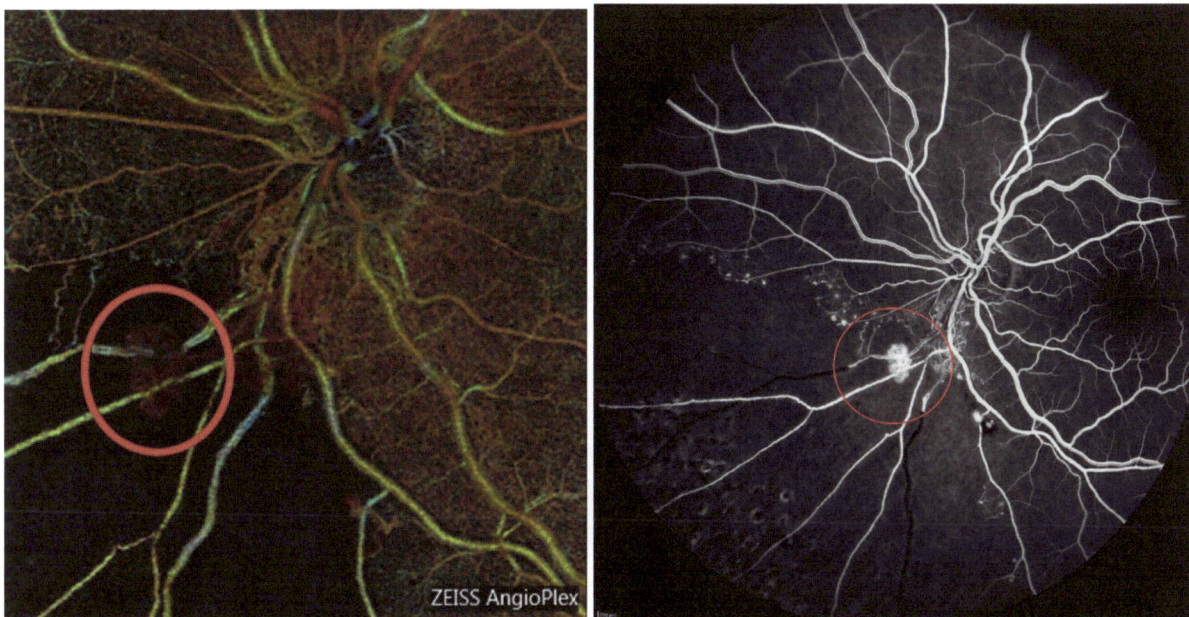

Pseudo-color depth encoded OCTA of a subject with a vascular occlusive disorder with NVE and diffuse area of impaired capillary perfusion. Fluorescein angiogram also shows the area of impaired capillary perfusion, as early leakage of neovascularization (red circle) as well as a small tuft of NVE just inferior and temporal to the red circle. Peripheral laser scars are visible in the lower left corner.

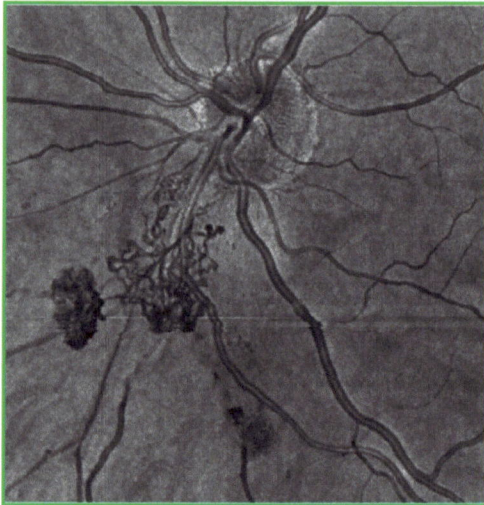

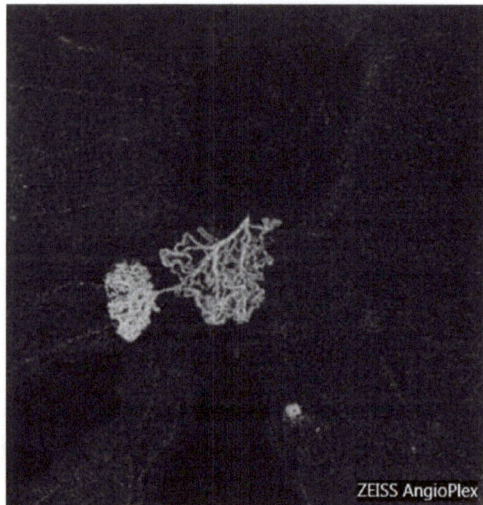

En face infrared image of NVE inferior to the disc (left). OCTA image of the vitreoretinal interface (VRI) of the same subject shows the NVE above the retinal plane and a small tuft inferotemporal to the larger NVE.

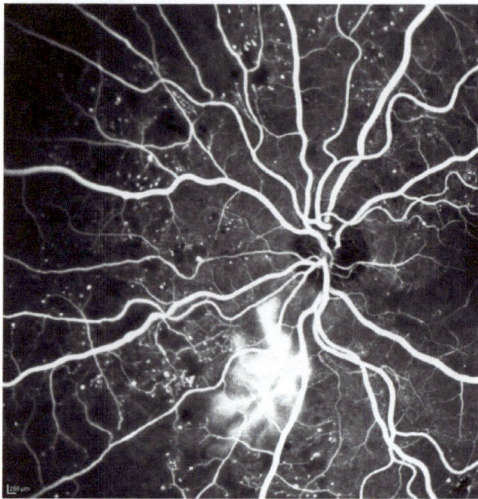

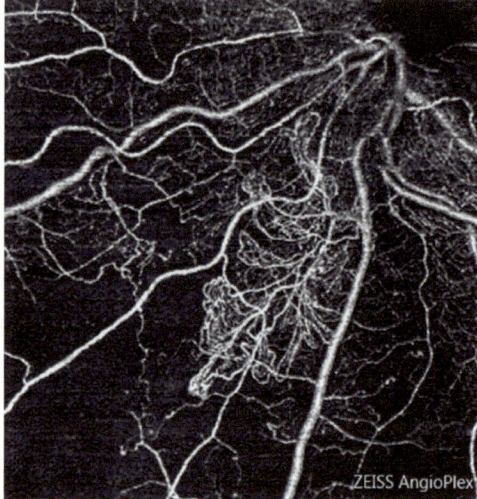

Fluorescein angiogram (left) and superficial level OCTA (right) of NVE and impaired capillary perfusion

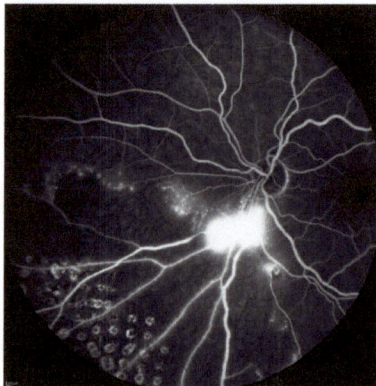

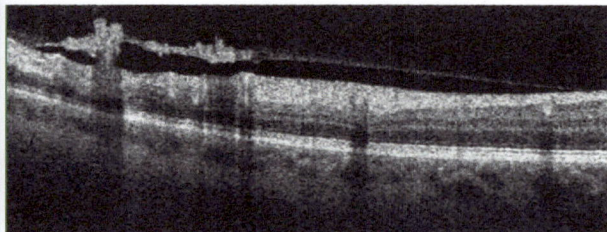

Late fluorescein angiogram showing leaking from the NVE. The B-scan OCT illustrates NVE growing along the posterior aspect of the hyaloid face (vitreous cavity).

Retinal Vein Occlusion

Branch Retinal Vein Occlusion

Retinal vein occlusion (RVO) is the most common retinal vascular disease after diabetic retinopathy, and macular edema is a frequent cause of vision loss in eyes with RVO. RVO is commonly caused by a thrombotic event that occurs at the crossing of a retinal artery and vein. In the case of Central Retinal Vein Occlusion (CRVO), this may occur in the central vein at, or posterior to, the lamina cribrosa. In Branch Retinal Vein Occlusion (BRVO), this happens at an arteriovenous crossing, which, as the name indicates, is where an artery crosses a vein. The artery may compress the vein and increase turbulent flow leading to thrombosis. This ultimately leads to either limitation or complete obstruction of flow. Hypertension is the strongest risk factor for retinal vein occlusion. Clinically, RVO appears with diffuse (CRVO) or sectoral (BRVO) findings including dilated and tortuous veins, diffuse intraretinal hemorrhages, and retinal edema in the acute phase. Chronic findings of RVO include inner retinal atrophy and neovascularization. OCT is an essential clinical tool for imaging the extent of macular edema caused by RVO, and quantifying change over time or after treatment. Fluorescein angiography is used primarily to evaluate the severity and extent of ischemia from RVO and to evaluate reperfusion of the vein(s). OCT angiography allows non-invasive visualization of ischemic macular regions in RVO and is at least equally as good at assessing the macular findings of RVO as fluorescein angiography. Fluorescein angiography is still necessary to assess the peripheral extent of ischemia and peripheral neovascularization. In fluorescein angiography, fluorescein dye typically presents in the central retinal artery ~10-20 seconds after intravenous injection and fills all the veins, between ~10-20 seconds in normal circulation. Any delay beyond this in a correctly performed FA suggests either a clinical or subclinical occlusion of the retinal vein or artery.

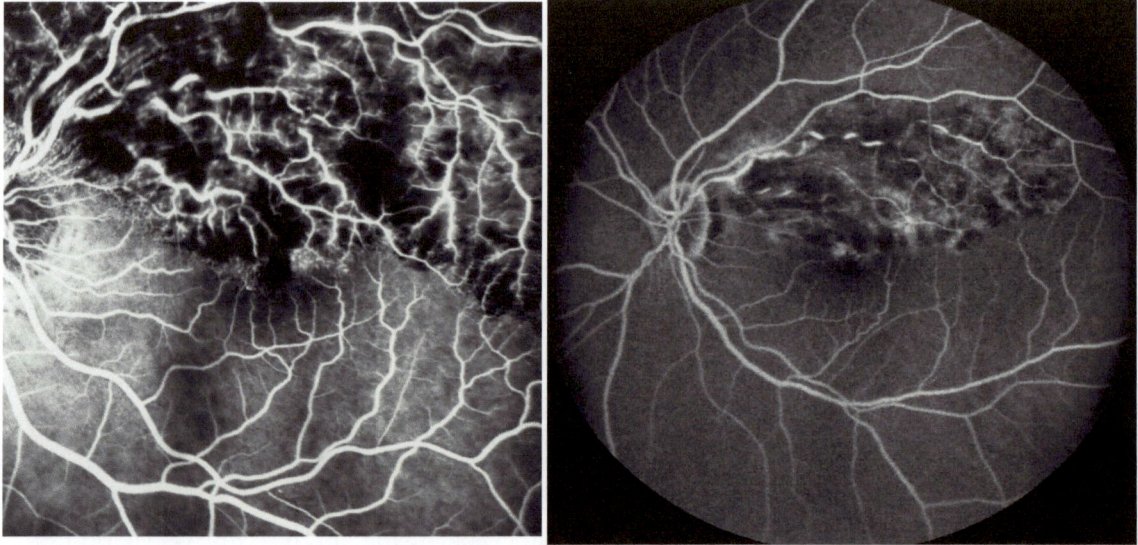

Two cases of branch retinal vein occlusion involving the superotemporal arcades on fluorescein angiography. Note the diffuse areas of intraretinal hemorrhage indicated by blockage of the fluorescein dye.

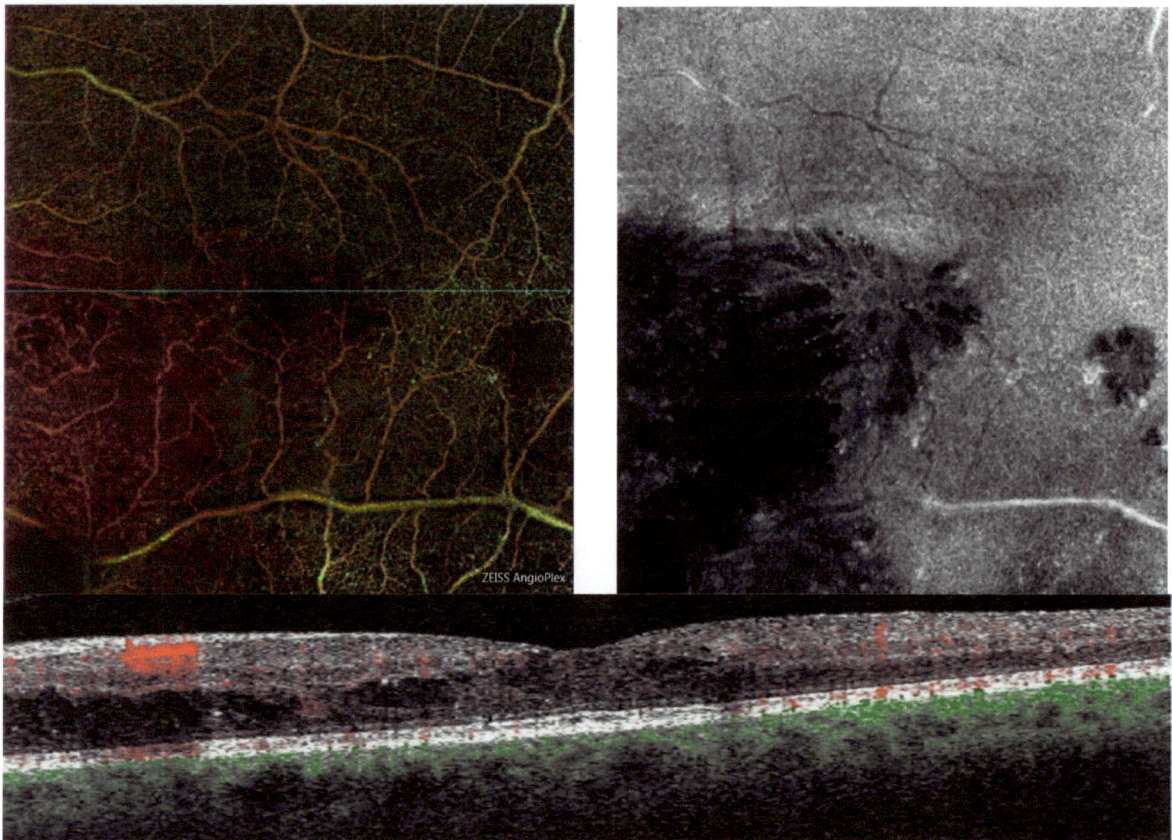

Depth encoded OCTA shows relatively intact superficial retinal perfusion (red) and attenuation of retinal perfusion in the deep retinal layer (lack of green) in the inferonasal quadrant of the macula. The enface intensity image demonstrates small pockets of hypo-intensity suggestive of intraretinal fluid in the deep retinal layer.

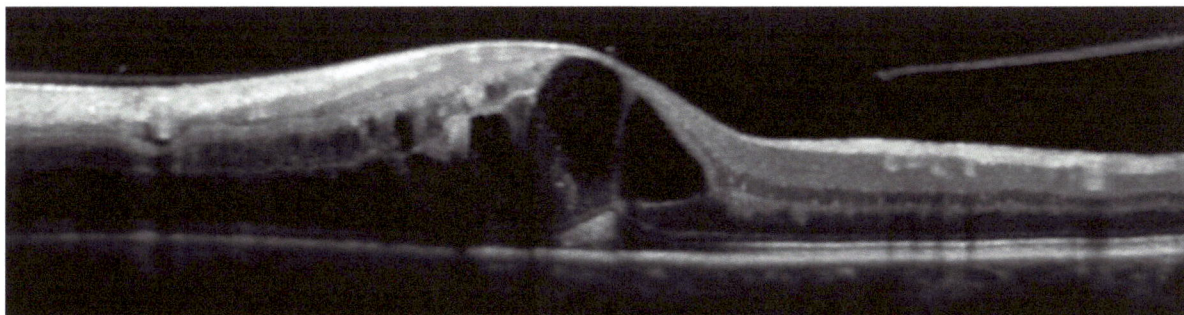

B-scan OCT of BRVO. Notice the large hyporeflective pockets that represent cystoid edema. The inner retina is hyperreflective and the whole retina is thickened on the left half of the image.

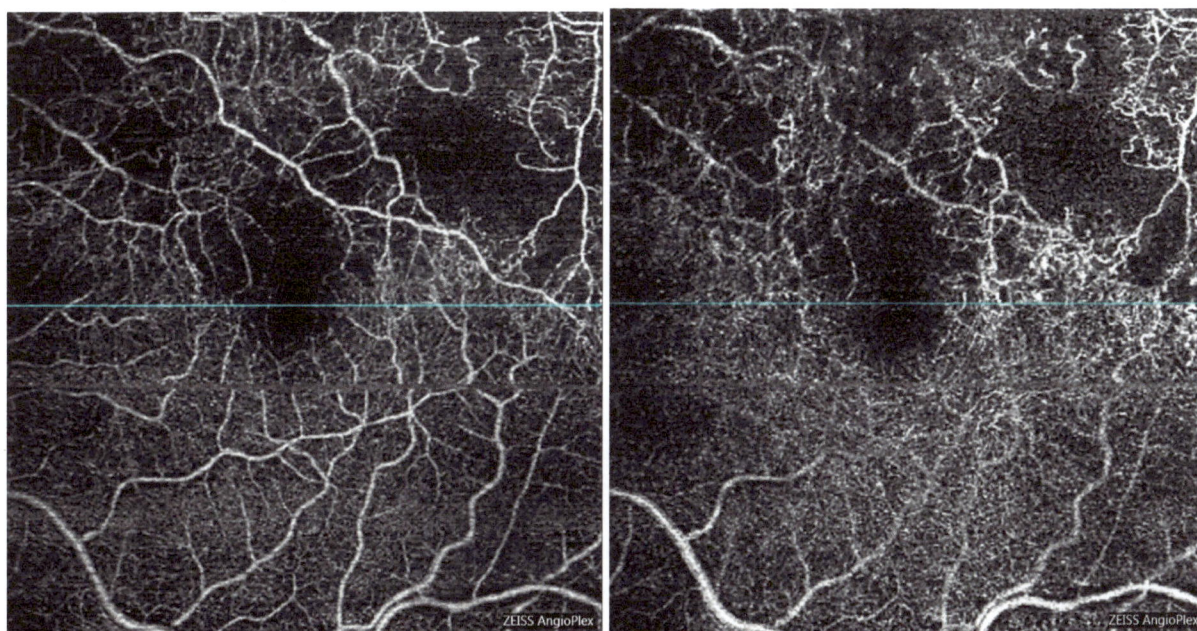

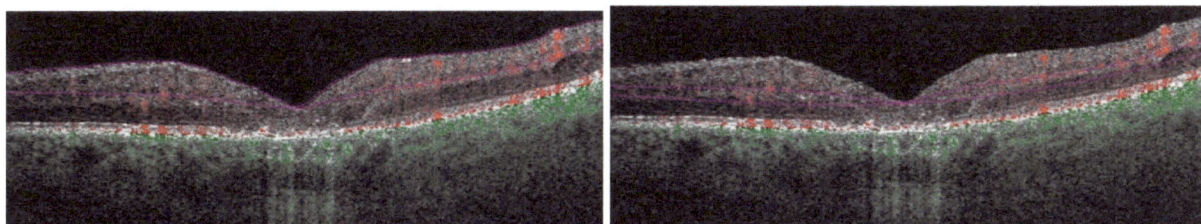

OCTA of a BRVO demonstrates areas of impaired retinal perfusion involving both the superficial retinal layer (left) as well as the deep retinal layer (right). Note the abnormal and dilated capillaries most prominent in the superficial retinal layer. The corresponding B-scans with OCTA signal show the superficial (left) and deep (right) retinal layers with red indicating retinal perfusion signal. Red areas that appear on the RPE are called "projection artifacts" and are not true perfusion.

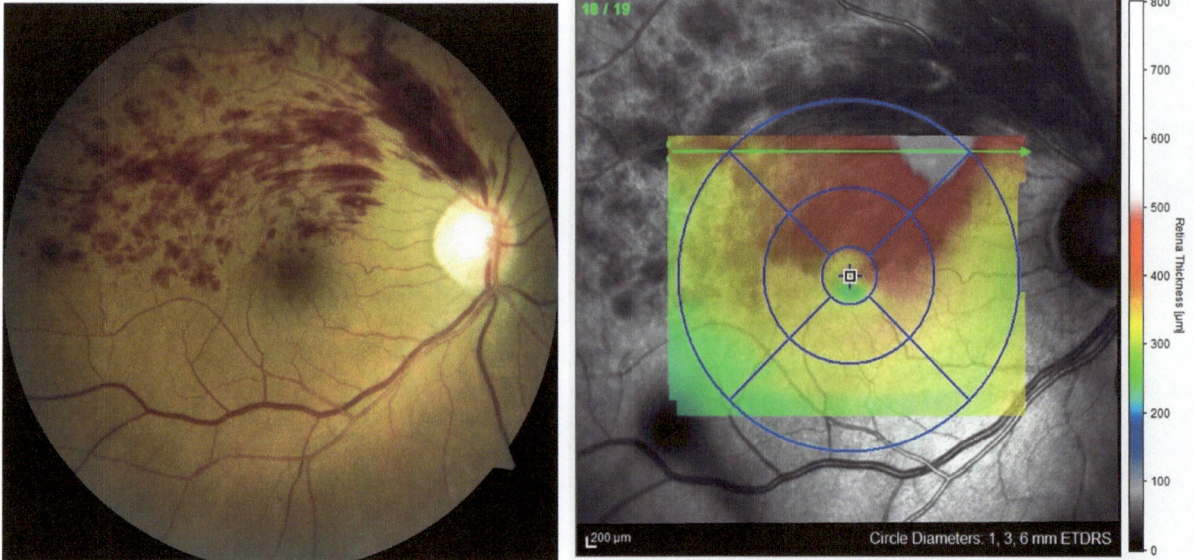

Color fundus image and volumetric OCT of a branch retinal vein occlusion involving the superotemporal arcade. Note the diffuse intraretinal hemorrhages. Volumetric OCT overlaid on the IR image demonstrates retinal thickening in the superior half of the macula corresponding to the area of the RVO. Note that the blood causes decreased intensity on the IR image. There is also a large floater along the inferotemporal vein.

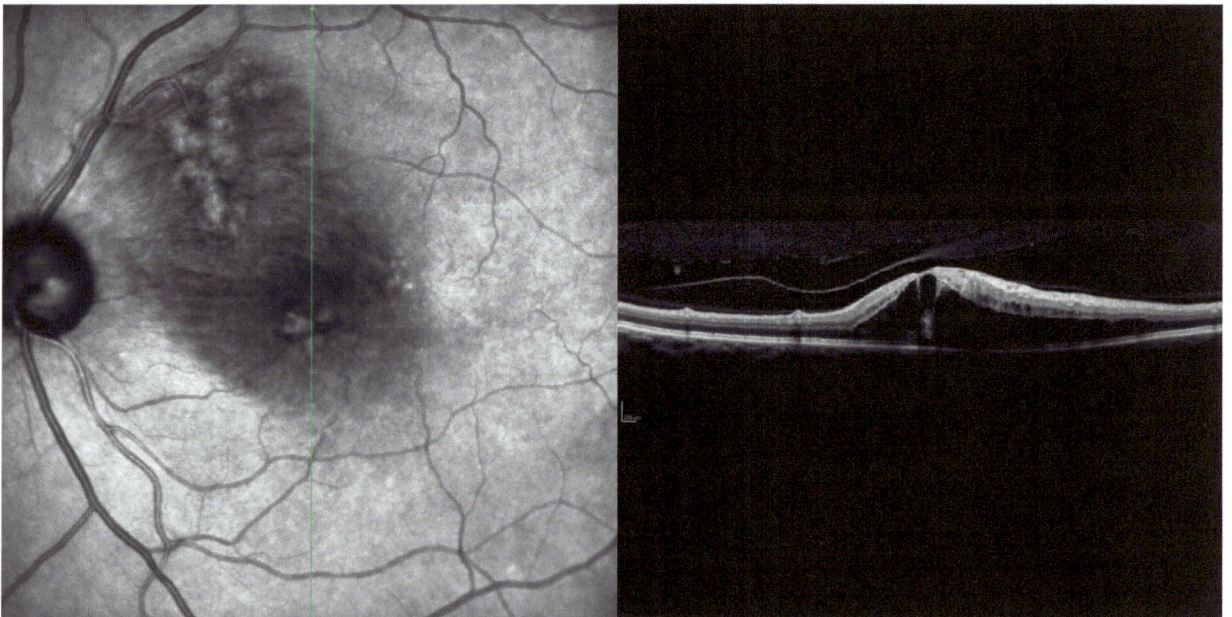

Vertical B-scan OCT through the fovea (right) demonstrates severe intraretinal edema and retinal thickening in the superior half of the macula corresponding to the area of decreased intensity on the IR image (left). Also note the overlying partial separation of the hyaloid face, which is unrelated to the RVO in this case.

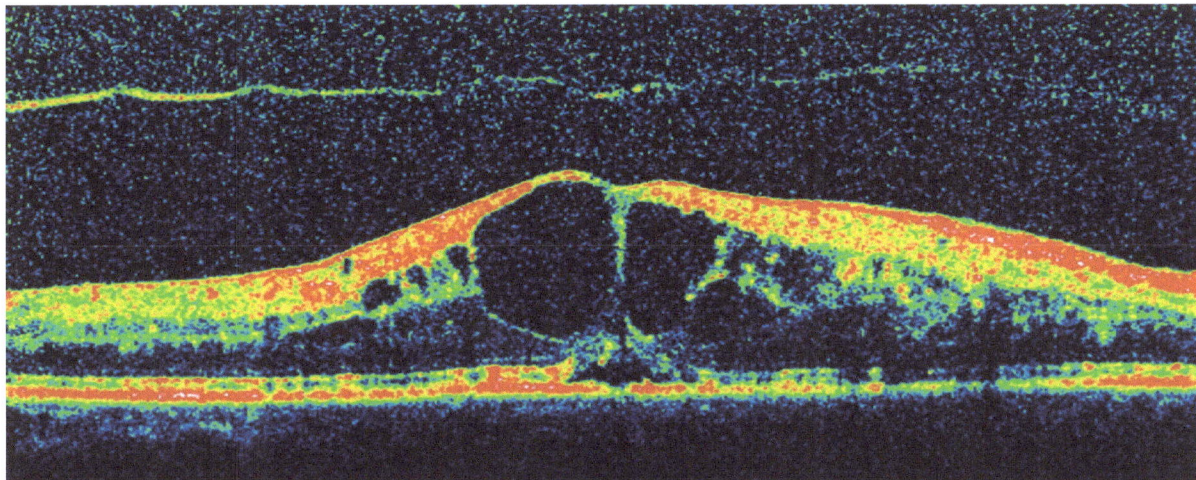

Pseudo-colored B-scan OCT demonstrates macular edema due to RVO. Note the overlying partial separation of the hyaloid face above the retina. This is unrelated to the underlying RVO.

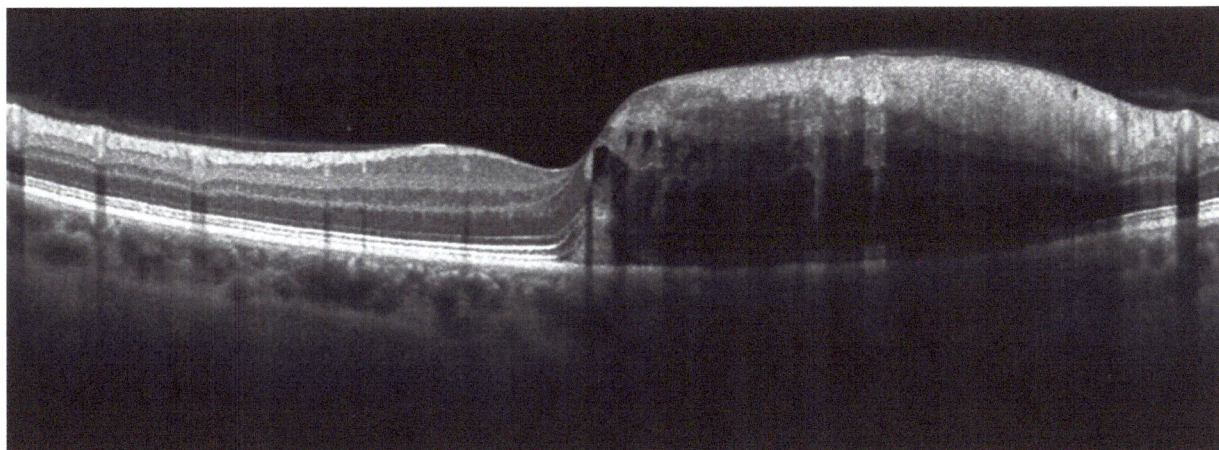

Vertical B-scan OCT showing edema in the superior macula with some distinct pockets of intraretinal fluid and overall severe retinal thickening.

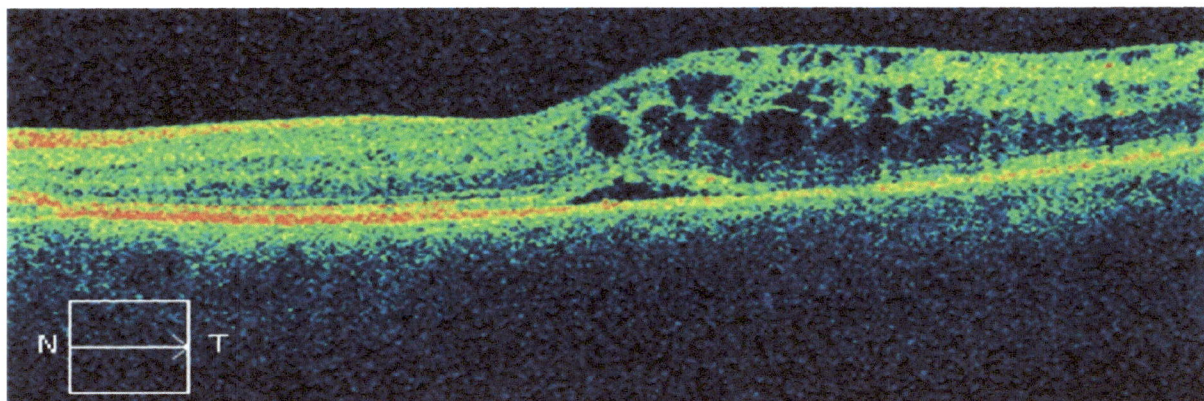

B-scan OCT image of temporal macular edema from RVO. Note the intraretinal fluid and subretinal fluid in this case.

In severe cases of RVO, intraretinal edema may be accompanied by subretinal fluid as well. By its name, retinal vein occlusions only affect retinal vasculature, so pathology from this condition will be present above the retinal pigment epithelium.

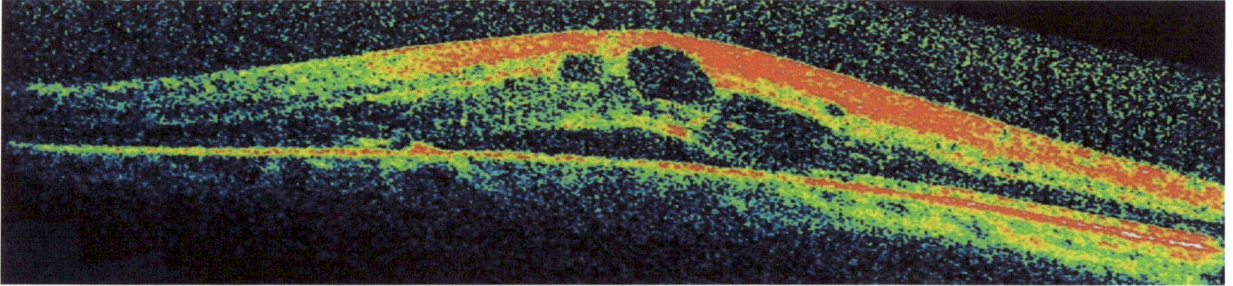

BRVO with intraretinal edema and sub retinal fluid

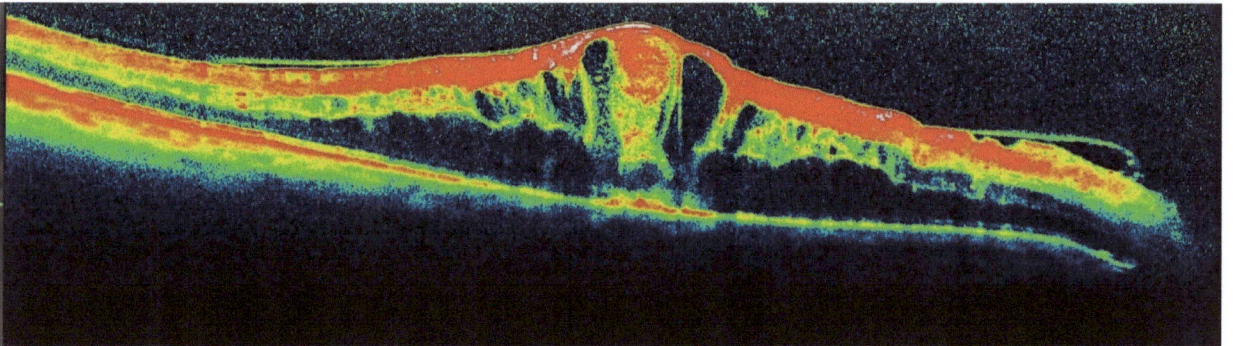

Severe intraretinal edema throughout the macula from RVO

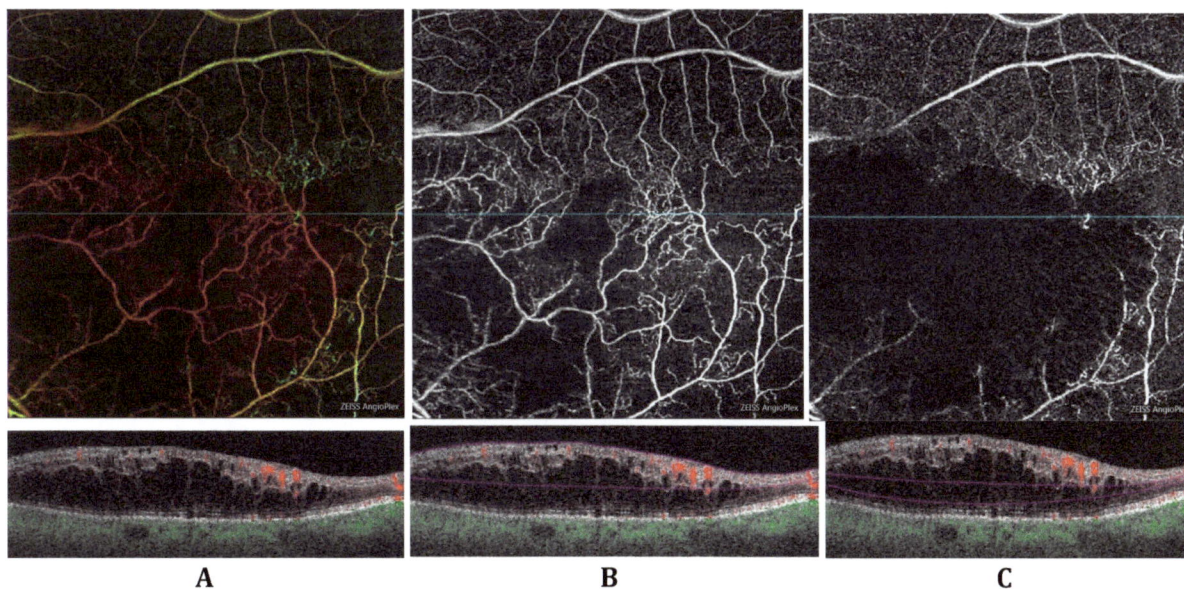

A   B   C

A. The depth encoded layer OCTA of BRVO demonstrates severe impairment of perfusion involving most of the inferior half of the macula. Note that there is some shunting of perfusion from the inferior to the superior macula and mild dilation of the retinal vessels along the horizontal raphe.

B. The superficial retinal layer on OCTA demonstrates diffuse areas of impaired perfusion along with abnormal and dilated retinal capillaries.

C. The deep retinal layer also shows diffuse areas of impaired perfusion more severe than the superficial layer. Because the segmentation of edematous retinal layers is not always accurate, care must be taken to correlate the changes on the en face OCTA with segmentation of the B-scan. In this case, the deep retinal layer is predominantly occupied by intraretinal fluid, which may account for at least part of the decrease in perfusion signal.

Central Retinal Vein Occlusion

As was discussed previously in the branch RVO section, arterio-venous crossing is a risk factor for developing retinal vein occlusions. In the case of a central retinal vein occlusion, the central vein, which is the culminating of the retinal venules and veins, is the vein that is occluded. This may happen at an intersecting point at the optic disc or within the optic nerve, and glaucoma is also a risk factor for central retinal vein occlusion. Once occluded, the pressure on the retinal venous system results in more diffuse and widespread hemorrhages and edema than BRVO.

CRVO may present as non-ischemic, which is the more common type, or ischemic, which may result in a bigger impact on vision. Ischemic CRVO can also lead to the formation of retinal neovascularization as a result of VEGF angiogenesis.

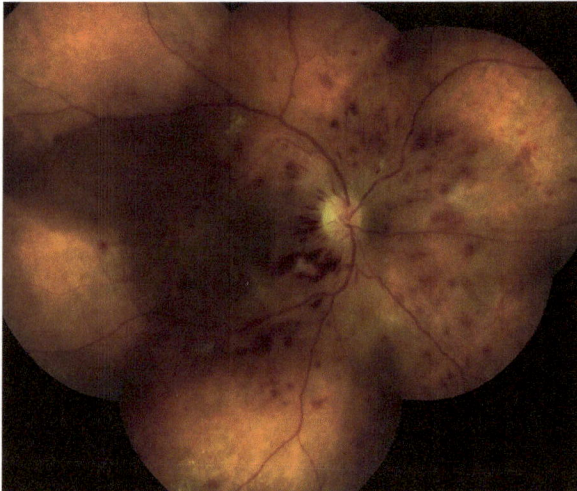

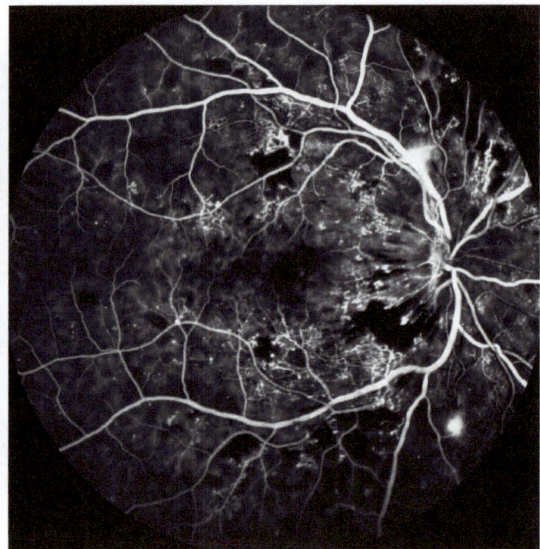

Color montage of CRVO (left) showing diffuse intraretinal hemorrhages. Note the hemorrhages are both flame shaped around the disc and "dot-blot" shaped in the periphery. Flame shaped hemorrhages are typically located in the nerve fiber layer. Dot-blot hemorrhages are located in the inner retina. Fluorescein angiogram (right) shows perfusion of the major arteries and veins, however there are several areas where the capillaries are "nonperfused" and appear black. There are also multiple hyperfluorescent lesions that are consistent with microvascular changes such as microaneurysms and telangiectasia. There are two very hyperfluorescent foci that are consistent with retinal neovascularization on the right side of the image.

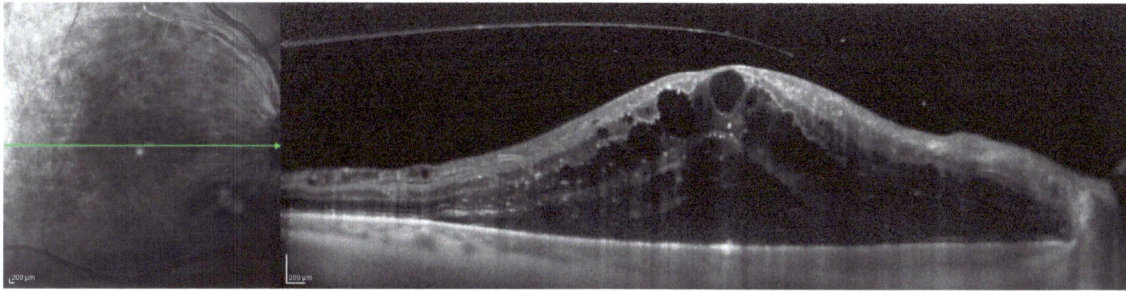

Horizontal B-scan OCT showing intraretinal and subretinal fluid. Note the large cystic spaces in the center of the image and within the retina. In this example the cystoid spaces are largely in the outer retina and extend into the inner retina. There is significant subretinal fluid elevating the retina most in the middle of the image where the fovea is likely located. The fovea is difficult to identify due to the diffuse thickening of the retina. The overlying white line in the vitreous demonstrates the partial detachment of the posterior vitreous.

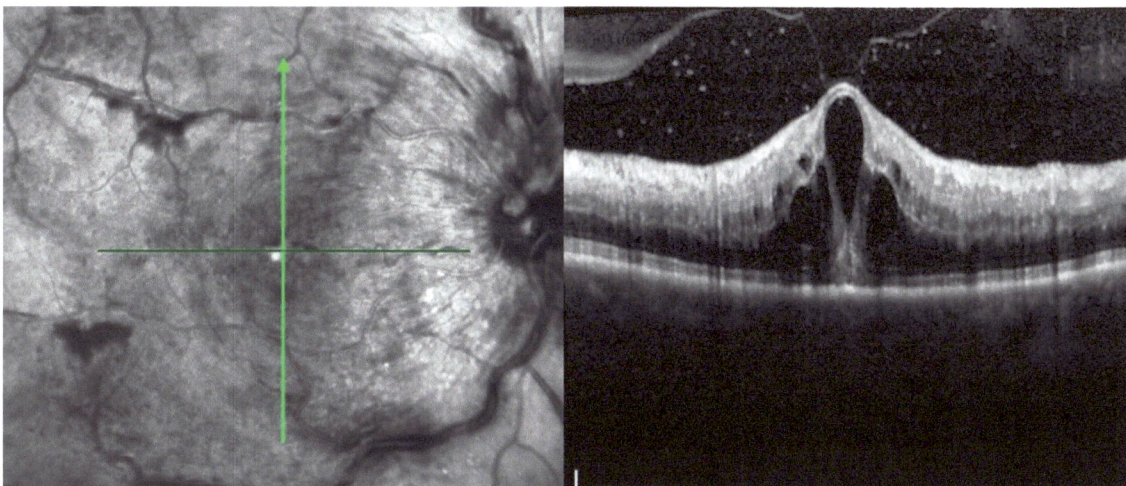

Infrared OCT image (left) and line B-scan OCT (right). Note tortuous and dilated veins in the fundus image, and classic intraretinal hemorrhages which appear dark. There is significant central cystoid macula edema with three large cysts located in and around the fovea. The fovea itself is completely distorted and "mountain" shaped due to the intraretinal fluid. Note the hyperintensity of the inner retina which is also common in CRVO but less intense than that observed in CRAO cases. The overlying white lines in the vitreous space demonstrate the partial detachment of the posterior vitreous with a focal attachment directly over the fovea.

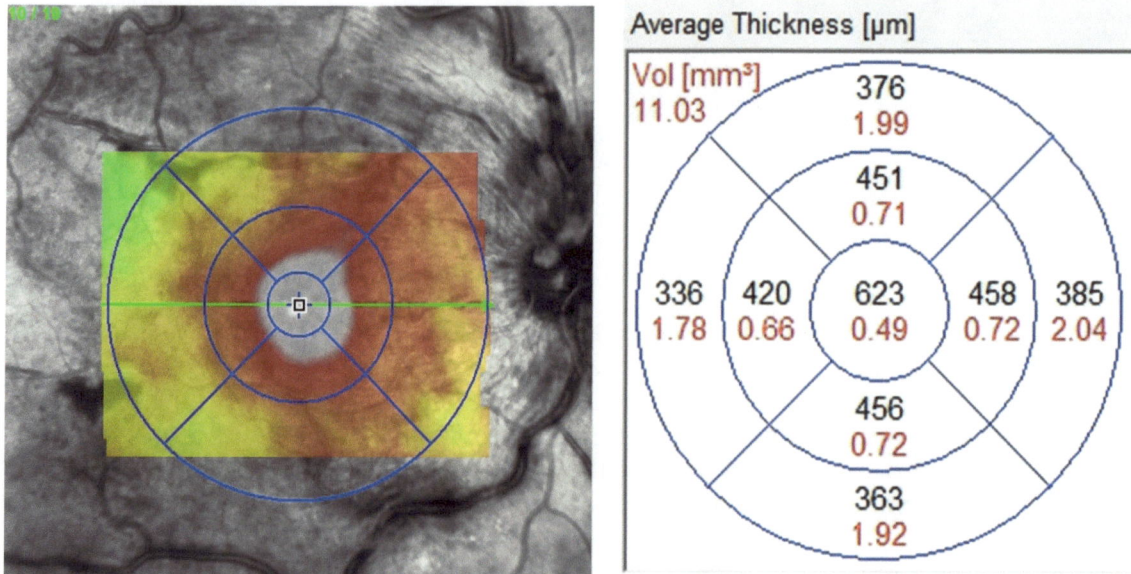

Volumetric OCT and average thickness map of the previous CRVO case. White and red pseudo-coloring indicates the severe thickening of the central macula. Green represents normal retinal thickness, which is almost completely absent in this case because of the diffuse edema.

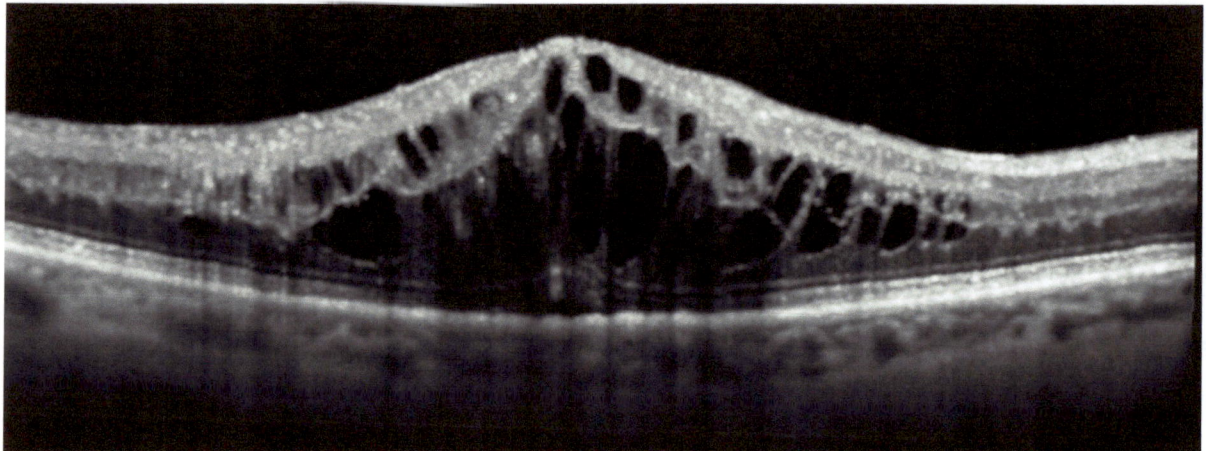

Typical intraretinal edema presentation of CRVO on B-scan OCT with a small pocket of subretinal fluid in the center of the image where the foveal depression is most likely to have been. In this case most of the edema is centered around the outer plexiform layer with significant amounts extending deeper into the outer nuclear layer and inner nuclear layer. Note the dark vertical bands, which project down from the large cystoid spaces onto the choroid. These represent "shadows" that are cast by the overlying cystoid spaces attenuating the OCT signal.

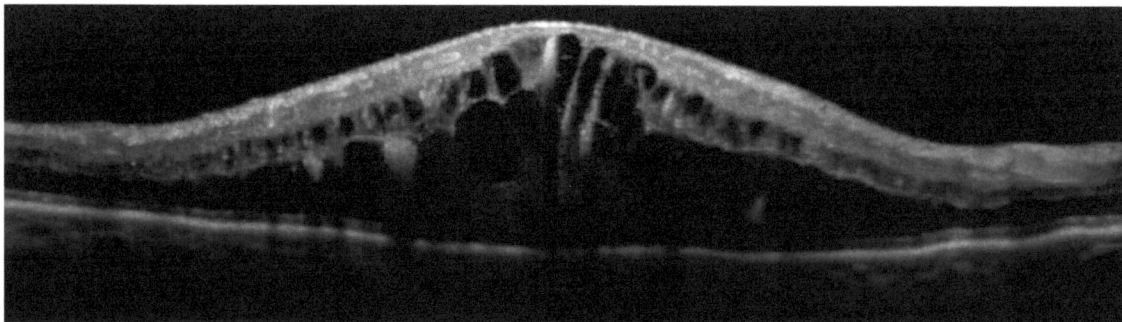

Line B-scan of CRVO with diffuse intraretinal fluid. Note that some of the intraretinal fluid spaces (cystoid spaces) are hyper-intense, while most are hypo-intense compared to the rest of the retina. The hyperintensity may be representative of the lipid or proteinaceous content of intraretinal cystoid spaces that are chronic or resolving, although the exact etiology is unknown.

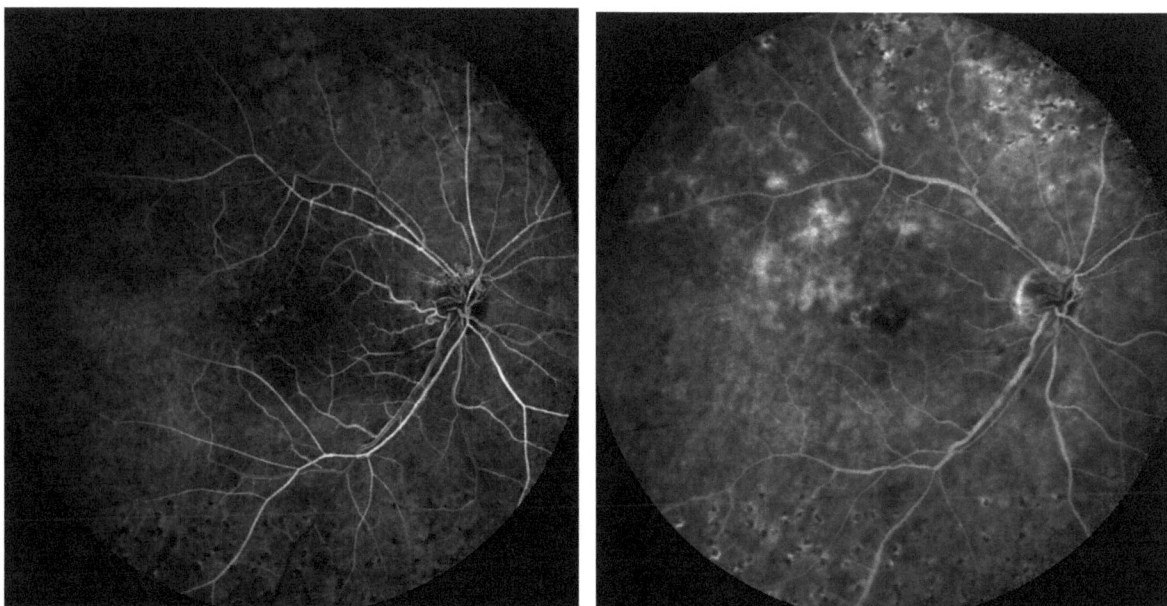

Mid and late wide-field fluorescein angiogram, illustrating poor venous filling, especially in the periphery. There are hypofluorescent regions in the periphery that may be consistent with previous laser photocoagulation. There are mild hyperfluorescent changes temporal to the fovea, that are not evident in the early phase, but leak in the late phase image (right) and suggest cystoid macular edema that is more prominent temporal to the macula and into the periphery.

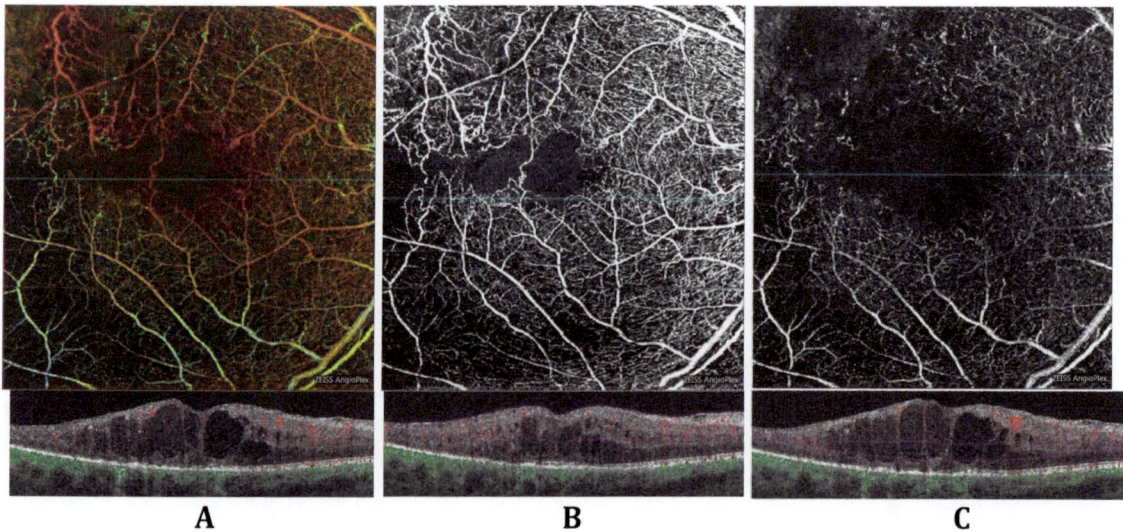

A B C

(A). Pseudo-colored, depth encoded OCTA of a subject with a retinal venous occlusion primarily affecting the temporal macula. The red pseudo-coloring indicates presence of perfusion in the superficial retina and the absence of green indicates the relative lack of perfusion in the deeper retinal layers. There are also prominent areas of impaired capillary perfusion ("capillary nonperfusion") especially temporal to the fovea. The foveal avascular zone is enlarged and irregular.

(B). The monochromatic image of the superficial retina clearly illustrates the extent of areas with impaired capillary perfusion. There are also small shunt vessels that extend across the horizontal midline of the retina, which is characteristic of retinal venous occlusion

(C). The monochromatic image of the deep retinal vessels further illustrates the extent of impaired capillary perfusion in the temporal macula.

Interpretation of pseudo-colored OCT angiograms can be easily confounded if the retina is edematous and retinal layers are thinner or thicker than they normally would be as shown in the B-scans above. The B-scan on the left **(A)** shows that there is less qualitative perfusion signal (red dots) throughout the whole retina surrounding the regions of edema than the regions without edema. The purple lines on the B-scans show the segmentation of the retina that is used to create the overlying en face OCTA. The B-scan in the middle **(B)** illustrates the segmentation that is used to generate the superficial retinal layer OCTA above it. Note that the segmentation of the superficial retina is not completely accurate in the center of the image. Nevertheless, there is less perfusion signal in the region with edema. The same applies to the B-scan on the right **(C)**, showing the segmentation lines for the deep retinal layer OCTA.

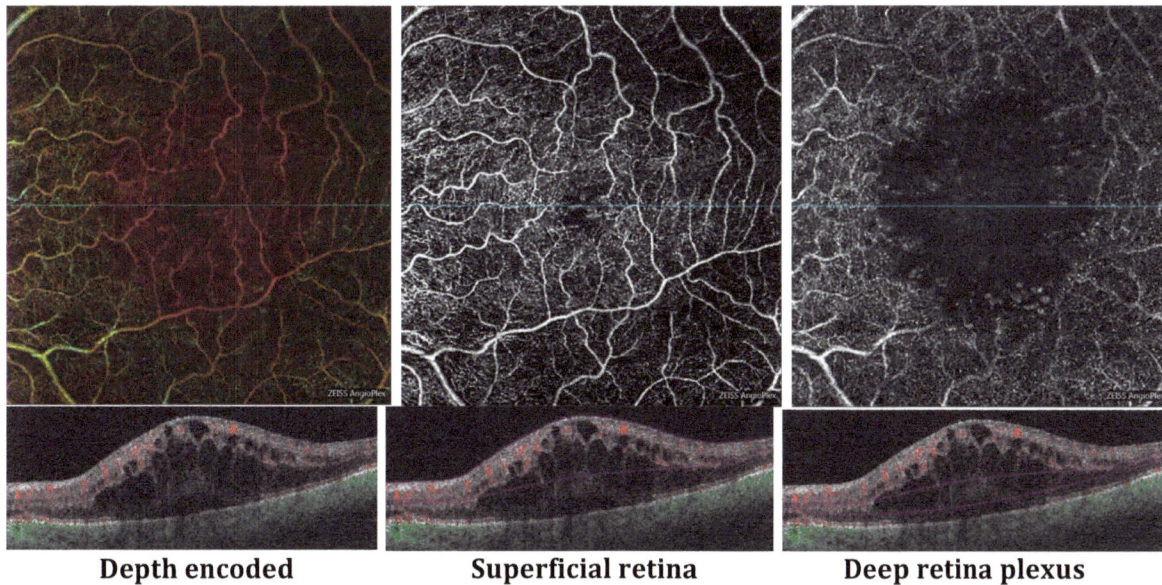

Depth encoded   **Superficial retina**   **Deep retina plexus**

The depth encoded en face OCT angiogram demonstrates preserved perfusion in the superficial retinal layer (red) and apparent lack of perfusion in the deep retinal layer (green) in the center of the macula. The B-scan on the left illustrates the perfusion throughout the whole retina with individual layers color-coded. The middle B-scan shows the segmentation lines for the superficial retinal layer. Note that the segmentation is not accurate in the region where the edema is the most severe. Due to the distortion of the retinal anatomy it is likely that the retinal vessels that would normally be in the deep retinal layer are now detected in the superficial layer. This makes the perfusion in the central macula appear to be artifactually more than in the periphery of the image (see en face OCTA in middle panel).

Retinal Artery Occlusion

Branch Retinal Artery Occlusion

Arterial occlusions are caused by blockage of either the central retinal artery (CRAO) or a branch of it (BRAO) by an embolus. These emboli block the flow of oxygenated blood, rendering the retinal tissue without the needed oxygen causing ischemia and tissue death. On ophthalmoscopy, the retina affected is white in appearance, and occasionally the embolus can be seen lodged in an artery. Fluorescein angiography is very helpful in identifying the location of the blockage and the affected downstream retinal areas. In the acute phase, the inner retina in the affected area will be thickened on OCT images.

Over time the inner retina will atrophy and will appear thinner than surrounding retinal tissue on OCT. This is a characteristic appearance of chronic arterial occlusions (and is also characteristic of chronic vein occlusions in some cases). In the case of central retinal artery occlusion, where the main artery entering the eye through the optic nerve is occluded, the entire retina will appear white and edematous except for the fovea. The appearance of the fovea is unchanged because it is comprised largely of the outer nuclear layer of the photoreceptors and derives its oxygen supply from the choroid. This gives the appearance of a "cherry red spot" in central retinal artery occlusions.

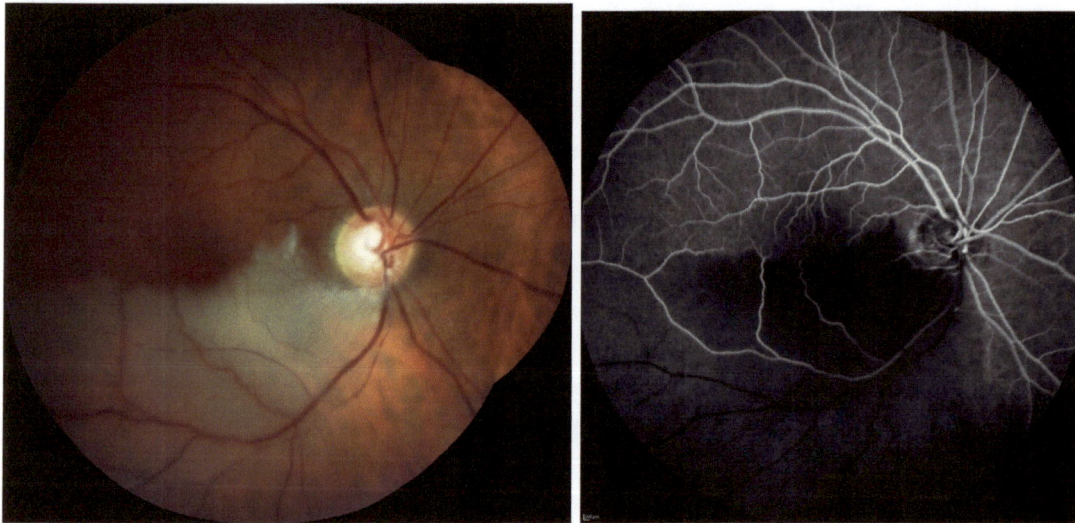

Color fundus image and mid-phase fluorescein angiogram of BRAO of the inferotemporal retinal artery with corresponding OCT below. Note thickening of the inner retina in the affected region. A very small amount of retrograde filling of the affected retinal arterioles is visible across the horizontal raphe.

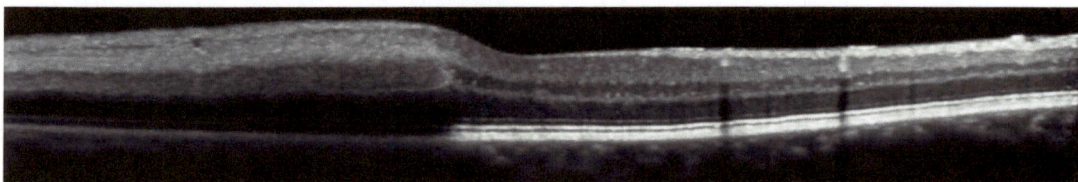

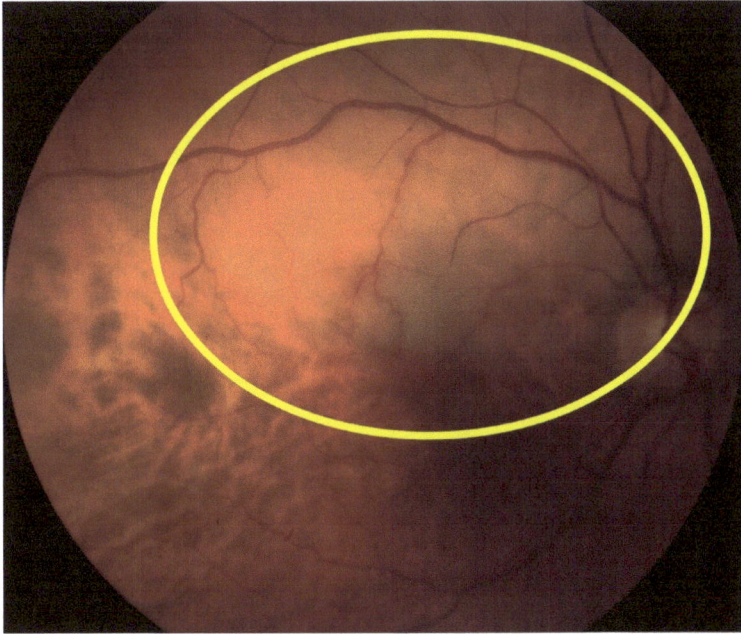

Color fundus image with occluded area (white appearing retina) in the yellow circle. Mid-phase fluorescein angiogram and corresponding vertical line B-scan OCT below. Note the retinal thickening in the right side of the OCT image (corresponding to the superior half of the retina in the FA). The attenuated OCT signal penetration through the thickened retina casts a shadow over the outer retina and choroid. There is a very fine ERM in this image as well.

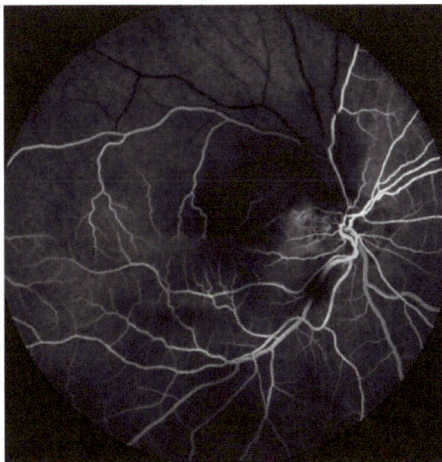

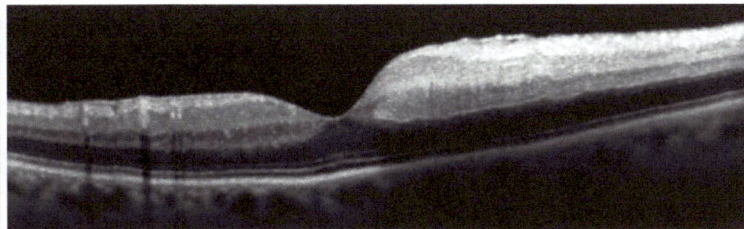

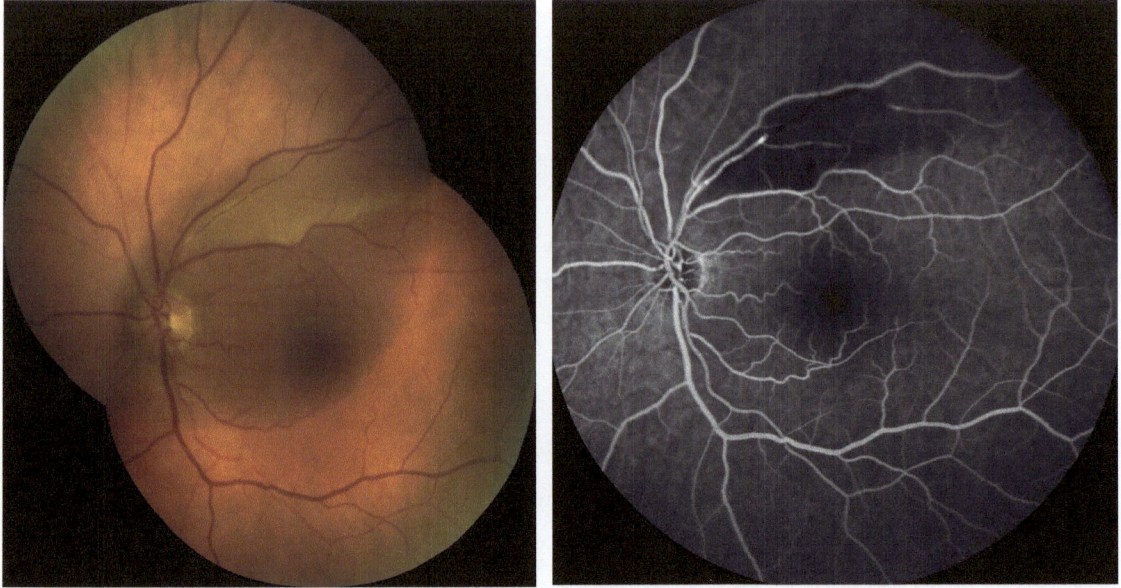

Color fundus image and late fluorescein of BRAO. The fundus image shows an area of retinal whitening along the superior arcades corresponding to the area of decreased fluorescence on the FA.

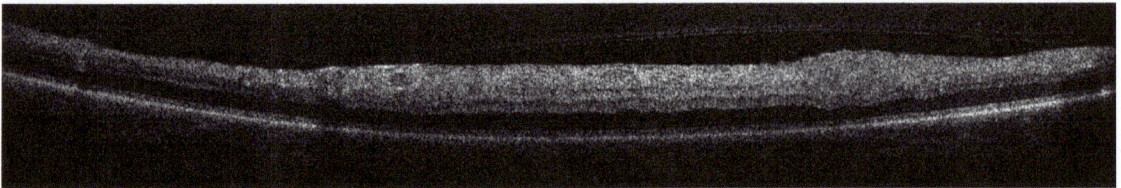

B-scan OCT through the retinal area that is in the distribution of the occluded artery. Notice the hyperreflectivity of the inner retina that represents inner retinal edema.

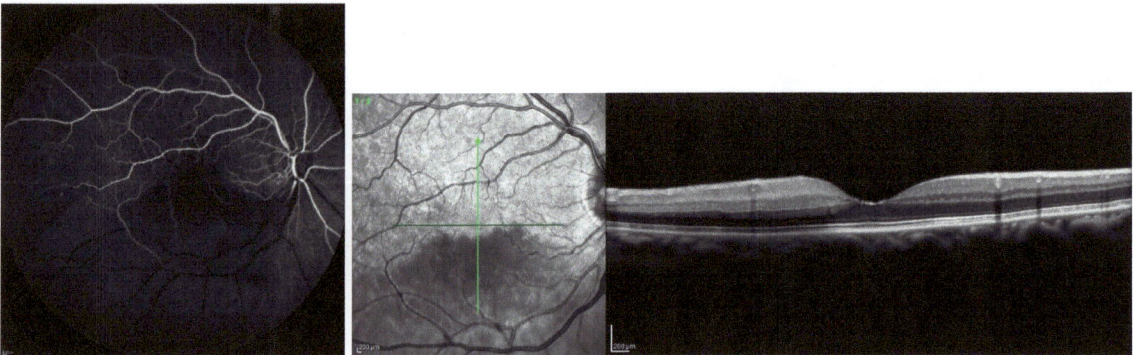

Early to mid-phase fluorescein angiogram of an arterial occlusion involving the inferotemporal branch retinal artery. The vertical B-scan OCT demonstrates the thickening and hyperreflectivity of the inferior retina. The infrared image shows attenuation of the IR intensity in the region of the BRAO.

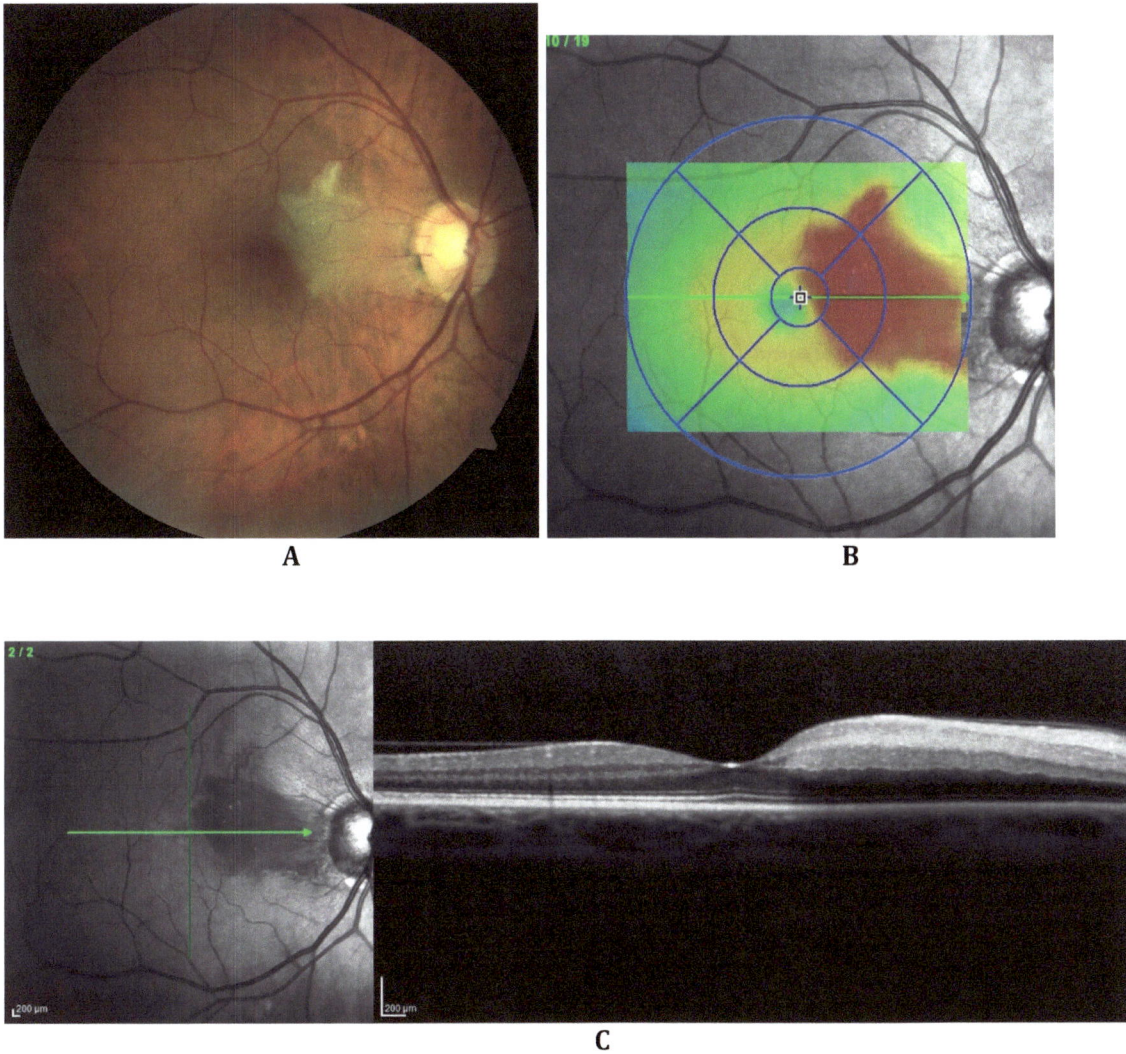

(A) Color image of a cilioretinal artery occlusion. This is a unique sub-type of arterial occlusion that only affects the distribution of the small cilioretinal artery that feeds the retina between the fovea and optic disc.

(B) Infrared fundus image and volumetric OCT shows thickening of the nasal retina in the distribution of the cilioretinal artery.

(C) Corresponding B-scan OCT. Note thickening and hyperreflectivity of inner retina nasal to the fovea.

Central Retinal Artery Occlusion

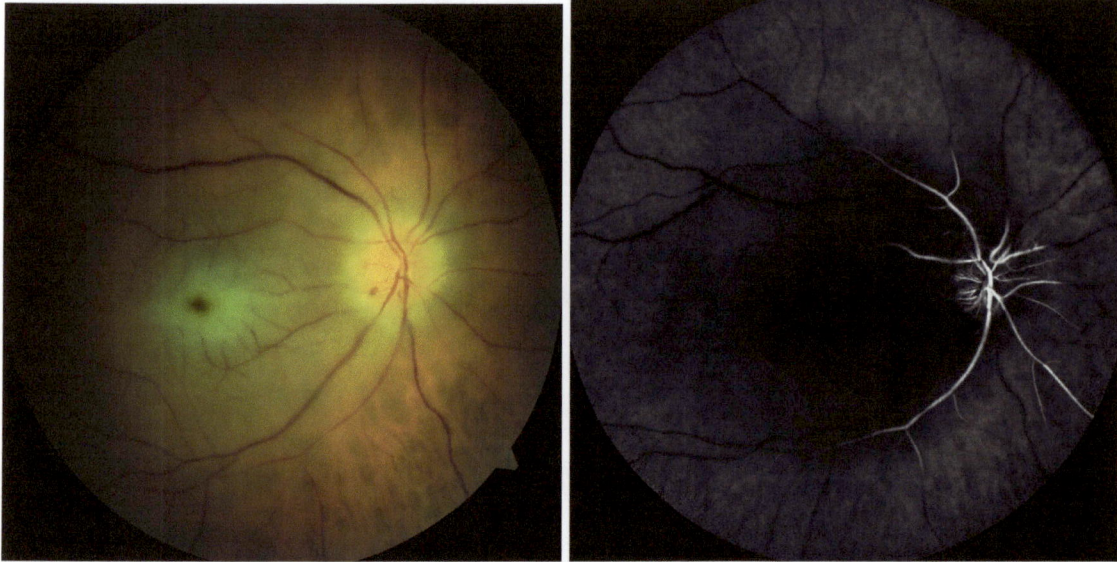

Color fundus image and early fluorescein angiogram of CRAO with corresponding OCT below. Color fundus image shows whitening of the retina and attenuation of the arteries. Note the loss of the choroidal detail as a result of inner retinal edema in the macula. The pigmentation of the fovea is preserved because there is no overlying inner retina at that location. The fluorescein angiogram illustrates very limited perfusion in the proximal segments of the retinal arteries. There is also significant attenuation of the fluorescein signal from the choroid in the central macula as a result of the overlying edema.

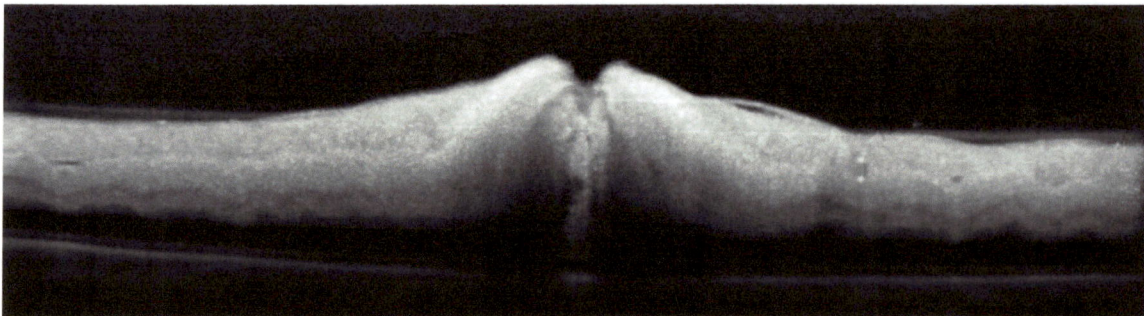

The B-scan OCT demonstrates the significant thickening of the retina that is predominantly in the inner retina.

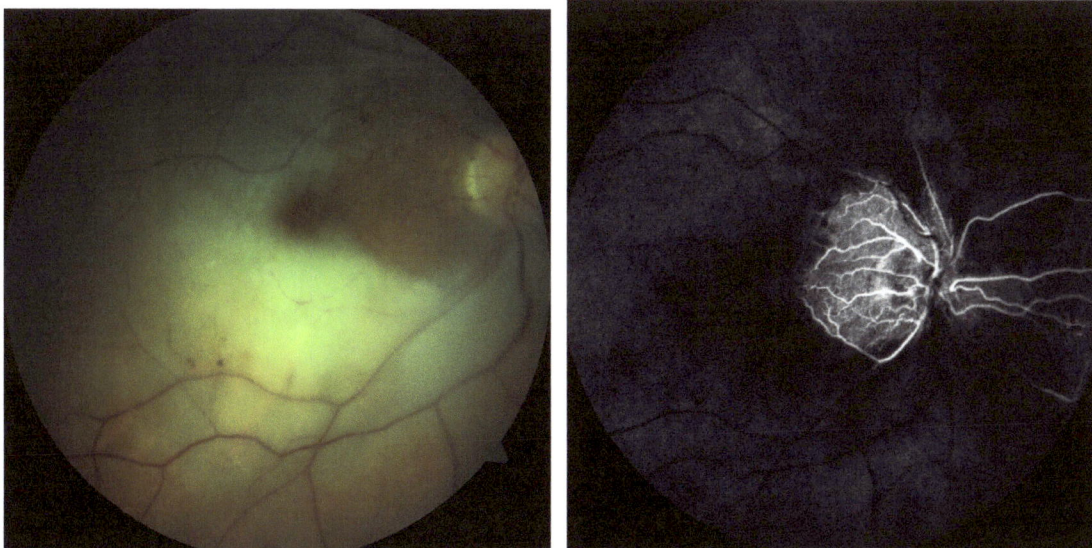

Color fundus image with early fluorescein angiogram of a CRAO with sparing of the cilioretinal artery. Note the diffuse whitening of the retina on the color image, which spares the region just temporal to the optic nerve head to the fovea. The fluorescein angiogram demonstrates perfusion of the spared region. This is a classic appearance of the distribution of perfusion from cilioretinal arteries. Cilioretinal arteries are supplied by the choroidal circulation and are therefore spared in central retinal arterial occlusions.

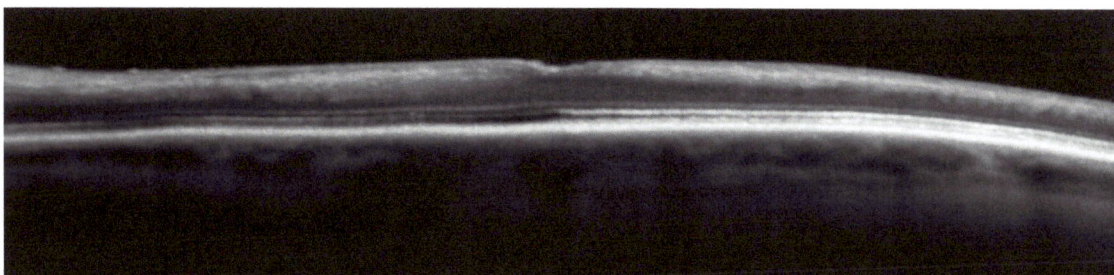

B-scan OCT of CRAO with relative sparing of the nasal macula corresponding to the distribution of the cilioretinal artery. Note the relative hyperintensity of the inner retina on the right side of the image (temporal) compared to the left.

Retinal Detachment (RD) and Retinoschisis (RS)

A retinal detachment is the separation of neurosensory retina from the underlying retinal pigment epithelium. This can occur in multiple retinal conditions and generally requires a clinical examination in combination with imaging findings for appropriate diagnosis. Retinal detachments can be focal and small or very large. Retinoschisis is a splitting of the neurosensory retinal tissue, usually in the outer plexiform layer. OCT imaging of the fovea is important to make the distinction of a "macula on" or "macula off" retinal detachment, which may add prognostic value to visual outcome of intervention.

Retinal Detachment

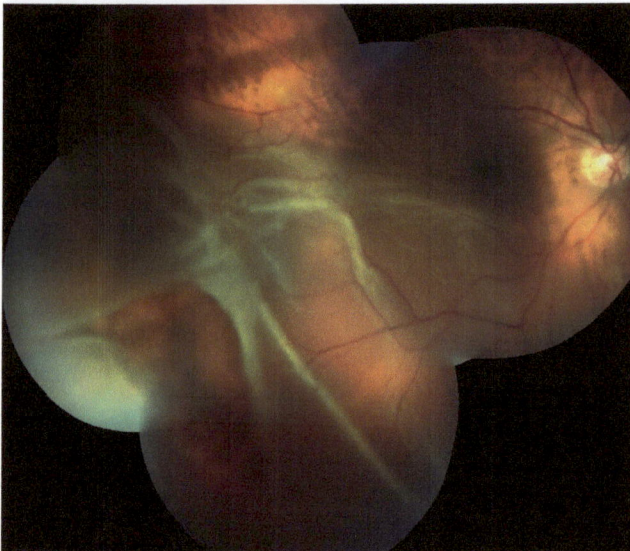

Color fundus image of retinal detachment extending into the macula. The white appearance of the retina and the loss of the underlying choroidal and RPE detail is characteristic of a retinal detachment. In this case the retinal detachment is caused by multiple retinal breaks that are visible in the lower left hand corner of the image.

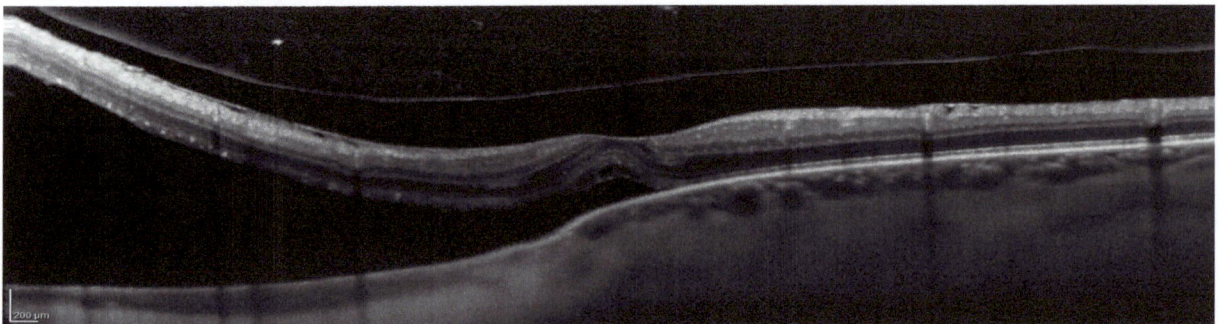

Subretinal fluid in this OCT extends into the sub-foveal space suggesting a macula-off retinal detachment. The overlying retina has an ERM evident in some regions as a bright hyperreflective line on the surface of the retina. The overlying white line in the vitreous represents the posterior hyaloid, which is partially separated in this case. The outer retina in the area of the detachment demonstrates elongated photoreceptor outer segments that appear as hyperreflective white regions in the outer-most aspect of the retina.

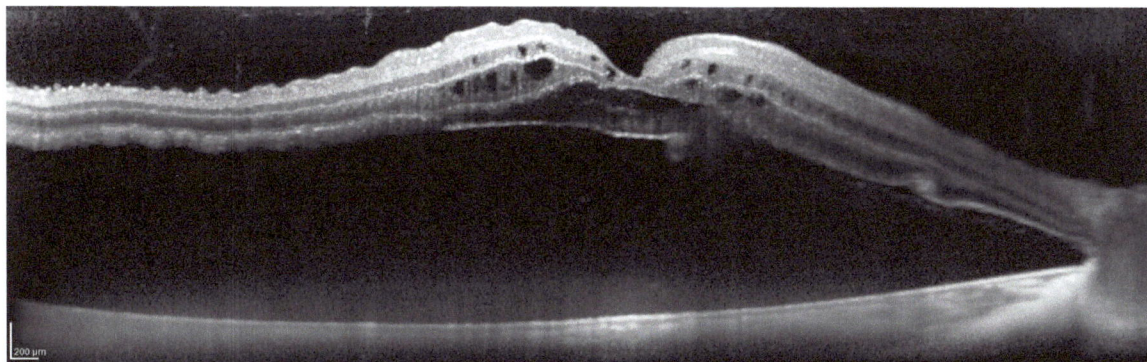

Complete retinal detachment of the macula from the RPE. Note that the subretinal fluid extends all the way to the optic nerve. The overlying retina has cystoid spaces in multiple layers, which suggests that this detachment is chronic.

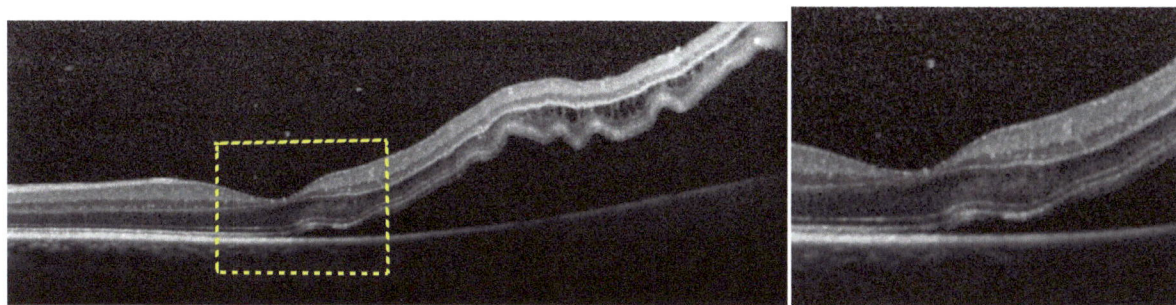

Retinal detachment that is extending into the sub-foveal space. The undulating contour of the detached retina is apparent both on the OCT here and in general on clinical examination. The accumulation of intraretinal cystoid spaces suggests that this retinal detachment is chronic.

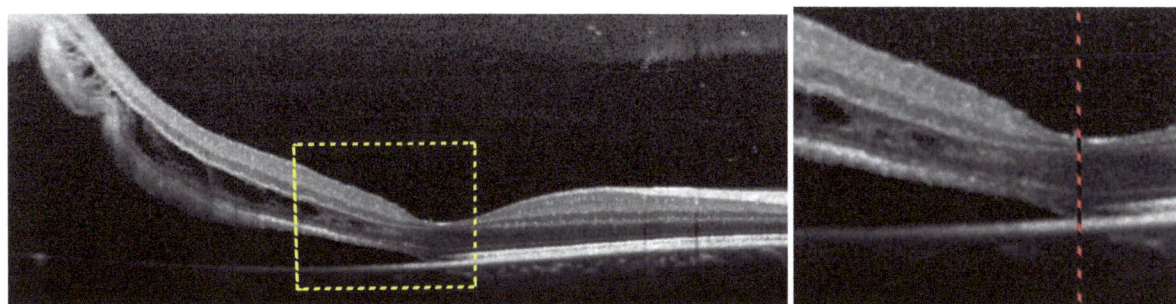

Retinal detachment with fluid extending into the subfoveal space. The accumulation of intraretinal cystoid spaces suggests a chronic detachment. The elongated outer segments of the photoreceptors appear as the thickened hyperreflective outer boundary of the detached retina. These findings also suggest a chronic retinal detachment.

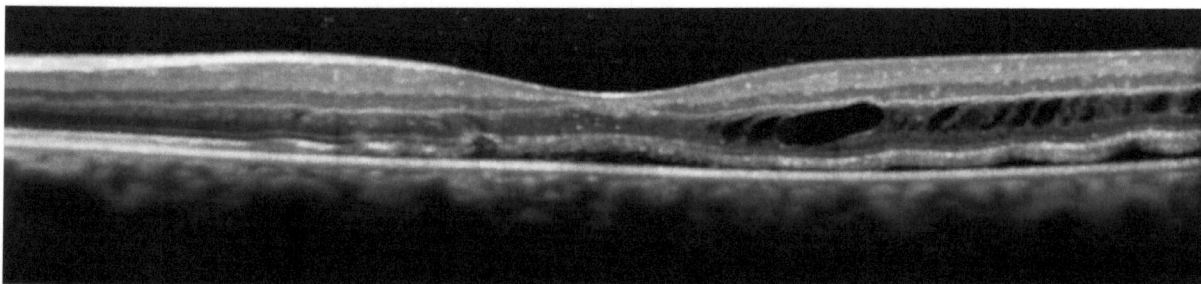

Residual subretinal fluid can be found on post-operative OCTs as in the above case. Sub-retinal and intraretinal fluid can take weeks or months to resolve after surgery.

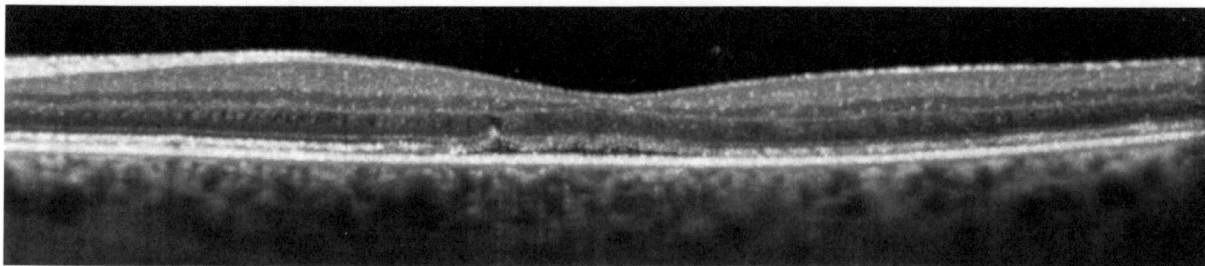

1-month post-surgical repair of RD with complete resolution of intraretinal fluid and slight disruption of the external limiting membrane and IS/OS segment.

Retinoschisis

Retinoschisis refers to the separation of retinal layers in several settings and usually implicates a mechanical process whereby retinal layers are being pulled apart. This is a distinct entity from accumulation of intraretinal fluid or subretinal fluid that we have described in other chapters. The clinical differentiation of retinoschisis, subretinal fluid and intraretinal edema can be challenging and the reader is encouraged not to solely rely on imaging results to make a determination of the condition. In some cases, retinoschisis is simply referred to as "schisis", and the spaces within the retina are also called "schisis cavities." Unlike retinal detachment, schisis cavities are not located between the neurosensory retina and the RPE. Retinoschisis is generally reserved for separation that occurs only within the retinal layers.

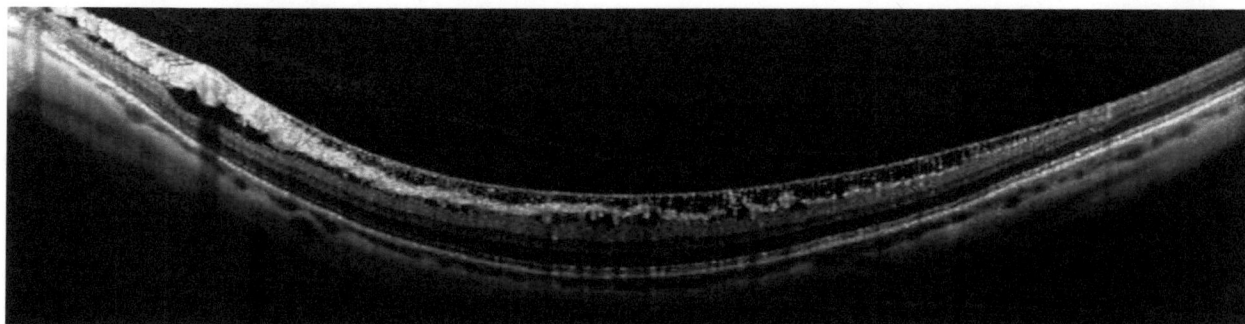

OCT of myopic eye with overlying ERM and attached posterior hyaloid, causing schisis cavities of the inner retina. In this case the schisis is largely limited to the space between the RNFL and inner plexiform layer.

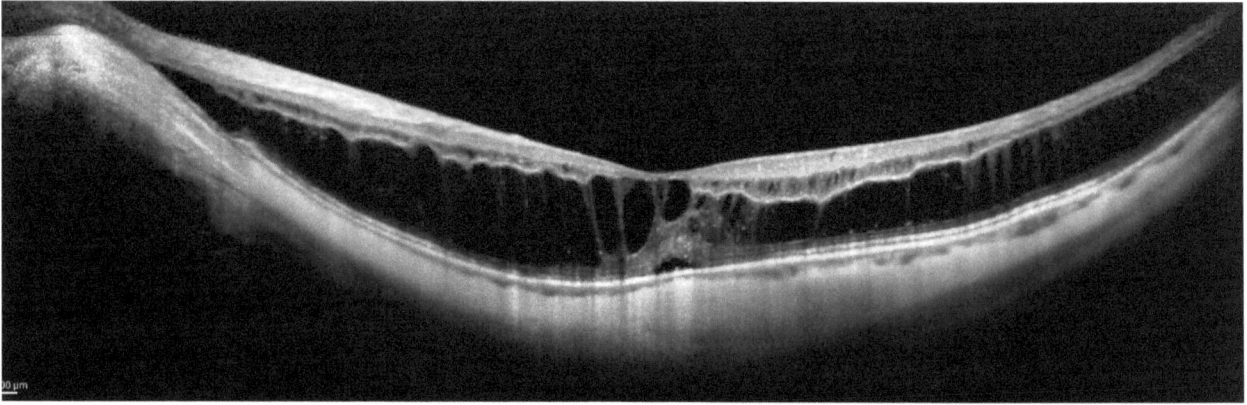

OCT of myopic eye consistent with myopic macular schisis. The exaggerated curvature of the posterior pole here is suggestive of a myopic eye. The schisis cavities appear as hyporeflective spaces that are most prominent in the outer retina. There are also small schisis cavities in the inner nuclear layer. There is a very small pocket of subretinal fluid in the center of the image. The foveal depression is completely blunted. Note the very thin appearance of the choroid, which is also consistent with a myopic eye.

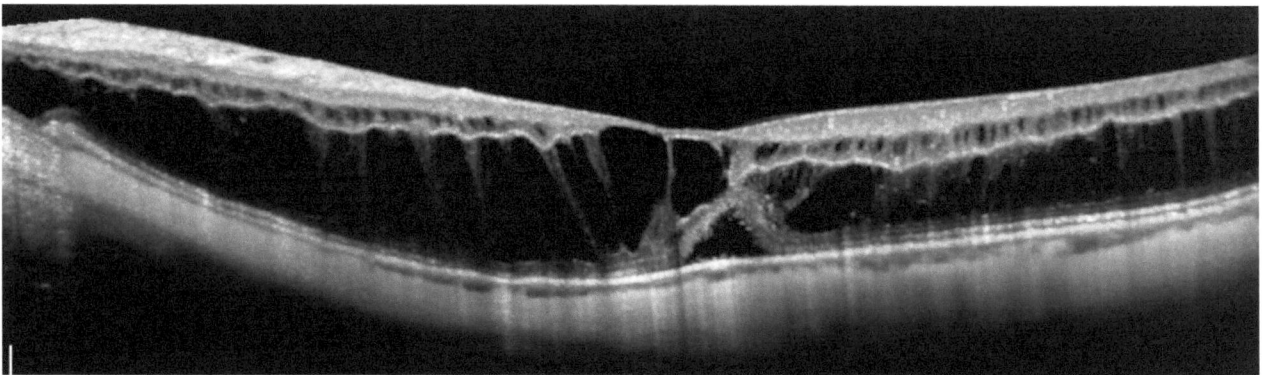

Another example of findings consistent with myopic macular schisis on OCT. Similar findings to the previous image are illustrated at slightly higher magnification.

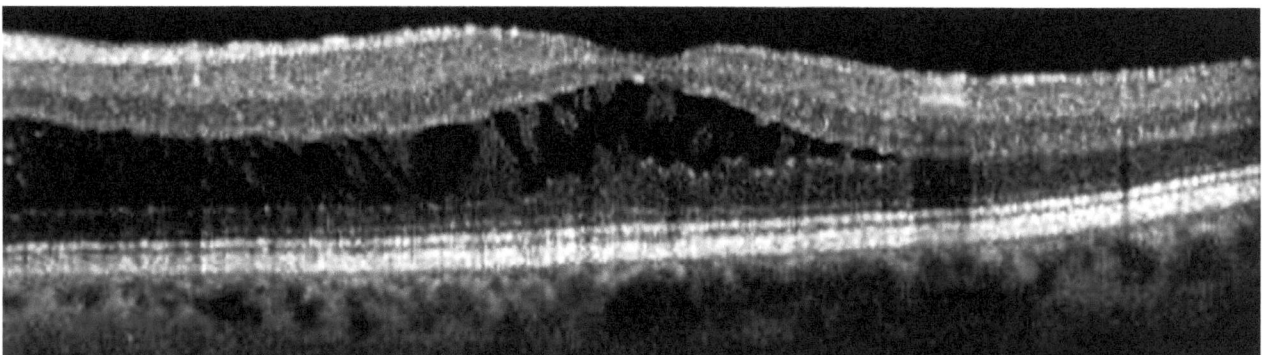

OCT of the macula with findings consistent with schisis of the retina. In this case the schisis is most prominent between the outer plexiform layer and the outer nuclear layer.

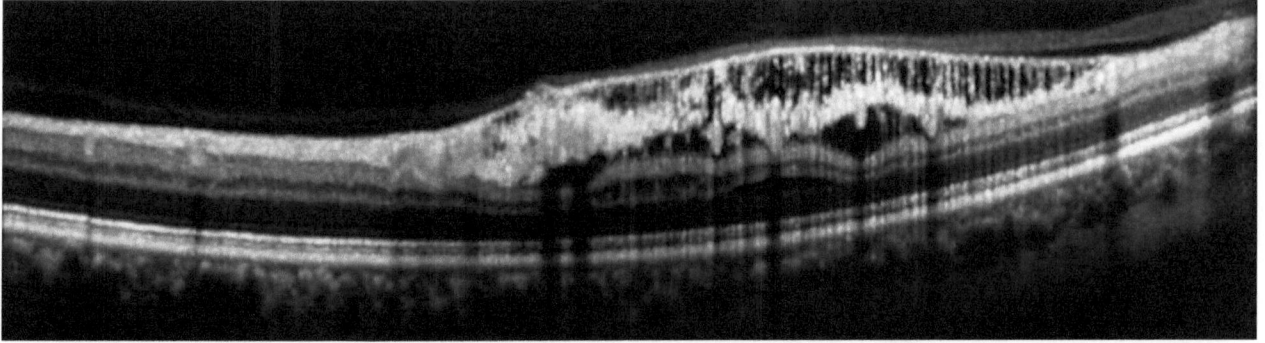

OCT image of a region of retina with attached overlying vitreous and separation of some of the retinal layers consistent with retinoschisis. There is separation between the ILM and the NFL, the NFL and the inner plexiform layer and a small separation between the outer plexiform layer and the outer nuclear layer.

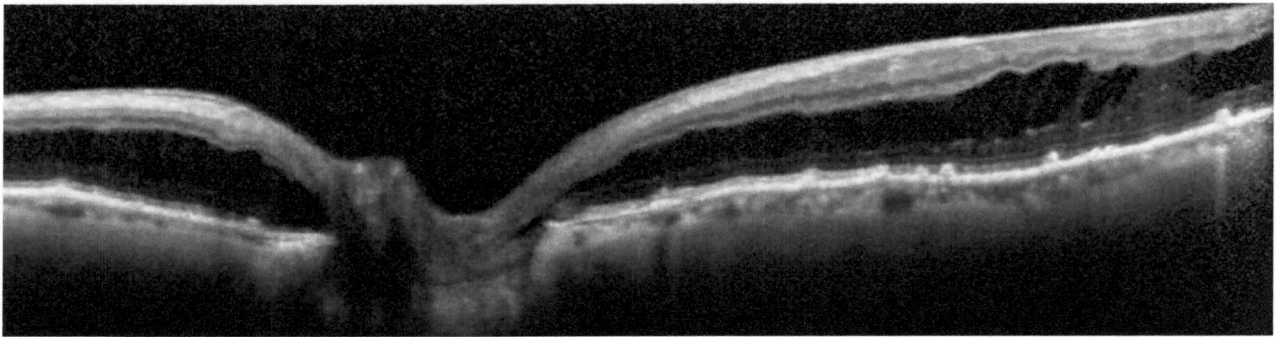

OCT centered on the optic nerve head demonstrates separation most apparent at the level of the outer retina on both sides. This finding is consistent with retinoschisis, although the close proximity to the nerve requires further evaluation to determine the cause of the schisis.

Sub-Retinal and Sub-Retinal Pigment Epithelium (RPE)

Retinal diseases that occur below the neuro-sensory retina and RPE, such as macular degeneration and central serous retinopathy, typically present on OCT as either low-density reflectivity (such as fluid) or high-density reflectivity (such as CNV, scar or drusen). OCTA is becoming a useful tool in detecting the presence of choroidal neovascularization (CNV), as well as distinguishing different categories of neovascularization, such as retinal angiomatous proliferation (RAP), Type 1 and Type 2 CNV, as well as polypoidal choroidal vasculopathy (PCV). OCTA images are not blocked by hyperfluorescence, which may obscure subretinal pathology on fluorescein angiography due to leaking or pooling of dye. However, visualizing subretinal or sub-RPE CNV can be tricky due to projection artifacts and segmentation artifacts on OCTA.

Dry Age-Related Macular Degeneration (AMD)

Age Related Macular Degeneration (AMD) is one of the leading causes of blindness and is a frequent disease that is imaged in ophthalmic practices. AMD is divided into two categories: dry AMD (non-neovascular or non-exudative) and wet AMD (neovascular or exudative). Currently, there is no cure for AMD. Anti-Vascular Endothelial Growth Factor (VEGF) injections are a very effective form of treatment for the wet form of AMD and no treatment is available for the dry type of AMD. Early stages of AMD may include hard and soft drusen, and the latter is an indicator of increased risk of progression to advanced AMD. Dry AMD can progress to RPE atrophy, loss of choriocapillaris and vision loss.

This loss of tissue defines the advanced form of dry AMD and is termed geographic atrophy. The thinning, or loss of RPE, allows for increased penetration of light into the choroidal layer resulting in a column of hyperreflectivity on OCT in the area of atrophy. This corresponds to the area of "window defect" that is commonly seen on fluorescein angiography.

Wet AMD is defined by the presence of choroidal neovascularization, which can occur either in the sub-RPE space (Type 1) or subretinal space (Type 2), and least commonly in the intraretinal space (Type 3 or RAP lesion). Type 1 and 2 vessels extend from the choroid and choriocapillaris through breaks in Bruch's membrane and infiltrate the sub-RPE and sub-retinal space. The origin and progression of Type 3 vessels are still controversial. Wet AMD is a progression from dry AMD- that is, AMD patients with neovascularization have some degree of the dry type of AMD. This is important to remember as treatment regiments may resolve the neovascular component of AMD, or the fluid from these vessels, but there is still degradation of retinal tissue due to the underlying dry AMD. Patients with wet AMD typically present with much more rapid decrease in vision than those with only dry AMD.

Retinal pigment epithelial detachment, (PED), is frequently found on OCT in patients with both kinds of AMD. Type 1 CNV may cause serous or fibrovascular PED. While serous PED appear hyporeflective on OCT, fibrovascular PED appear both hyper- and hyporeflective and may have both findings within a single lesion. With the advent of new treatments for wet AMD, OCT imaging has played a critical role in clinical decision making for physicians. With the advent of OCT angiography, visualization of distinct retinal and subretinal layers will allow even more detailed detection and classification of CNV. OCT is an essential clinical tool for the baseline evaluation of AMD, as well as on-going serial imaging for the treatment of choroidal neovascularization in AMD. Current treatment of CNV typically requires monthly OCT evaluations to determine the need for retreatment.

Drusen

Drusen are typically yellow deposits under the RPE but above Bruch's Membrane and can be classified as soft or hard. However, reticular drusen are located in the subretinal space. Drusen can vary in size from small (<63 microns), medium (63-125 microns) to large (>125 microns). Very large drusen are called drusenoid PED and are typically > 250 microns in diameter.

Soft drusen have indistinct borders, tend to be larger, and are a definite precursor to macular degeneration. Soft drusen can appear, disappear and even coalesce so the shapes vary greatly. Soft drusen are essentially a type of PED that occur in Dry AMD.

Hard drusen have distinct borders and tend to be smaller than 63 microns.

Reticular drusen have indistinct border and occur in the subretinal space typically between the inner and outer photoreceptor segments. These are typically difficult to observe on color fundus images, but appear distinct on OCT and IR imaging.

Drusenoid PED are essentially soft drusen that are defined by their very large size. As drusenoid PED collapse, they generally result in regions of geographic atrophy (RPE loss).

Drusen typically appear moderate to hyperreflective on OCT, but their appearance on color and fluorescein imaging can vary even more, as drusen can vary from white to yellow in color. About 50% of drusen will stain with fluorescein and some will stain with ICG (hard drusen), while others may stain minimally or not at all (soft drusen and reticular drusen).

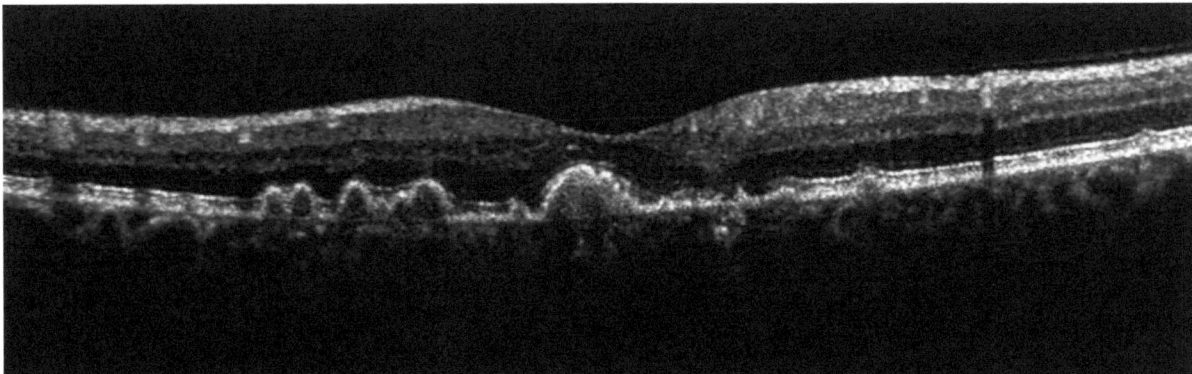

In this case, there are multiple drusen throughout the macula, with a large druse under the fovea.

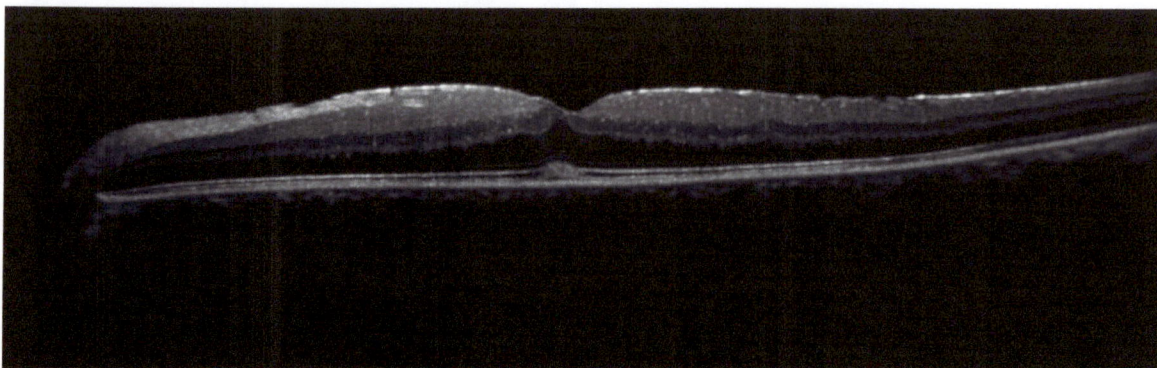

Note the hyper reflectivity of the RPE and interdigitation zone under the fovea. This is typical of the RPE appearance under the fovea and is not a druse.

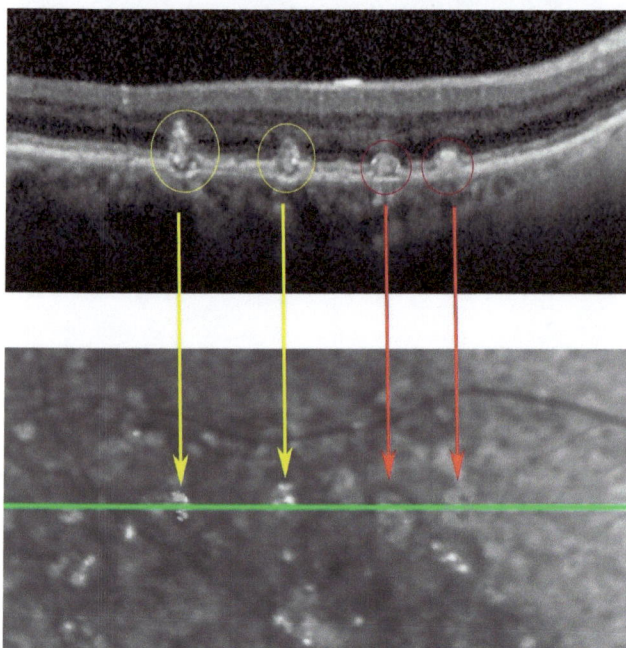

Hard drusen represented by yellow arrows, soft drusen represented by red arrows.

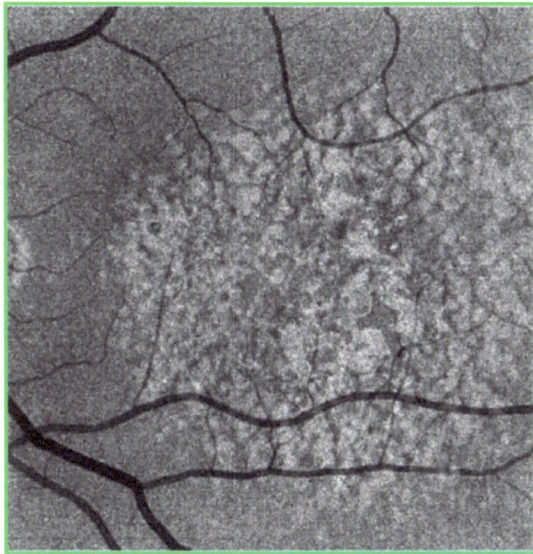

A

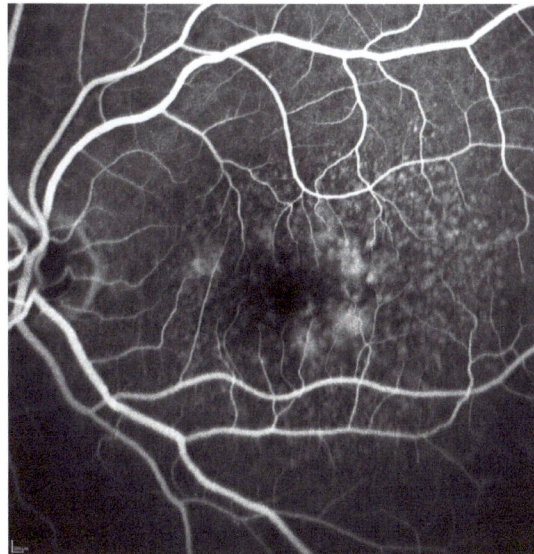

B

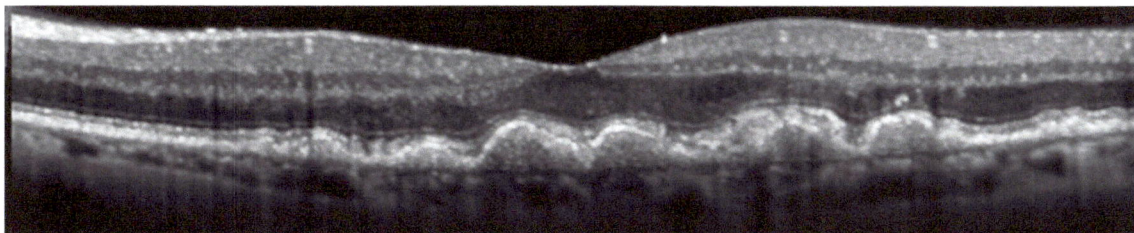

C

Infrared imaging **(A)** illustrates drusen very well. On fluorescein angiography **(B)**, drusen will stain differently depending on their biochemical composition. Not all drusen will stain as illustrated by the difference between the number of drusen on the IR versus FA images. OCT **(C)** of the same patient with soft drusen.

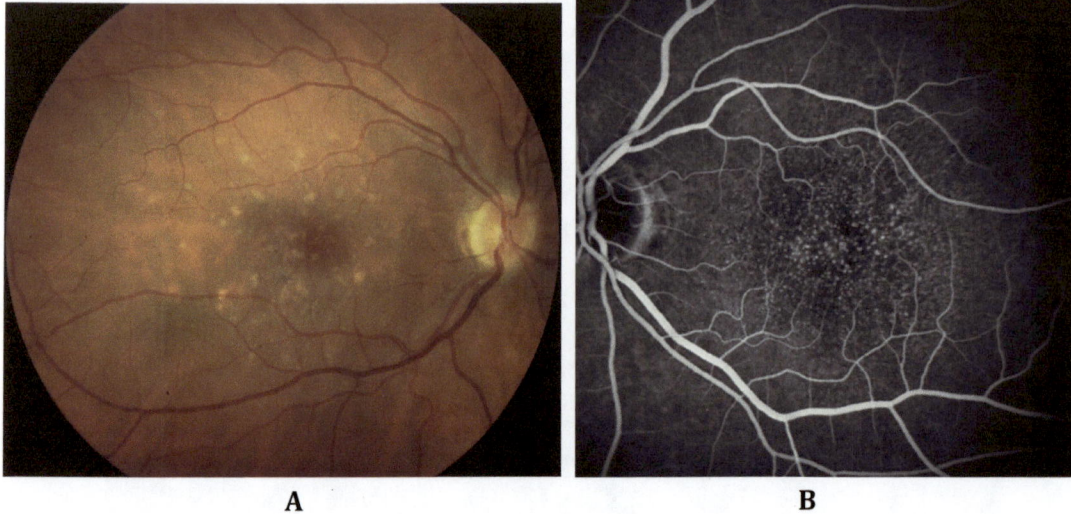

Color fundus image of soft drusen **(A)**. Fluorescein angiogram showing appearance of small hard drusen **(B)**.

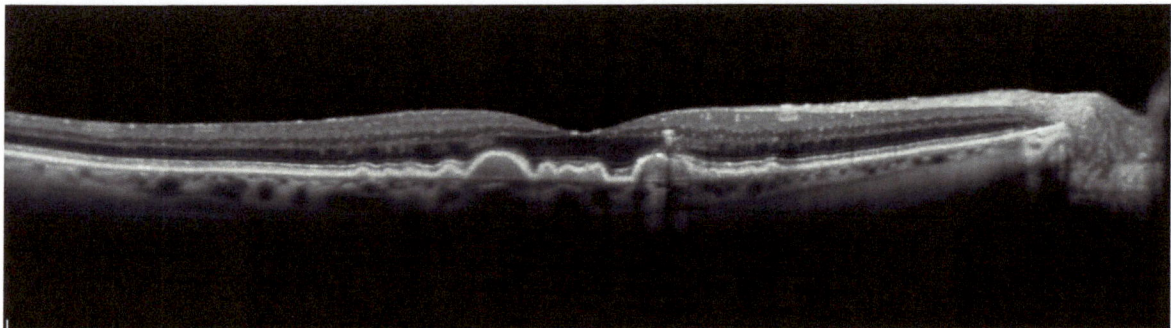

Drusen can have moderate to hyperreflectivity on OCT imaging. The reflectivity of the internal components can help distinguish drusen from serous PED and fibrovascular PED. Also note the pigment migration overlying the drusen on the far right.

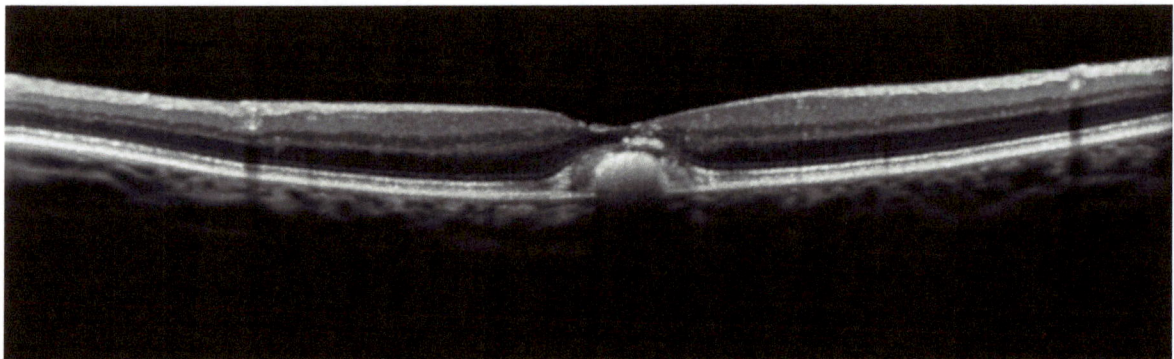

The internal appearance of drusen may vary significantly from moderate to hyperreflective (as in this case). Note that in this case the overlying RPE is altered and migrating into the intraretinal space within the fovea.

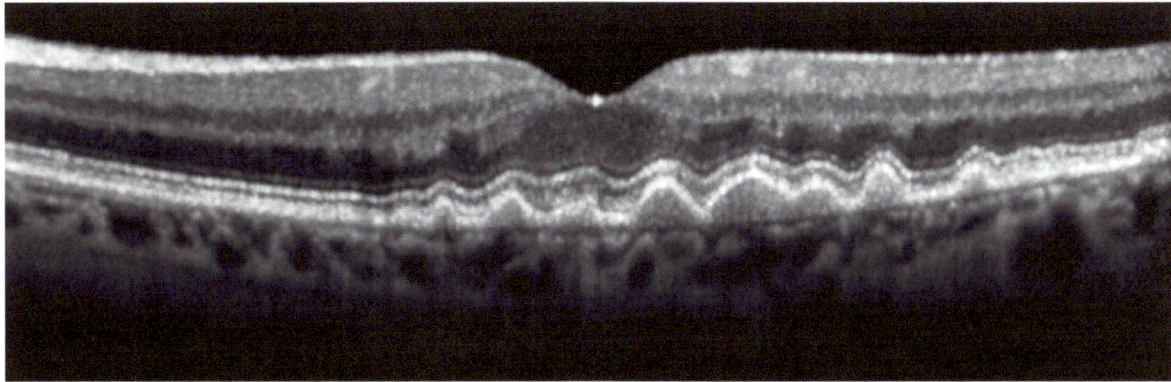

Multiple drusen

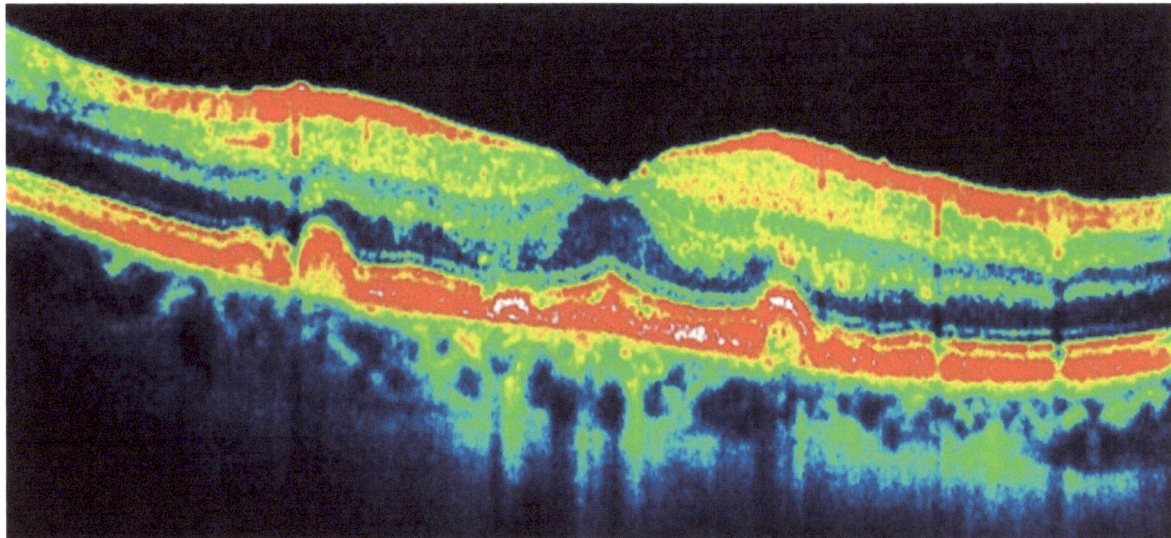

Multiple drusen

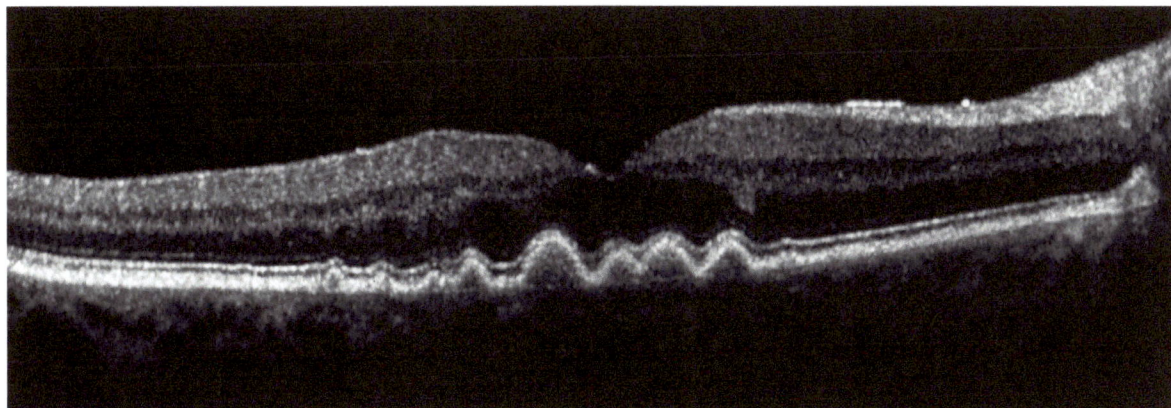

Multiple drusen

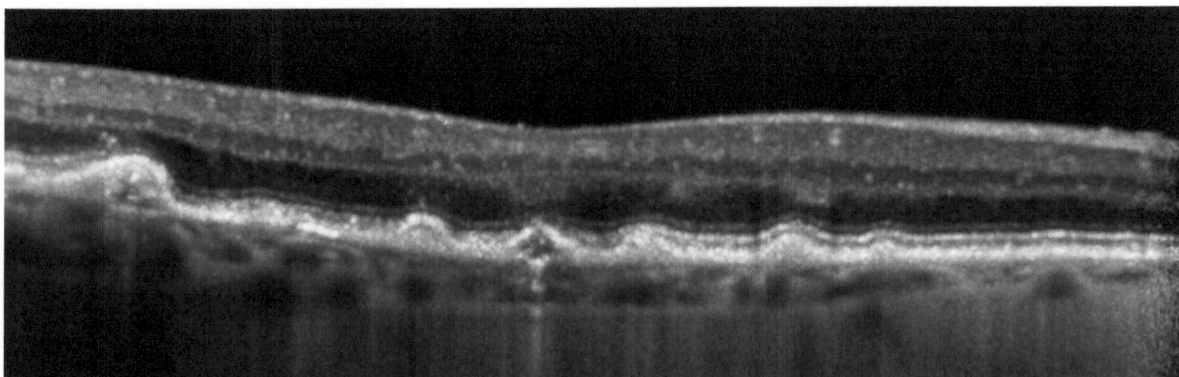

Multiple drusen appear on this image. Note the central drusen has hyporeflective internal components and a break in the overlying RPE. This suggests the druse may be collapsing and the overlying RPE may likely atrophy. Also note the absence of the ELM overlying the collapsing drusen.

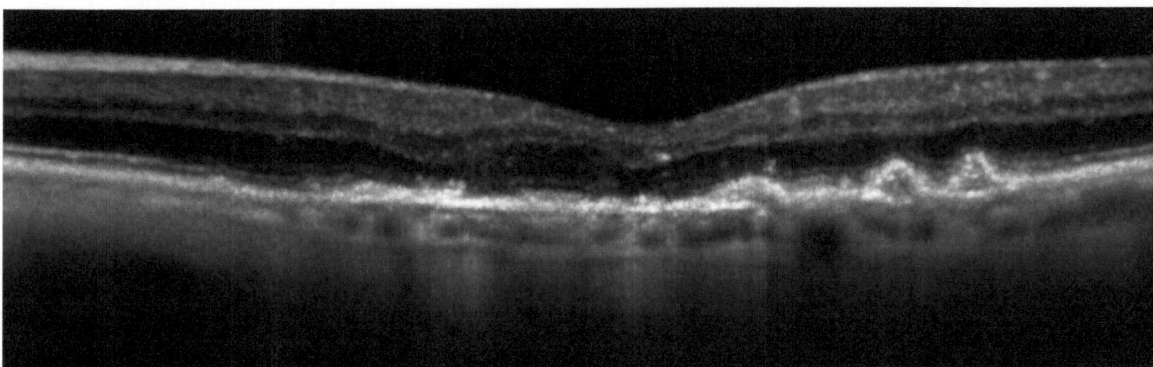

Multiple drusen are located on the right side of this image. Note the absence and irregularity of the outer retinal bands in the center of the image. There are also areas of RPE loss suggestive of early geographic atrophy and overlying ONL atrophy.

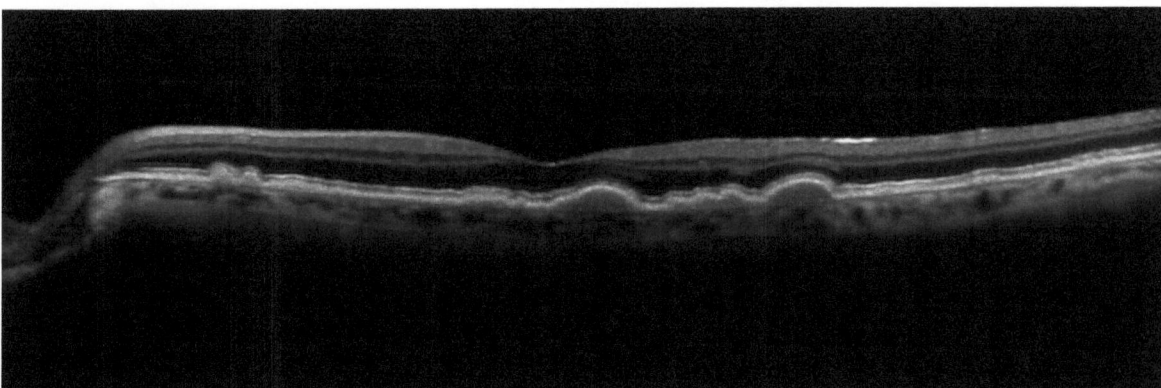

Several large drusen in the center of this image are starting to coalesce. The central drusen may qualify as a drusenoid PED if it measured more than 250 microns in diameter.

Reticular Pseudodrusen

Reticular pseudodrusen are also known as just "pseudodrusen," "subretinal drusenoid deposits" or "reticular drusen." Reticular pseudodrusen are best imaged either with the blue light, red free images or fundus autofluorescence images. In contrast to typical drusen, pseudodrusen appear as hyperreflective material above the RPE and in the sub retinal space on OCT. Pseudodrusen are often not visualized on color images or fluorescein angiography.

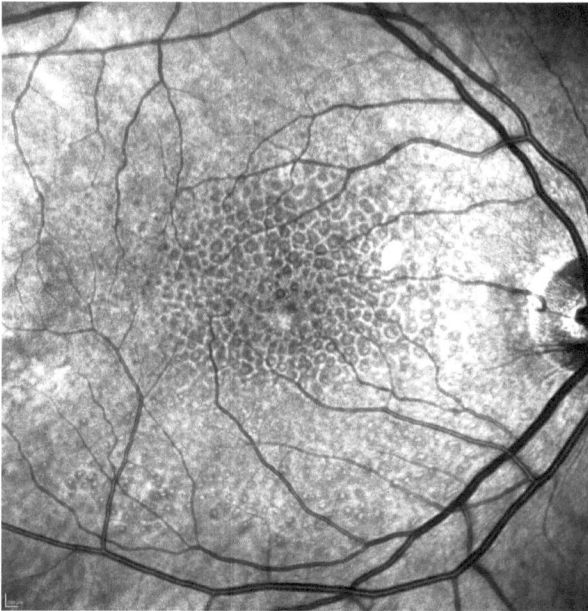

IR image of pseudodrusen with corresponding B-scan below. Note the speckled pattern of drusen throughout the macula.

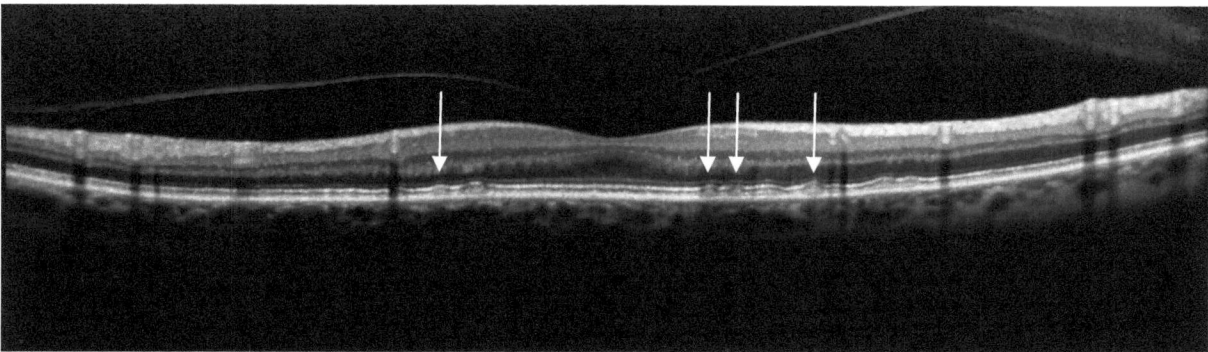

Reticular pseudodrusen appear between the RPE and the boundary between inner and outer segments of the photoreceptors (arrows).

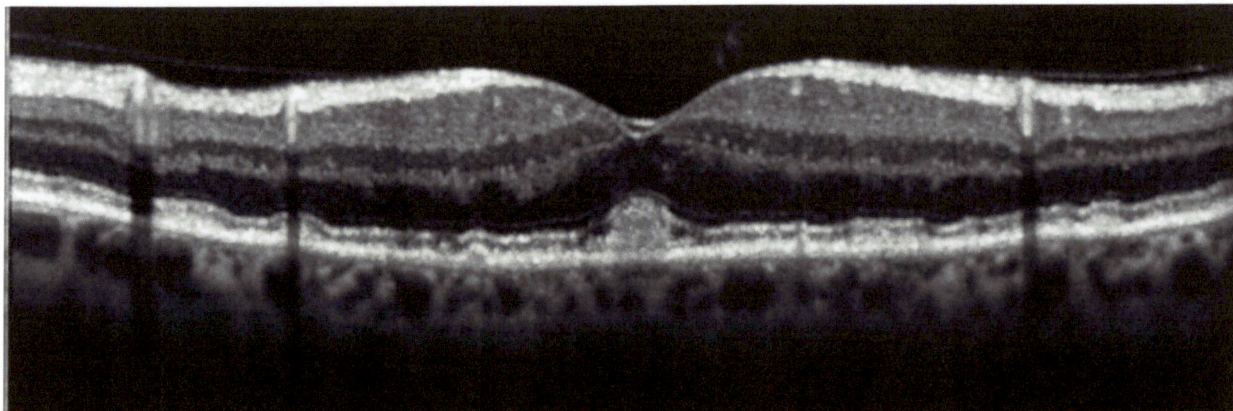

Reticular pseudodrusen are dispersed throughout the subretinal space here. There appears to be a "vitelliform" type deposit directly underneath the fovea in this case. As this case illustrates, the difference between a reticular pseudodruse and a vitelliform deposit is not well defined.

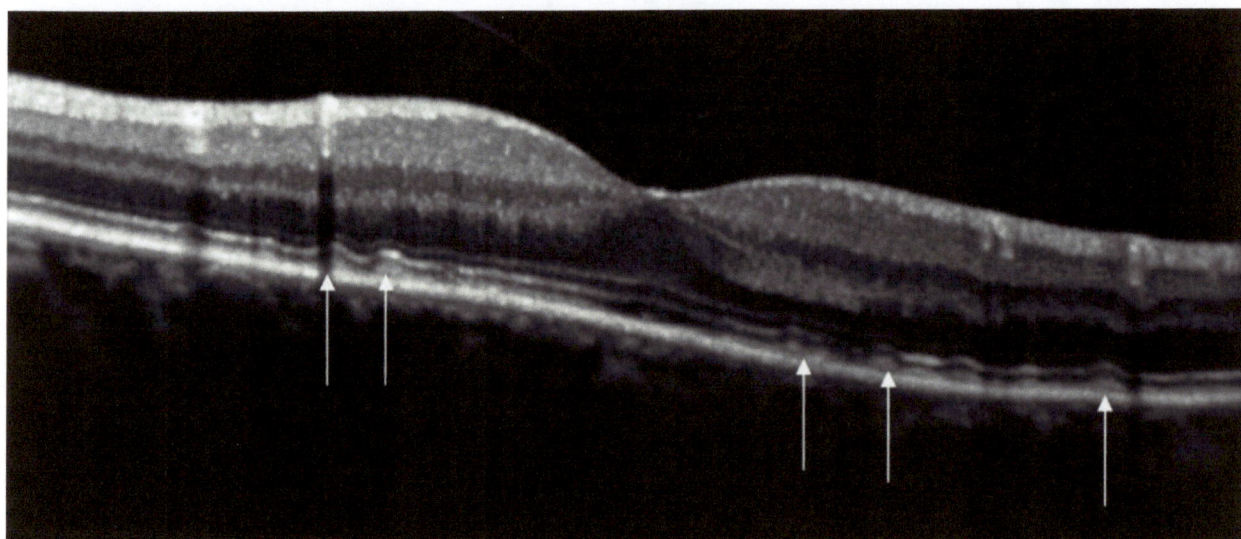

Reticular pseudodrusen (arrows) are clearly located above the RPE and in this case exclusively below the ellipsoid band of the outer retina.

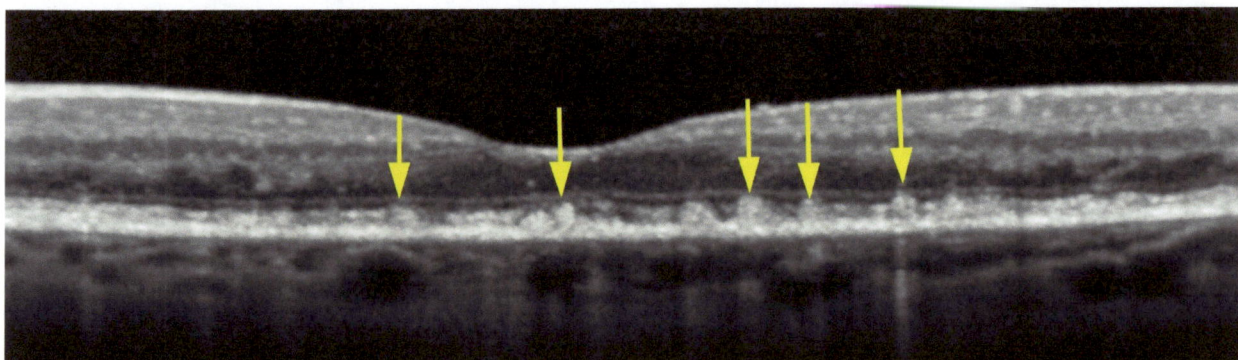

Reticular pseudodrusen (yellow arrows) are present in the above image above the RPE and below the ellipsoid band of the outer retina.

Geographic Atrophy

Geographic Atrophy (GA) refers to an area with loss of retinal pigment epithelial (RPE) cells. Areas of GA often have atrophy of the underlying choriocapillaris as well as varying degrees of atrophy in the overlying retina. GA is commonly the defining feature of Advanced Dry Age Related Macular Degeneration and can be associated with severe vision loss.

GA is visualized very well on OCT as well as a number of other imaging modalities. The loss of the RPE in the region of GA creates several characteristics of GA on OCT images. First, because there is no RPE in the area of GA, the underlying choroid appears hyperreflective compared to the surrounding areas. This is because the RPE in the normal surrounding areas attenuates the OCT signal from the underlying structures. Second, GA lesions are commonly associated with very thin underlying choroid and choriocapillaris. Third, the retina overlying the area of GA is usually sunken in appearance and various degrees of atrophy can be seen in the outer retinal layers.

GA is also visualized well on fundus color images, fluorescein angiography, fundus autofluorescence (FAF) images and en face OCT images. FAF utilizes an excitation wavelength of either blue or green light and detects the emission of naturally occurring fluorophores in the RPE that are found in lipofuscin (a metabolic byproduct of cell function). Regions of GA do not have RPE and therefore appear black on FAF due to the absence of any light emission.

GA appears as a "window defect" on fluorescein angiograms. The lack of RPE in the area of GA allows clear visualization of the underlying choroid through a "window defect" of the RPE.

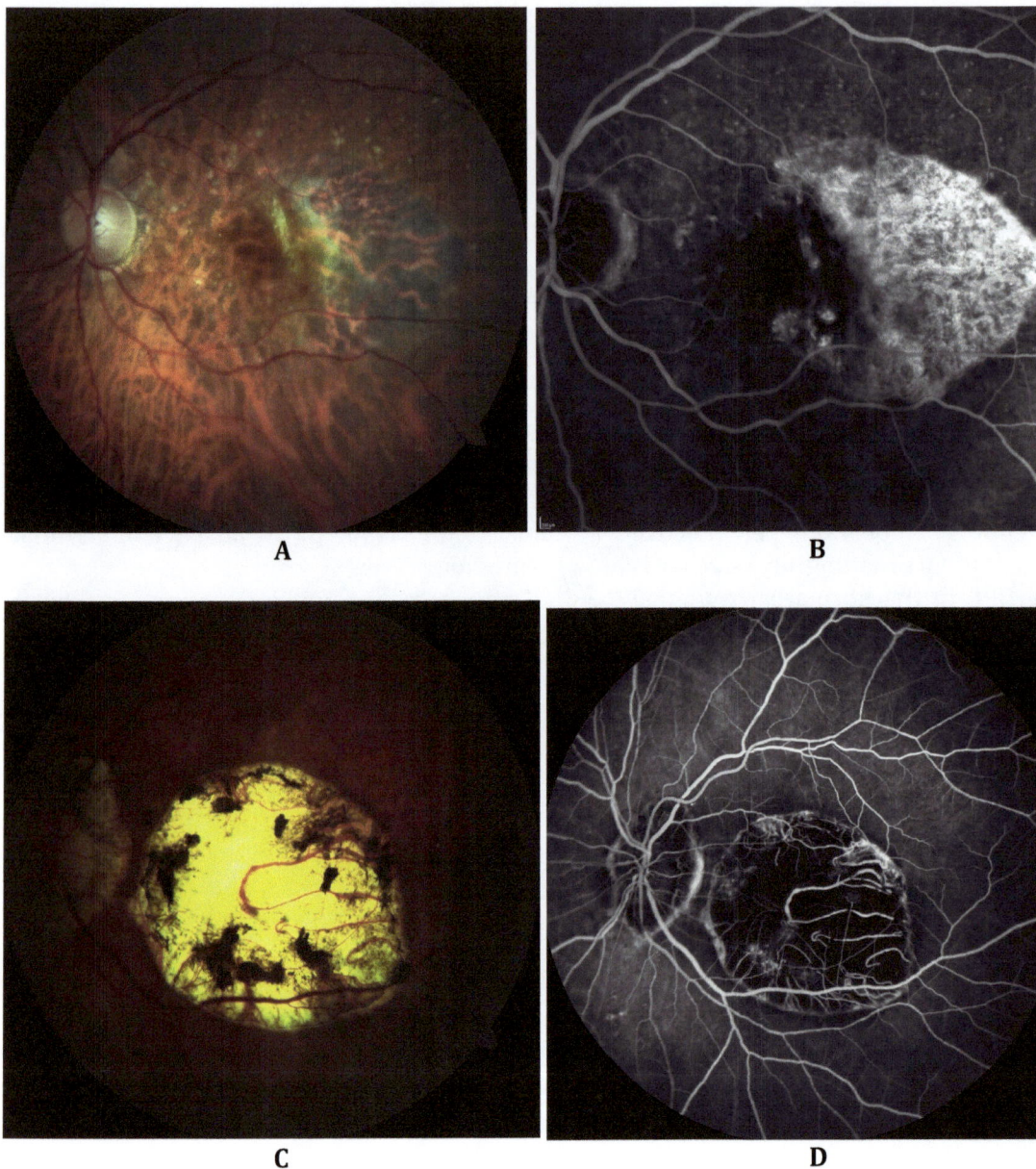

Color image **(A)** showing a large region of GA temporal to the fovea. There are numerous small and medium size drusen throughout the macula, and a very small amount of intraretinal hemorrhage at the inferior nasal border of the GA lesion and some subretinal fibrosis (white) at the superior nasal edge. Fluorescein angiogram **(B)** shows temporal window defect corresponding with the region of GA seen in the color image. In another case, color image **(C)** shows a large area of central geographic area, encompassing most of the macula. Pigment clumps are seen as well as large choroidal vessels. Fluorescein angiogram **(D)** demonstrates a circular "window defect" of the RPE through which the choroidal vessels are clearly visible. The grayish appearance of the area surrounding normal retina is due to the fluorescence of the choroid that is filtered through the RPE.

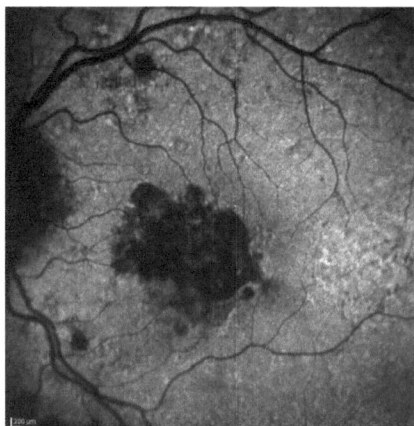

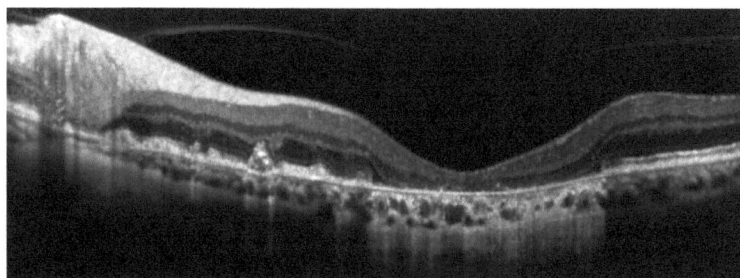

Fundus autofluorescence image demonstrates an area of hypoautofluorescence in the central macula that is consistent with GA. The corresponding SD-OCT shows absence of the RPE in the center of the image. In addition, there is loss of the outer retinal structures including the outer nuclear layer. The overlying retina appears sunken into the area of GA. The underlying choroid in the area of GA appears hyperreflective compared to the surrounding choroid because of the lack overlying RPE. The bright line in the vitreous is the posterior vitreous, which is partially detached over the macula but still attached at the nerve.

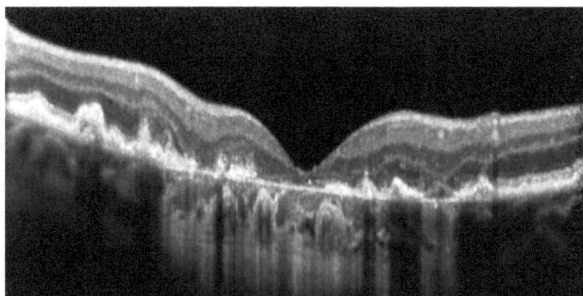

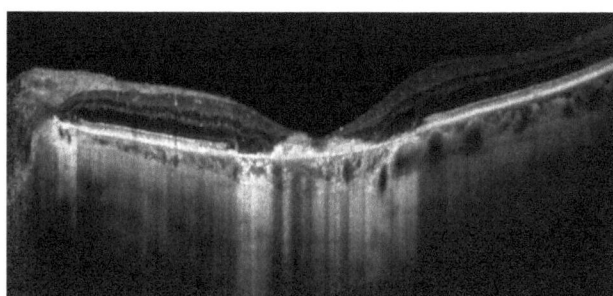

Two examples of GA on B-scan OCT. Note the partial or complete loss of the RPE layer and the sunken appearance of the overlying retina. Also, the hyperreflectivity of the underlying choroid compared to the surrounding choroid is clearly demonstrated in both cases. The case on the bottom demonstrates some hyperreflective material in the subretinal space that is consistent with old fibrosis.

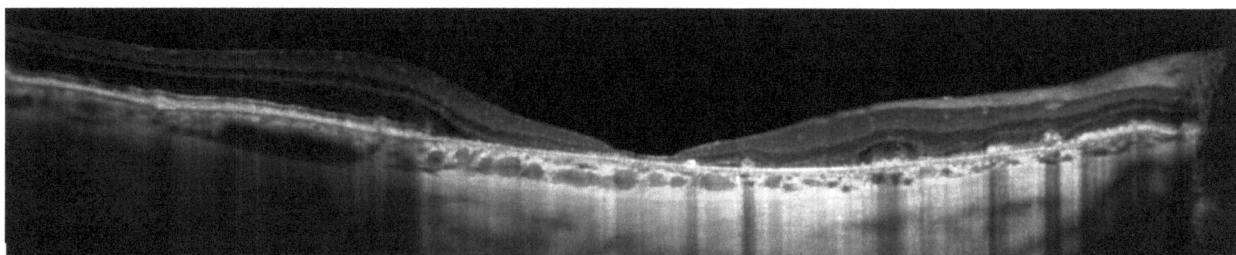

Large area of GA: Again, note the loss of the RPE layer, the sunken appearance of the overlying retina on the right half of the image and the hyperreflective choroidal structures underneath the area of GA.

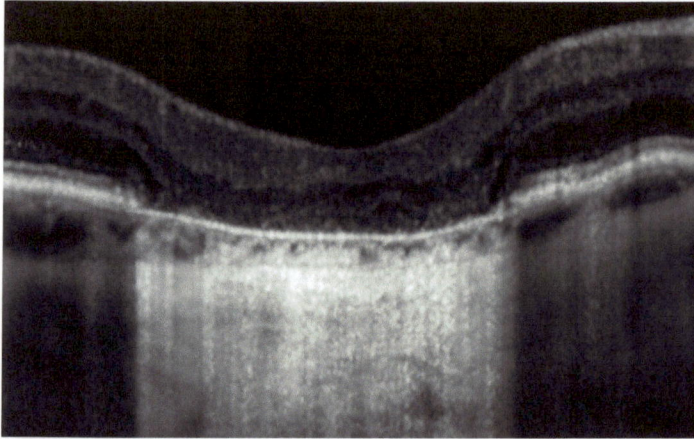

With the loss of RPE and the overlying retinal tissue support, intraretinal tissue collapses, as demonstrated on this B-scan.

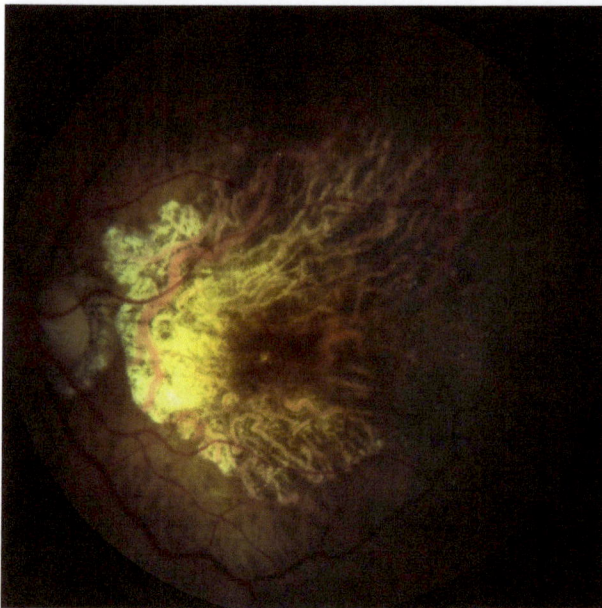

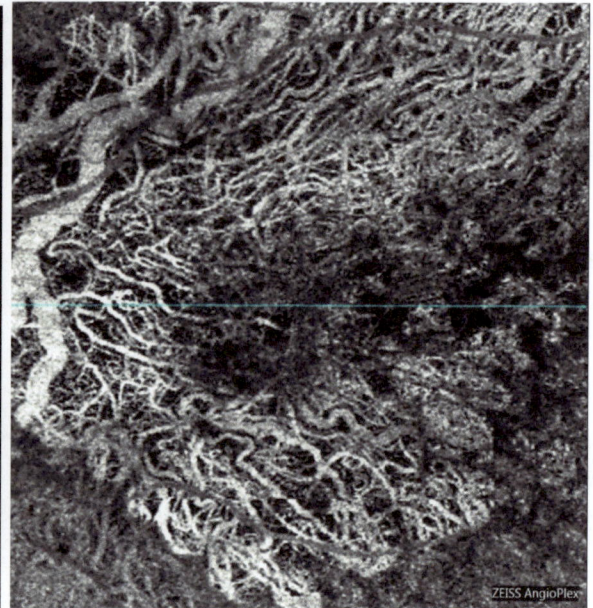

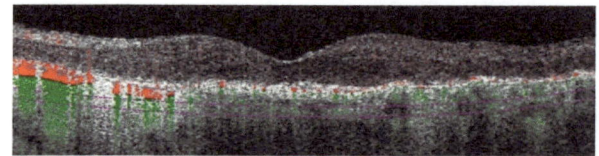

Color fundus image shows a large area of RPE loss consistent with geographic atrophy. A large choroidal vessel is visible in the region of the atrophy. Choroidal level OCTA with corresponding B-scan shows the choroidal and some choriocapillaris vessels in the area of RPE loss. The impact of the RPE on OCTA signal is clear in this case.

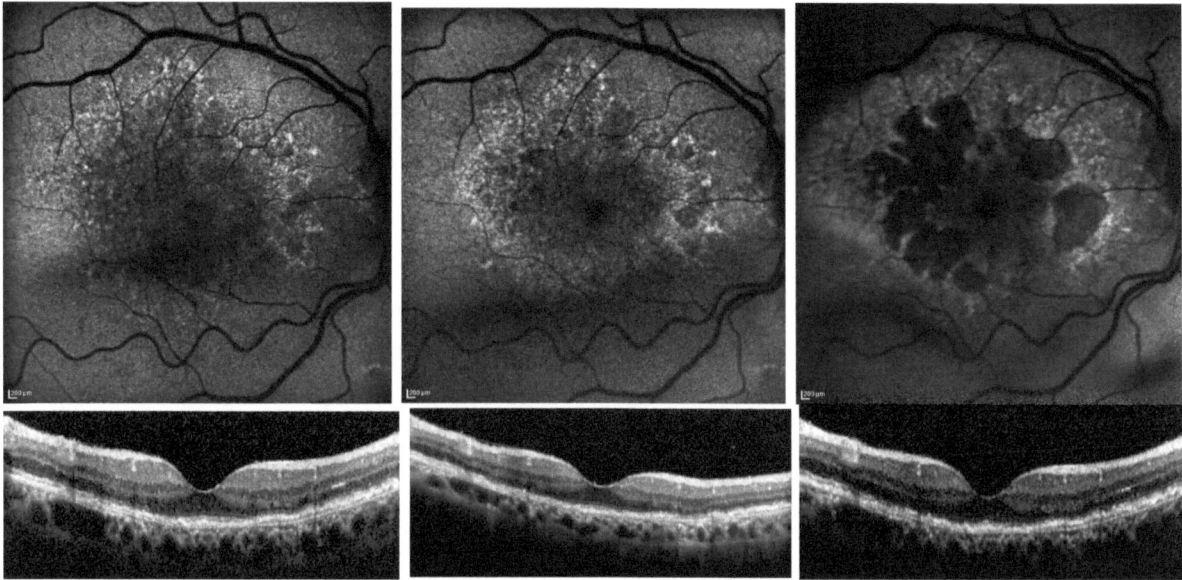

Fundus autofluorescence images with corresponding B-scans taken annually over a 3-year period. Left image shows numerous areas of hyper-autofluorescence and generalized hypo-autofluorescence throughout the macula. The middle panel shows increasing hyper-autofluorescence. The left panel shows large areas of intense hypo-autofluorescence surrounding the fovea. Each of these areas is surrounded by a hyper-autofluorescent ring. The OCT images below show that the RPE in the central macula is still intact. These B-scans do not cross any segment of GA in the above images, but note slight thinning of the choroidal thickness as time progresses.

Outer Retinal Tubulation (ORT)

In advanced cases of AMD, especially dry AMD, degenerating photoreceptors may become arranged in an ovoid manner within the outer retina. These processes are frequently found above the RPE, in the outer nuclear layer, and the round or ovoid structures have a definite border with hyporeflective spaces. The identification of ORT is important to differentiate from intraretinal or subretinal fluid.

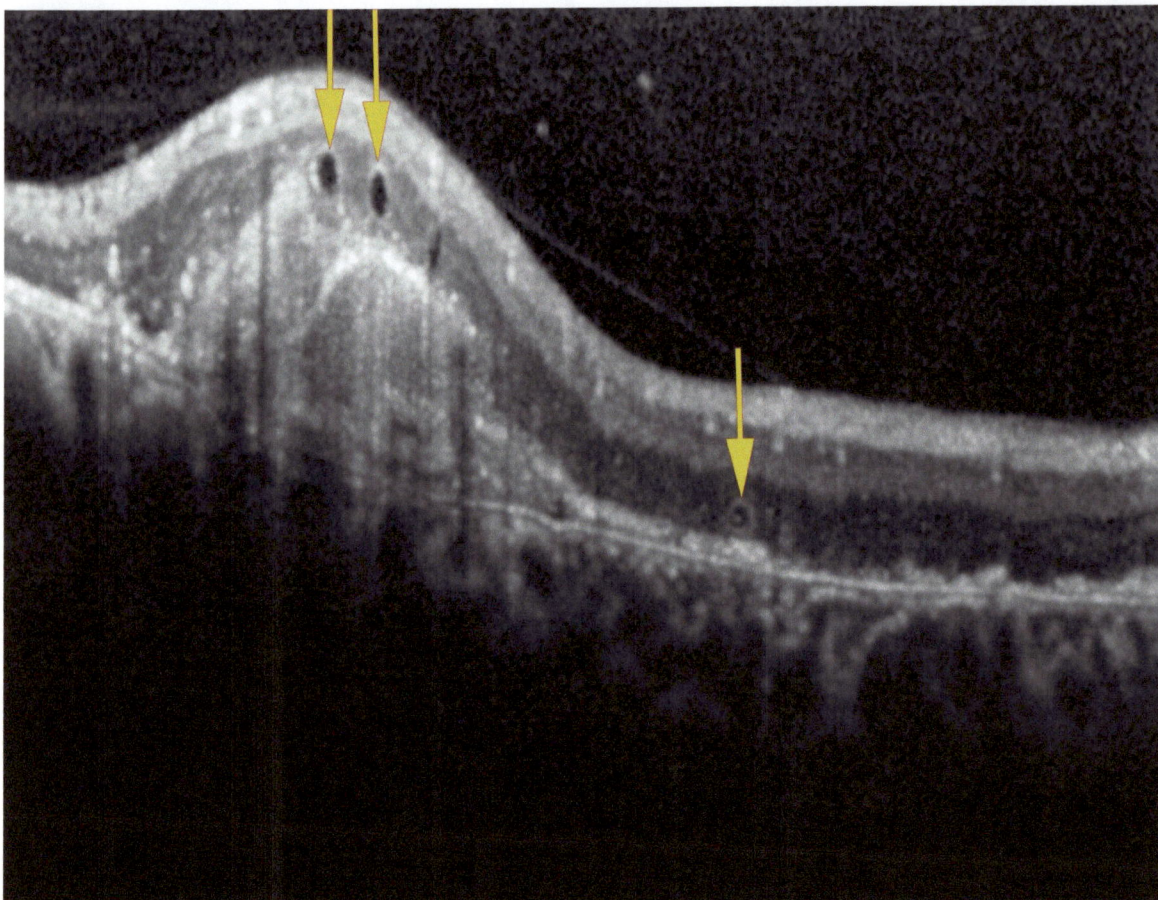

ORT seen on OCT in advanced AMD. Note the hyper reflective border and hypo reflective space in the center. There is prominent elevation of the retina due to a large pigment epithelial detachment that is consistent with choroidal neovascularization. ORT are not intraretinal fluid and it is important to differentiate them from intraretinal edema. ORT have hyperreflective borders that are not present in intraretinal cystoid spaces, and are also usually located in the outer retina and overlying areas of geographic atrophy or inactive CNV (subretinal fibrosis).

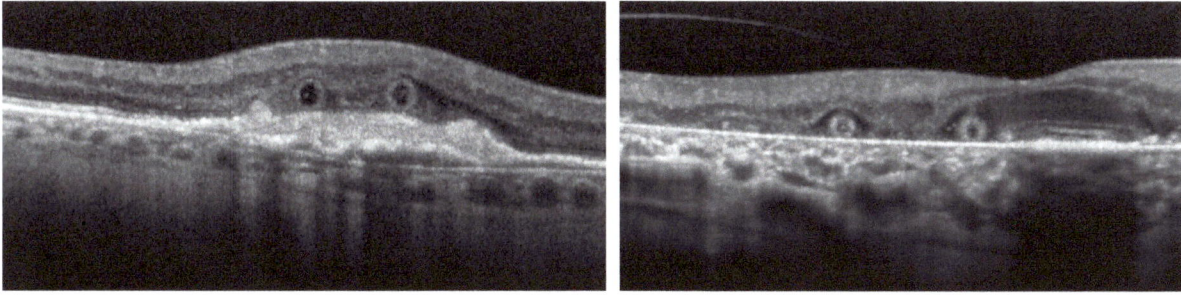

ORT on OCT in dry AMD. Note the absence of RPE and collapse of intraretinal tissue between ORT, which is indicative of GA. The RPE throughout most of the retina here is missing. The choroid appears hyperreflective in the areas without RPE when compared to the segment on the right side of the image with RPE.

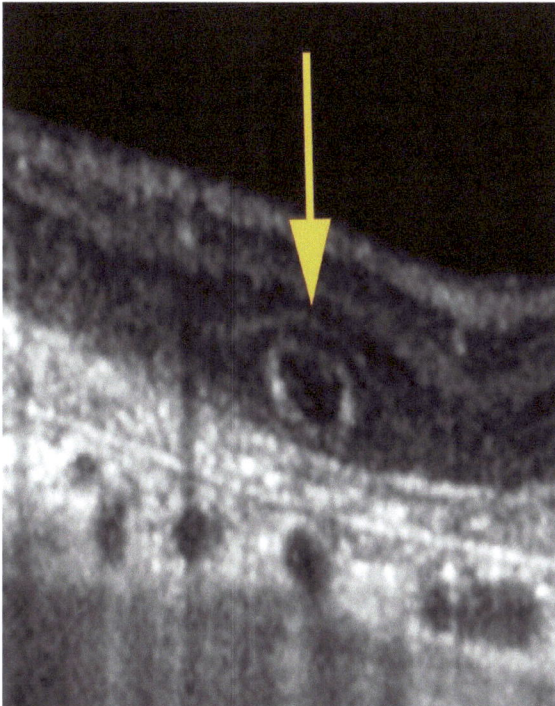

High magnification image of outer retinal tubulation on OCT

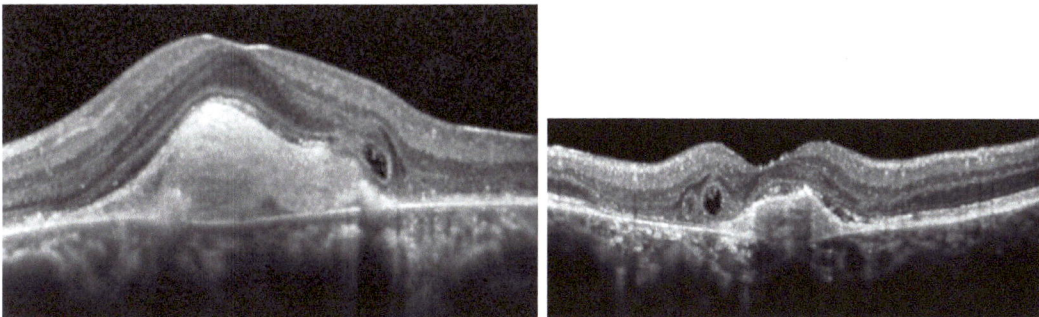

ORT on OCT in cases of fibrovascular PED

133

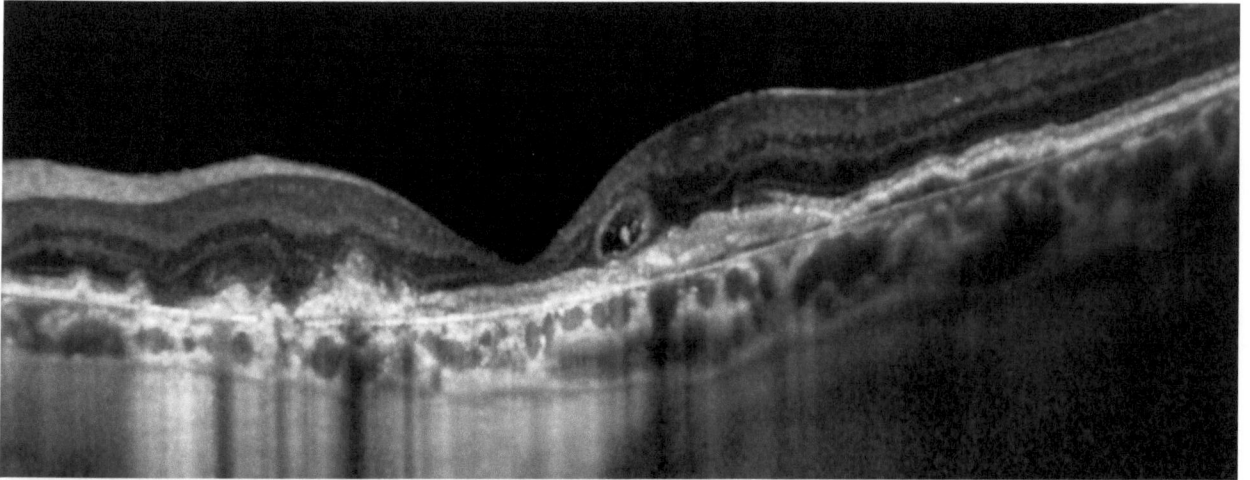

ORT on OCT in advanced AMD with subretinal fibrosis

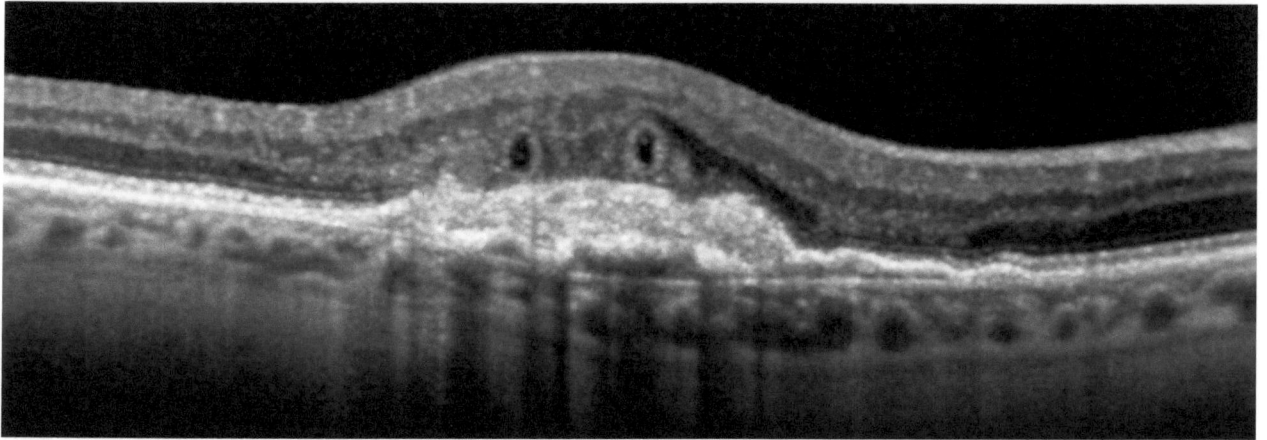

ORT on OCT with fibrovascular PED

Neovascular Age-Related Macular Degeneration (Wet AMD)

Choroidal Neovascularization

Neovascular Age Related Macular Degeneration is also known as "Wet AMD" or "Exudative AMD." The term neovascular refers to the presence of abnormal blood vessels that are collectively called "choroidal neovascularization" or CNV.

CNV originate from the choroidal circulation and grow into the sub-RPE (occult CNV) or sub-retinal (classic CNV) space. These vessels can cause subretinal or sub-RPE hemorrhage as well as macular edema. Occult CNV are also called Type 1 CNV, and classic CNV may also be called Type 2 CNV.

CNV that grow under the RPE (occult) can cause either serous, hemorrhagic or fibrotic pigment epithelial detachments (PED). PEDs appear as dome shaped or irregular elevations of the RPE on OCT. The type of PED is largely determined by the fluorescence and reflectivity properties of the lesion on fluorescein angiography (FA) and OCT. CNV in the subretinal space can cause subretinal or intraretinal fluid that is referred to as macular edema.

The best way to visualize CNV has traditionally been fluorescein angiography (FA).

Because the abnormal vessels do not have mature endothelial lining, the fluorescein dye tends to leak from them and this helps identify the region where the CNV is located on FA images.

Indocyanine angiography (ICG) has also been used to identify CNV and is better for demonstrating CNV that occurs under the RPE. This tends to leak from them and this helps identify the region where the CNV is located on FA images. is because the pigmentation of the RPE tends to absorb or block the fluorescence signal from fluorescein dye but not Indocyanine green dye. Additionally, ICG is more highly bound in the plasma of blood and therefore "leaks" less.

OCT angiography presents a unique opportunity to improve our ability in detecting and understanding CNV. Because OCT angiography detects the movement of RBCs rather than the flow and extravasation of intravenous dye, it can be very sensitive in detecting the actual abnormal vessels in CNV. While this is not always true, there are many cases where OCTA images can reveal the extent of the CNV with amazing resolution. Keep in mind that visualizing the actual CNV vessels on FA or ICG is very difficult because as the dye extravasates, it also obscures the vessels surrounding it.

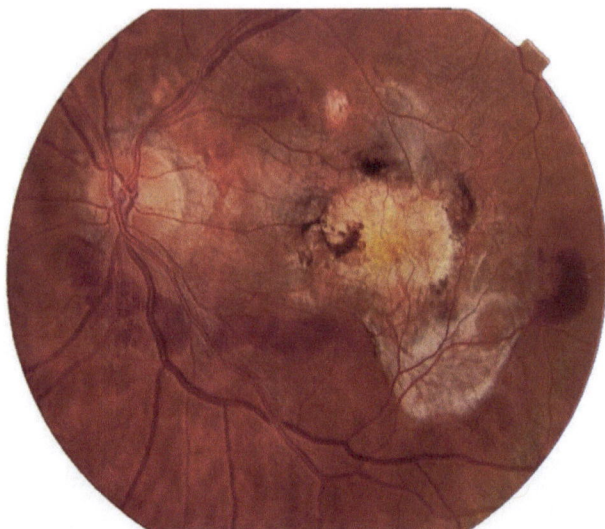

Color fundus photo of a patient with exudative (wet) macular degeneration. Note the numerous areas of subretinal and intraretinal hemorrhage. The focal areas of hyperpigmentation are consistent with RPE disturbances and hyperproliferation. The white appearing subretinal material is consistent with the fibrosis of CNV that occurs as the vessels sclerose and leave residual fibrotic tissue.

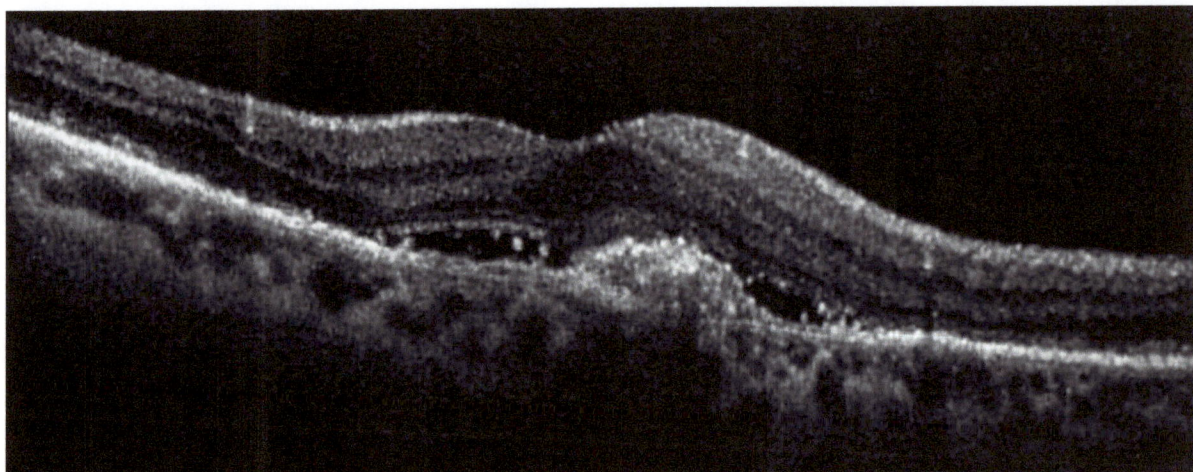

OCT shows a subretinal hyperreflective lesion consistent with a PED. It is not clear if the lesion is completely sub-RPE or both sub-RPE and sub-retinal. There is a focal area of subretinal fluid (exudative neurosensory detachment or retinal detachment) on both sides of the lesion. The underlying choroid is obscured by the lesion, and the overlying retinal contour is irregular and elevated over the PED.

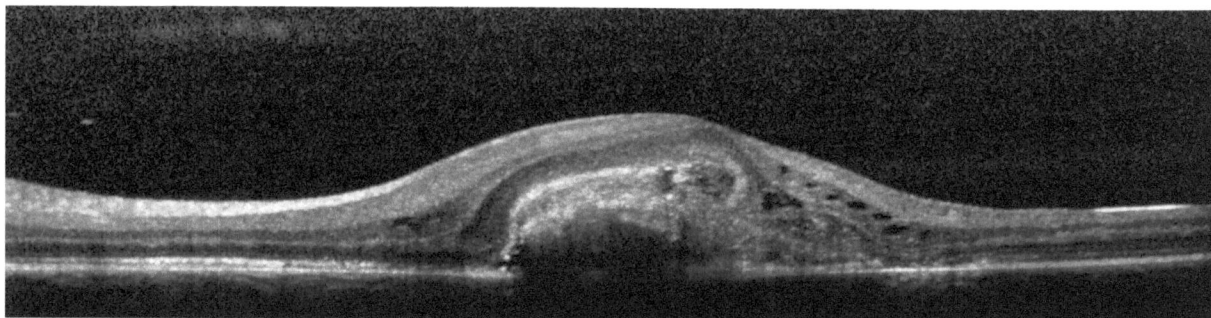

OCT with large subretinal lesion that appears to be both subretinal and sub-RPE and is consistent with either a PED or RPE rip (or both). The details of the center of the lesion are not visible because of the lesions size and attenuation of the OCT signal. The more hyperreflective aspect of the lesion may represent blood. There are several pockets of intraretinal fluid that appear as cystoid spaces to the right of lesion.

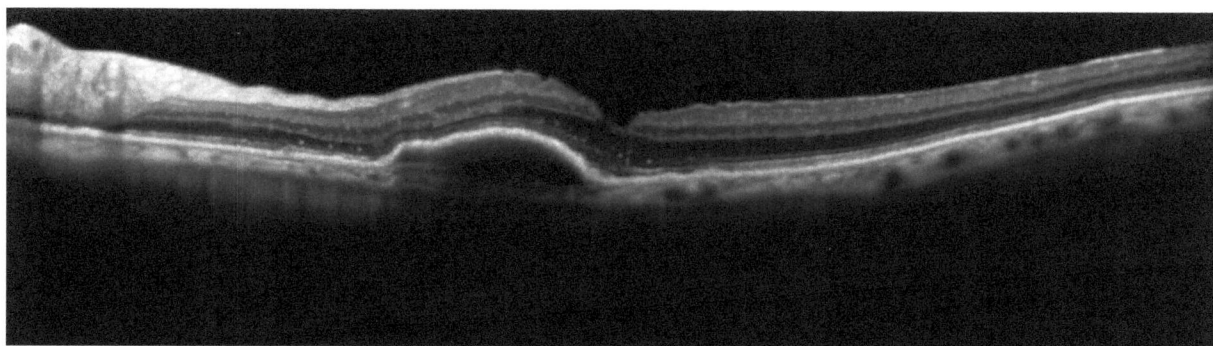

OCT consistent with a large PED. The internal reflectivity of the PED varies from hyporeflective to mild hyperreflectivity suggesting that it is a fibrovascular PED.

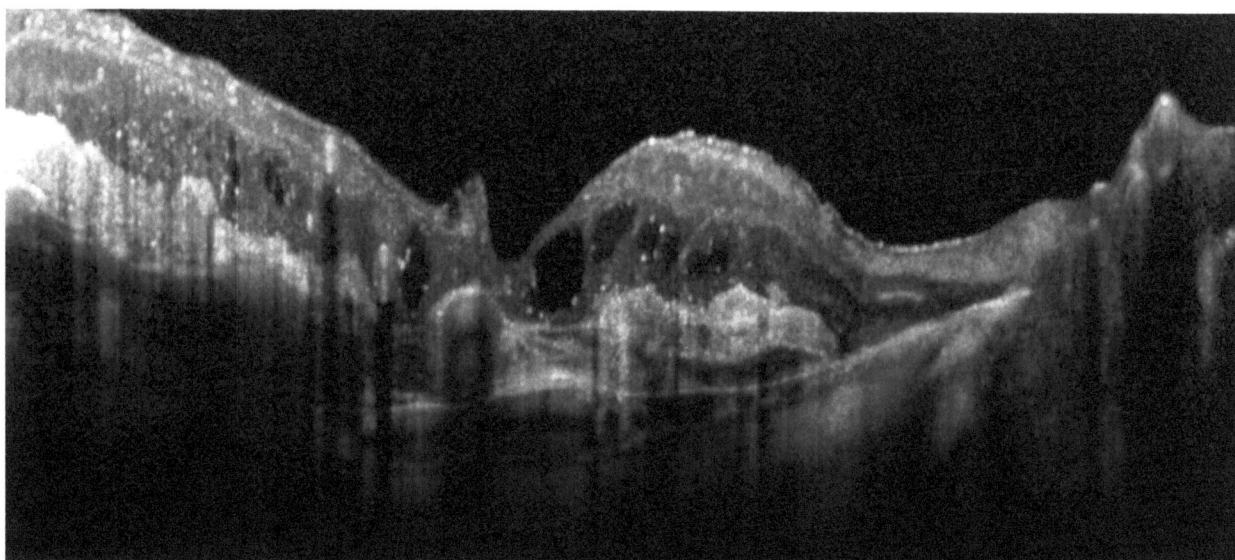

OCT demonstrates severe retinal and subretinal changes. There are numerous areas of intraretinal cystoid spaces consistent with macular edema. The hyperreflective material in the subretinal space is consistent with fibrovascular debris or active CNV. The choroidal detail is poor in the above image using the standard OCT imaging protocol. Use of EDI (next page) demonstrates significantly more choroidal and subretinal detail. The prominent shadows of major retinal vessels are visible as dark columns extending towards the bottom of the image.

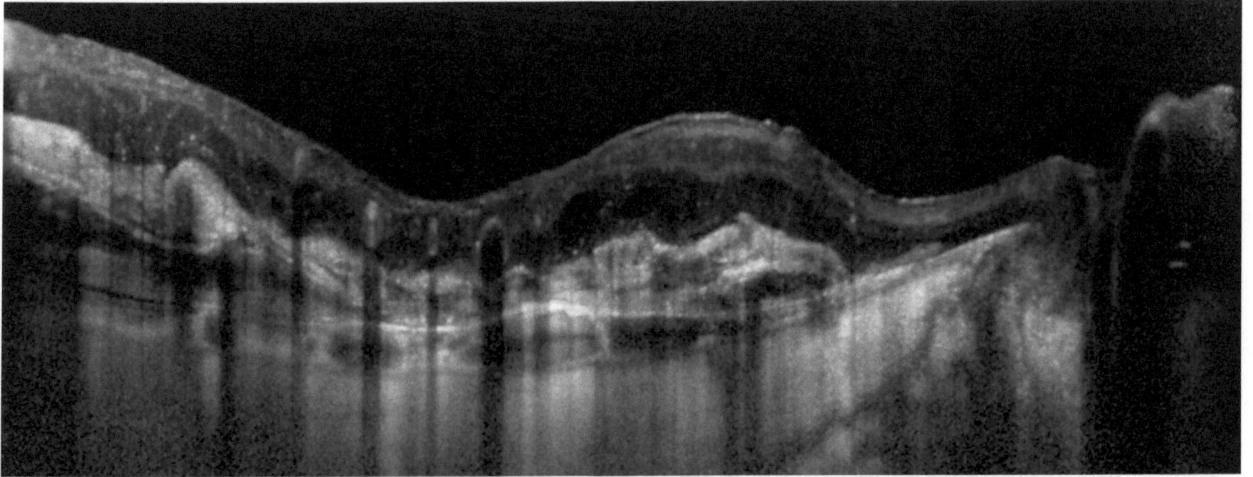

EDI OCT of previous patient

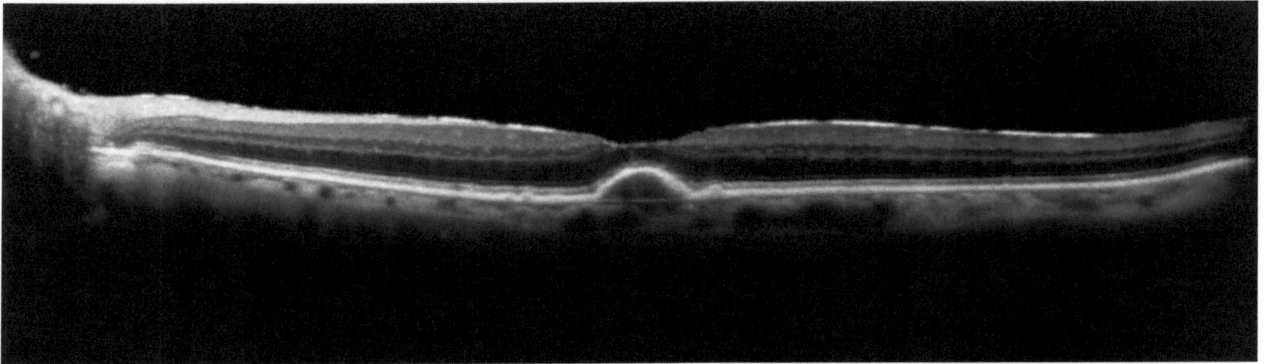

OCT with ERM and subfoveal PED. The PED demonstrates moderate internal hyperreflectivity and is most consistent with a large druse. There is no overlying intraretinal fluid.

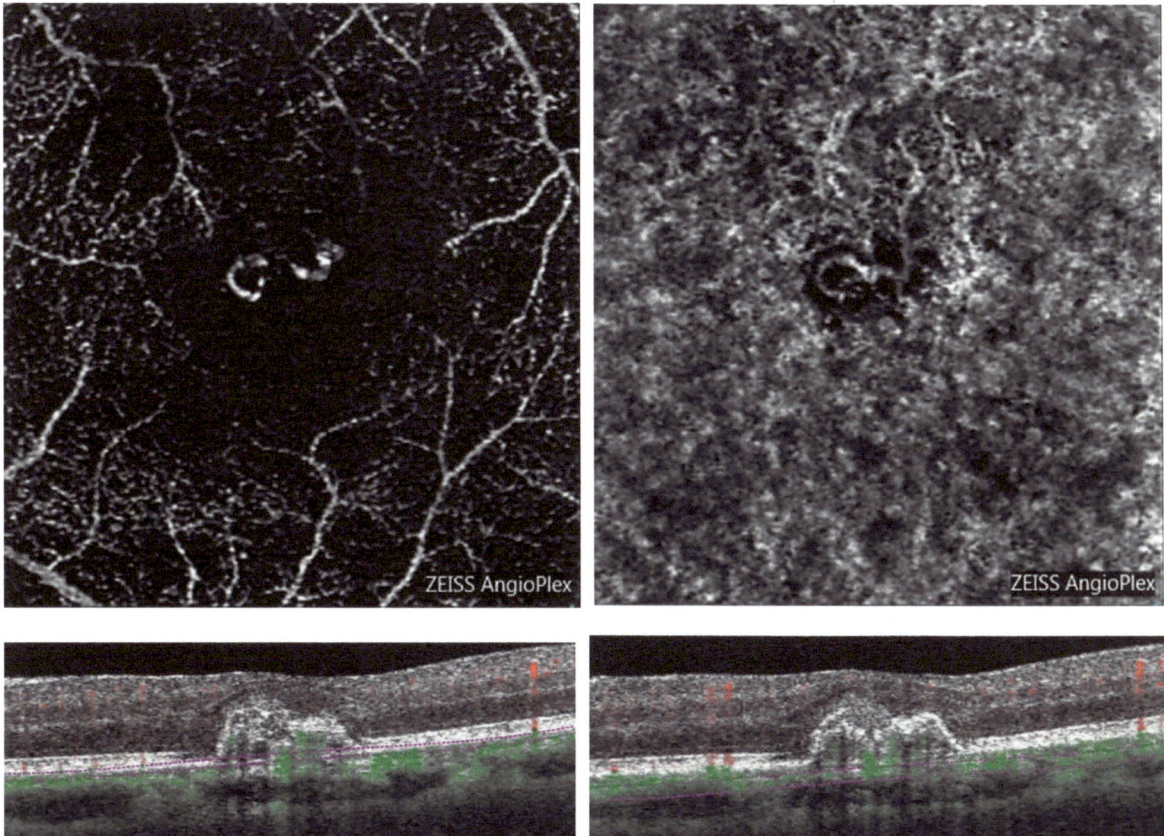

OCTA of CNV. There are vessels in the outer retina consistent with CNV (left) and there is loss of choriocapillaris in the same region (right) on the choriocapillaris slab. The corresponding B-scans show shows subretinal lesions with choroidal perfusion (green) indicating that the lesion contains CNV.

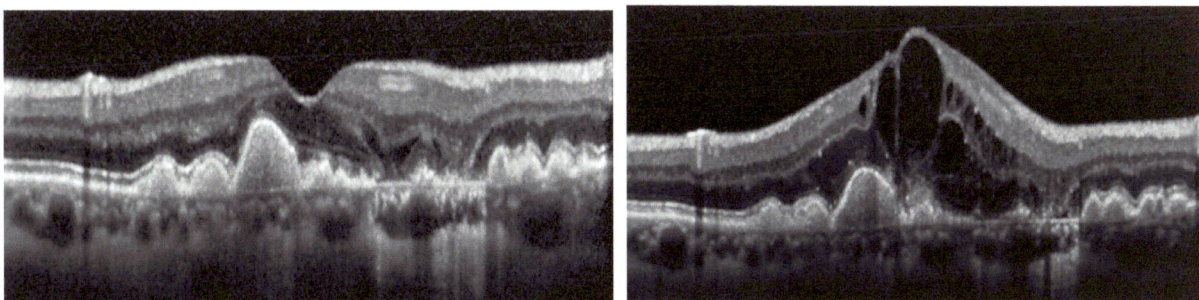

OCT on the left illustrating a macula with numerous large PED (drusen). There is a focal area of RPE loss and outer retinal distortion to the right of the fovea consistent with early geographic atrophy. Note the area of hyperreflectivity in the choroid underlying the area of RPE loss. The same retina is illustrated after conversion to neovascular AMD (right). Note the presence of several large intraretinal cystoid spaces and macular edema.

Macula Thickness : Macular Cube 512x128

OD ● | ○ OS

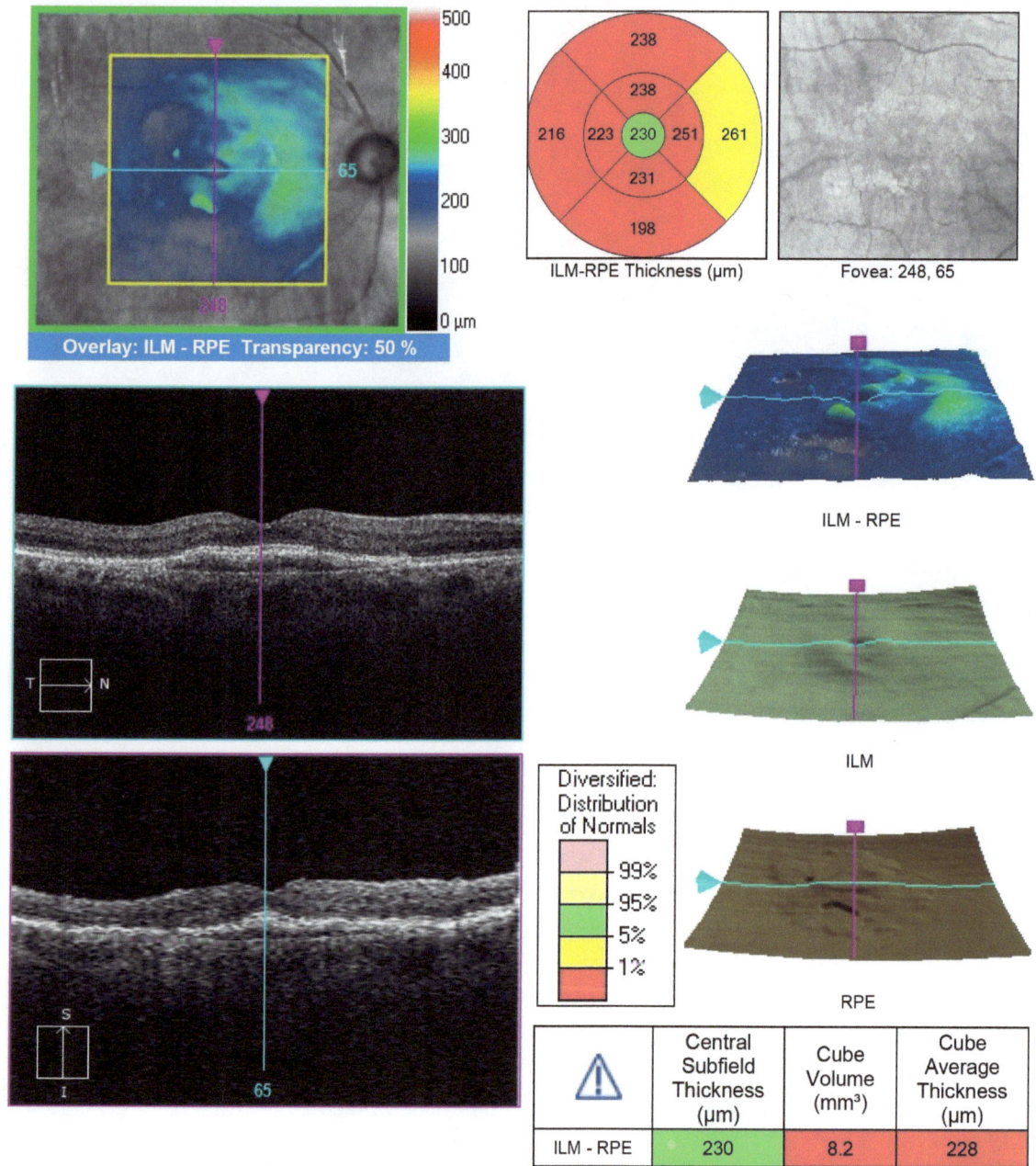

Overlay: ILM - RPE Transparency: 50 %

ILM-RPE Thickness (µm)

Fovea: 248, 65

ILM - RPE

ILM

RPE

Diversified: Distribution of Normals

- 99%
- 95%
- 5%
- 1%

	Central Subfield Thickness (µm)	Cube Volume (mm³)	Cube Average Thickness (µm)
ILM - RPE	230	8.2	228

Macular thickness scan and report of a patient with neovascular AMD. The RPE map on the bottom right of the image shows the elevation of the RPE that corresponds to the PED on the B-scan.

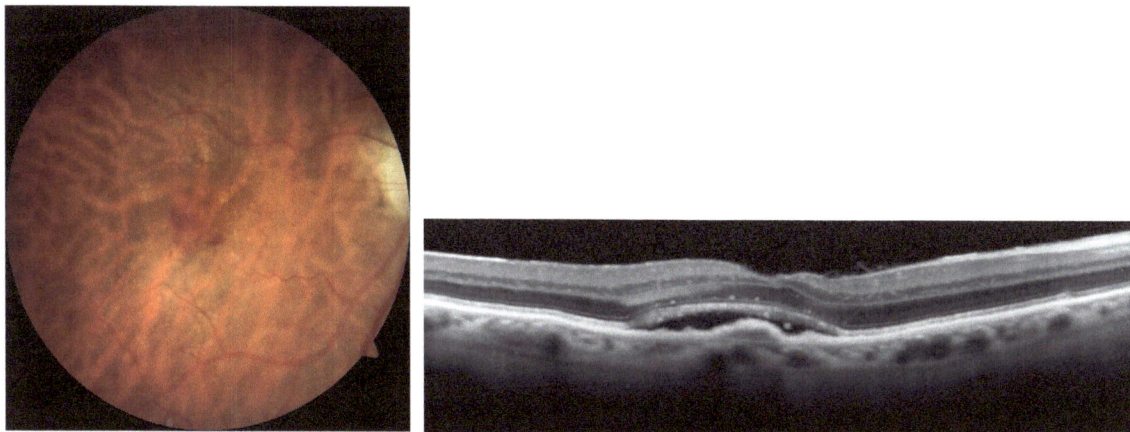

Color fundus image of neovascular AMD with intraretinal hemorrhage and few drusen. Corresponding OCT demonstrates hyporeflective subretinal region consistent with subretinal fluid. There is an irregular elevation of the RPE that is consistent with a fibrovascular PED. The PED has moderate internal hyperreflectivity. (Corresponding fluorescein and OCTA below).

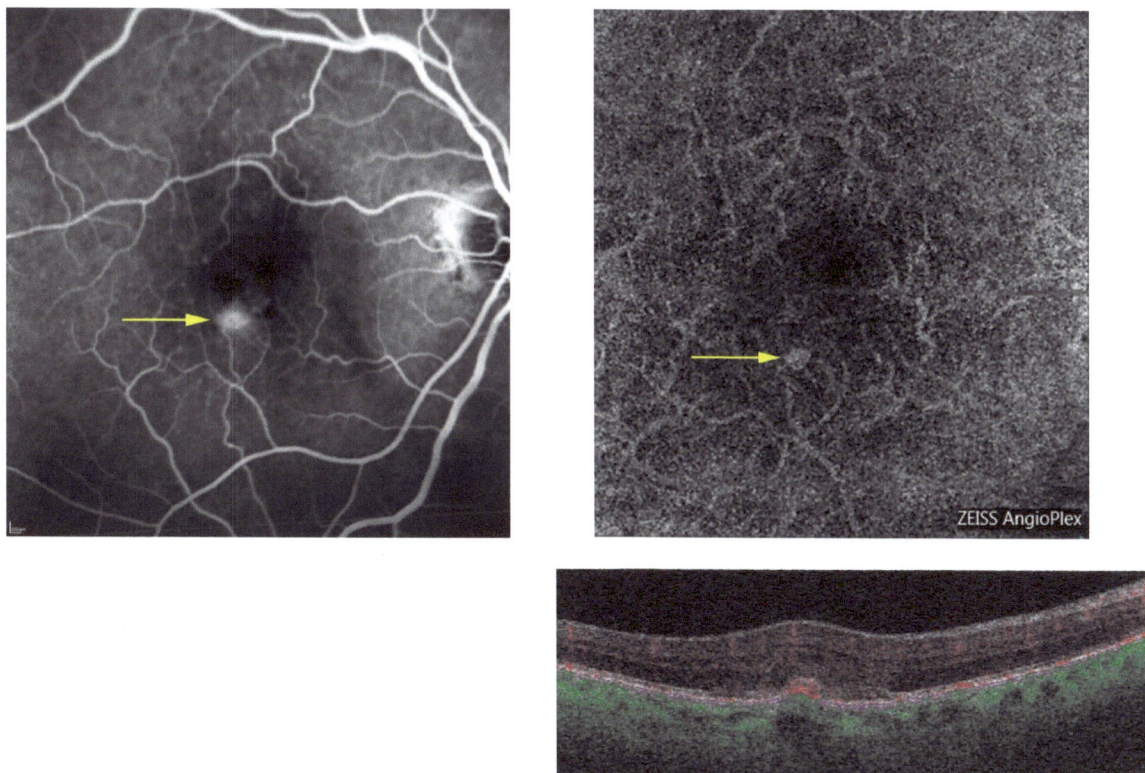

Fluorescein angiogram shows several microaneurysmal lesions and an area of blocking temporal to the fovea and inferior to the fovea corresponding to the intraretinal hemorrhages. There is also a hyperfluorescent lesion inferotemporal to the fovea that leaks on this late phase image and corresponds to the PED. OCTA of the avascular layer shows a region that corresponds with the PED and appears to have perfusion on the B-scan. This is consistent with CNV that is within the PED.

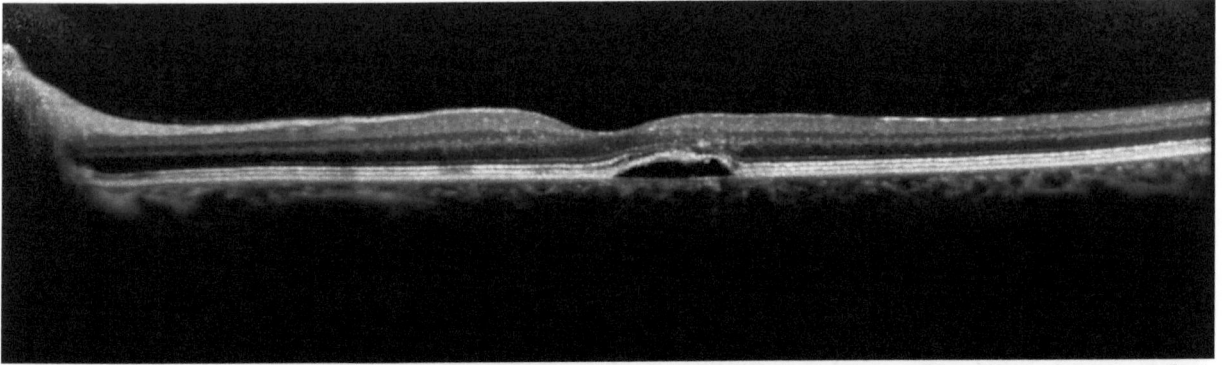

OCT demonstrates an isolated serous PED that is hyporeflective internally. There is some abnormality of the overlying outer retinal structures, and there is no intraretinal fluid.

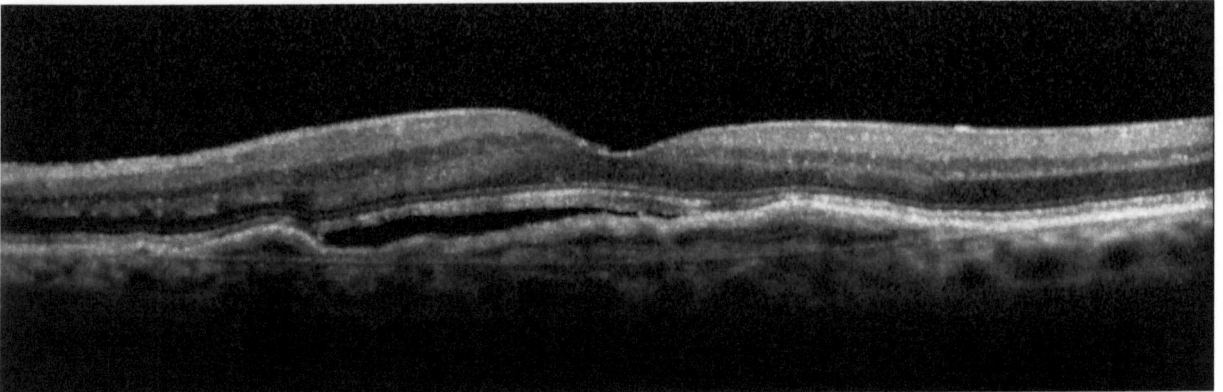

OCT scan demonstrates a PED with moderate to high internal hyperreflectivity that is consistent with fibrovascular PED. The overlying subretinal hyporeflectivity is consistent with subretinal fluid. This overall lesion would be consistent with choroidal neovascularization.

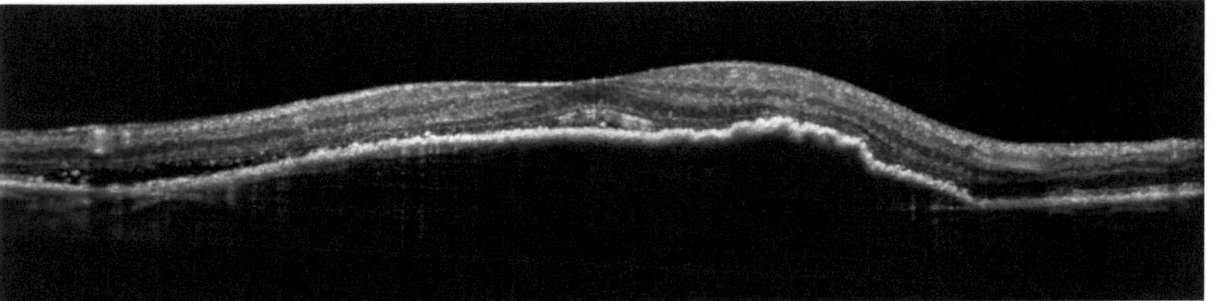

OCT demonstrates a very large PED that has low to moderate internal hyperreflectivity. The alternating light-dark appearance within the PED is consistent with a fibrovascular PED. There is a small area of subretinal hyporeflectivity consistent with subretinal fluid on the far left edge of the image.

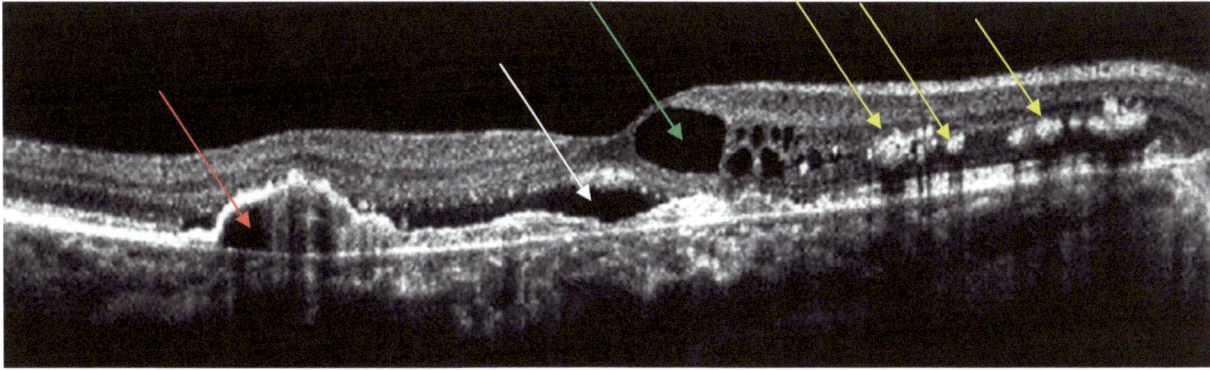

OCT of a lesion with multiple components throughout the retina and subretinal space. There is a PED (*red arrow*) with areas of hypo- and hyperintensity that is consistent with a fibrovascular PED. There is hyporeflectivity in the subretinal space consistent with subretinal fluid (*white arrow*). The intraretinal cystoid spaces are hyporeflective in appearance (*green arrow*) and demonstrate macular edema. The intraretinal hyperreflective lesions are most consistent with hard-exudates (*yellow arrows*).

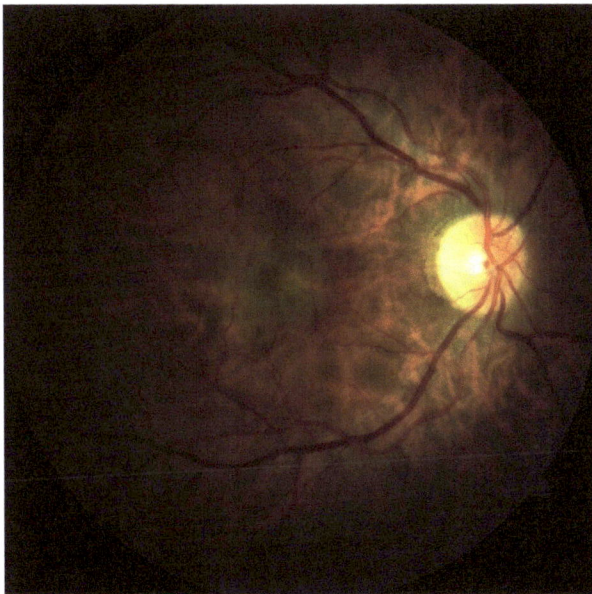

Color fundus image of CNV

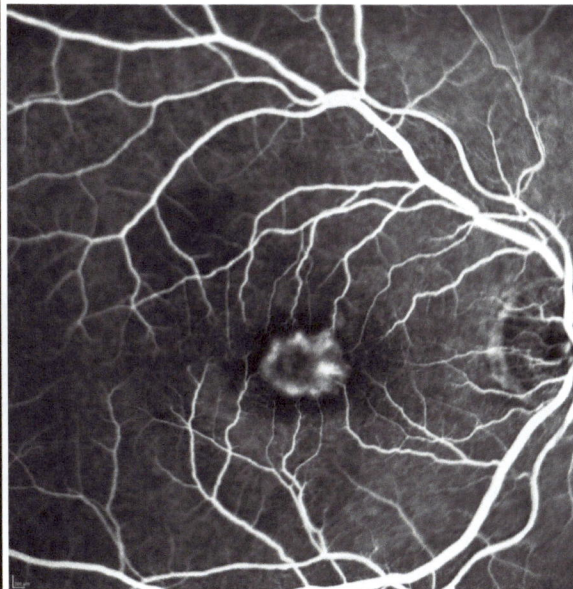

Mid phase FA of CNV

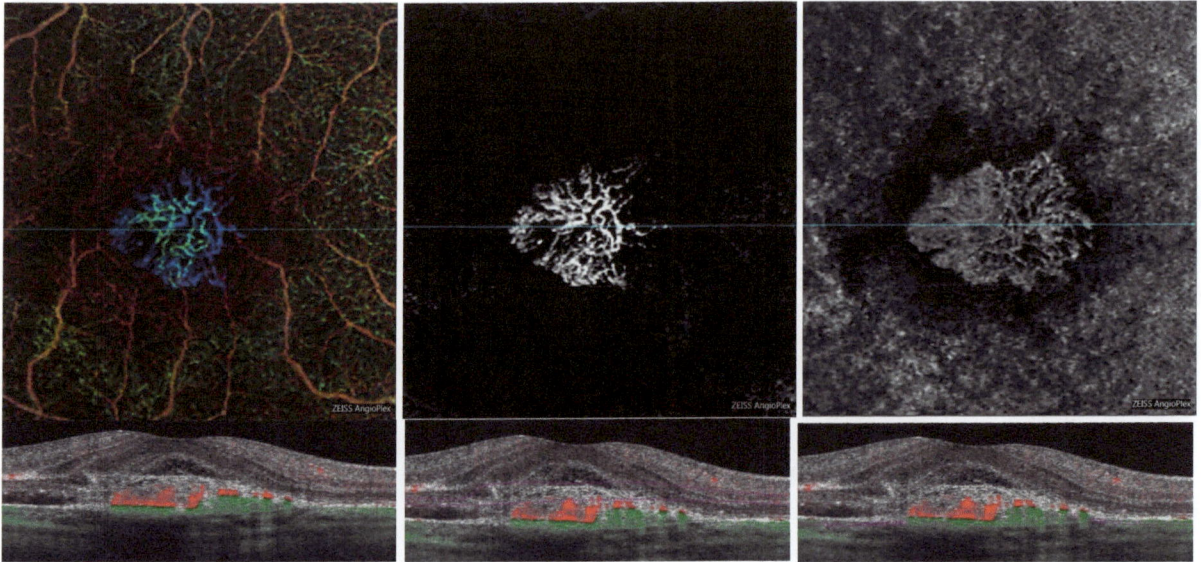

| Depth encoded OCTA | Avascular layer OCTA | Choriocapillaris layer OCTA |

Color image shows discoloration of the macula consistent with a subretinal lesion. There is a small intraretinal hemorrhage temporal to the fovea. The mid-late phase fluorescein angiogram shows a hyperfluorescent lesion that corresponds to the macular lesion. Depth encoded OCTA shows impairment in the deep retinal perfusion in the temporal macula as well as the presence of perfusion in the avascular layer (blue). The avascular layer slab (middle image) demonstrates a neovascular complex that extends in to the choriocapillaris slab (right image) as well. The corresponding B-scans show the depth location of the perfusion signal.

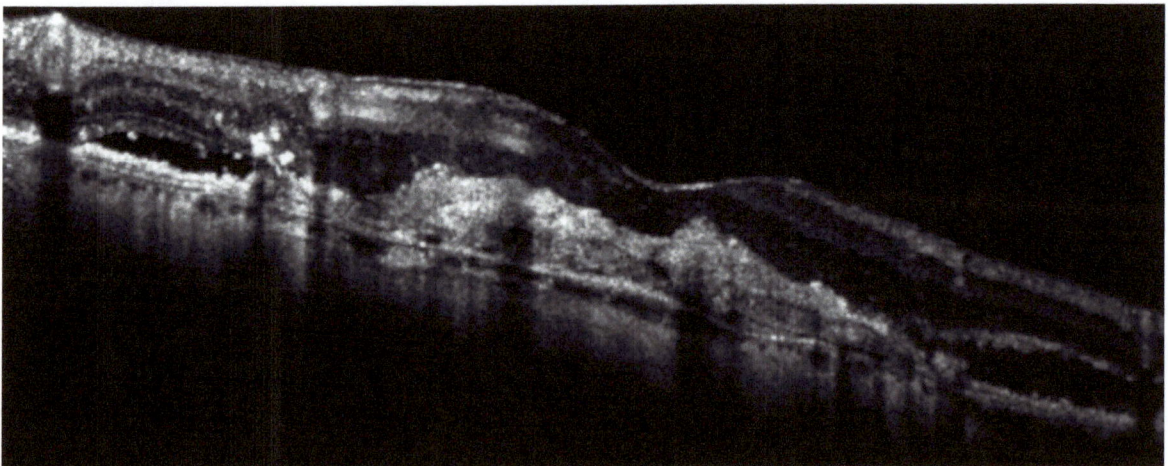

There is a large lesion in the subretinal space with high hyperreflectivity in the center of the image. This lesion has consistently high hyperreflectivity throughout, suggesting that it is largely fibrosis. There are areas of subretinal hyporeflectivity on either side of the lesion that are consistent with subretinal fluid, and small intraretinal cystoid spaces throughout the retina consistent with macular edema. The choroid also appears very thin.

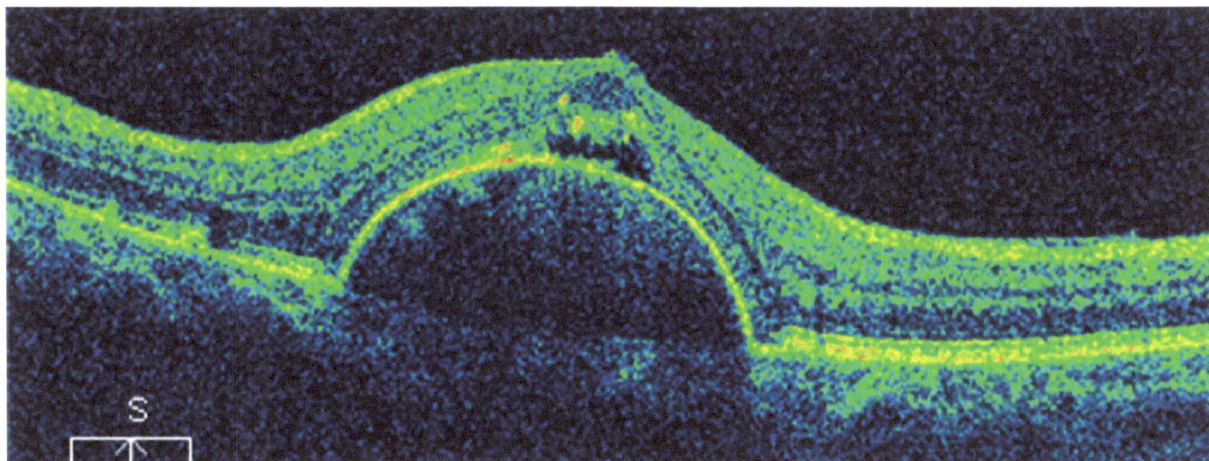

Pseudo-colored OCT line B-scan shows a large PED with moderate amount of internal hyper-reflectivity. There is an area of subretinal hyporeflectivity directly above the PED that is consistent with subretinal fluid.

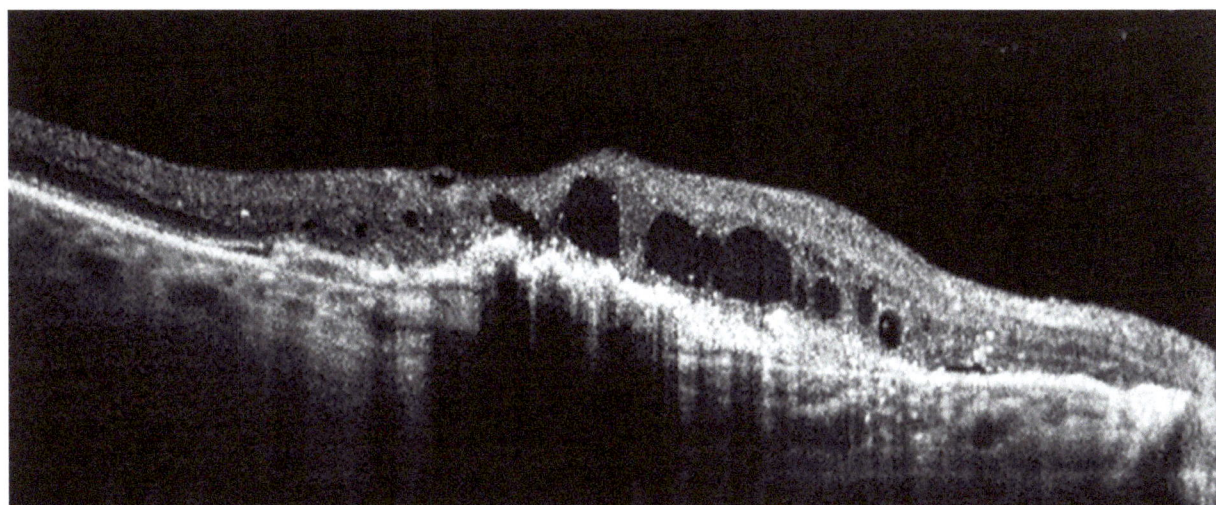

An OCT line B-scan shows severe abnormalities in both retinal and subretinal anatomy. There are large cystoid spaces within the retina consistent with macular edema. A large sub-retinal lesion appears to be largely underneath the RPE and is consistent with a PED, there is significant shadowing of the underlying choroid in the center of the image due to the sub-retinal lesion.

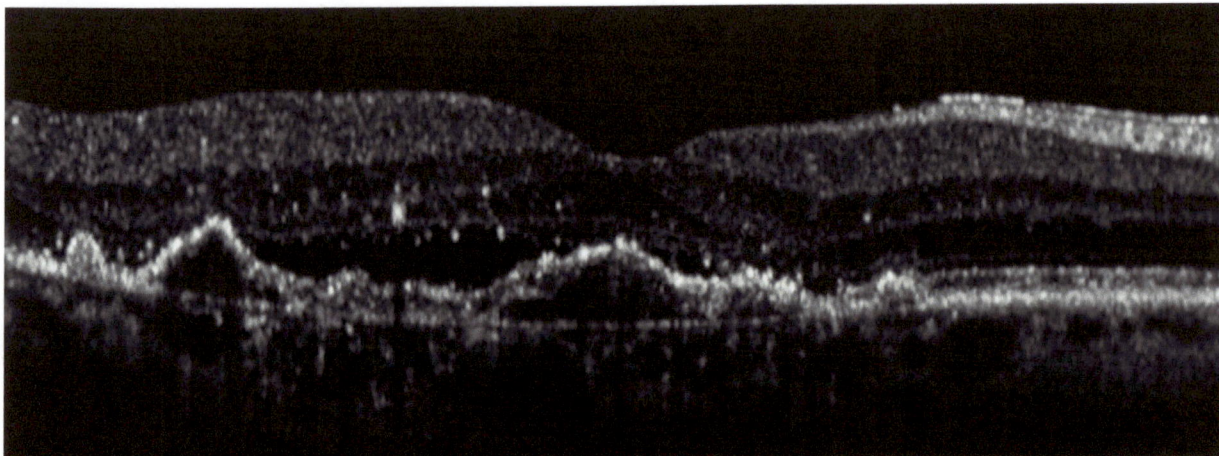

An OCT line B-scan shows numerous hyperreflective spots within the mid and outer retina. These foci are thought to be migrating RPE or other cells, although the exact etiology is unknown. There is an irregular elevation of the RPE from the middle to the left side of the image with variable reflectivity. There is subretinal fluid overlying some areas of the PED suggesting an underlying CNV complex.

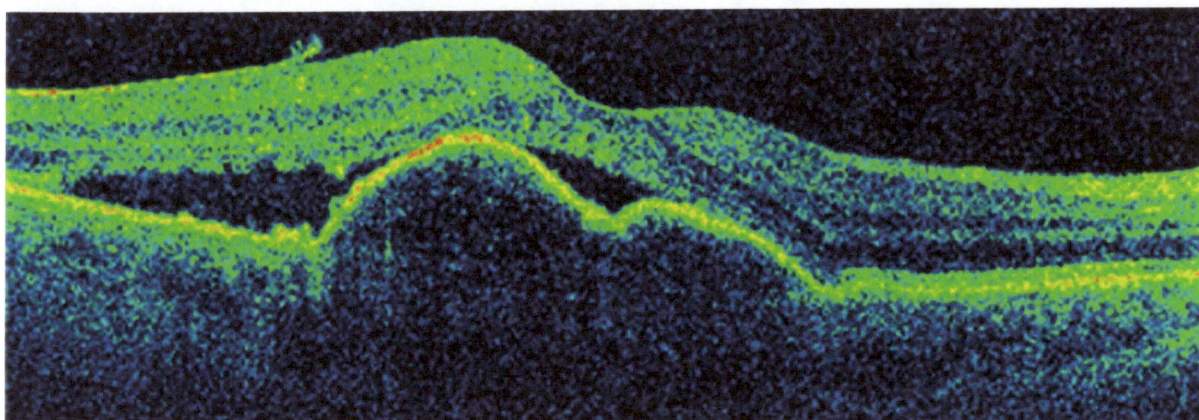

A large multi-lobulated PED appears under the fovea with two areas of subretinal fluid overlying it. The PED appears to have a homogenous hyporeflective internal consistency.

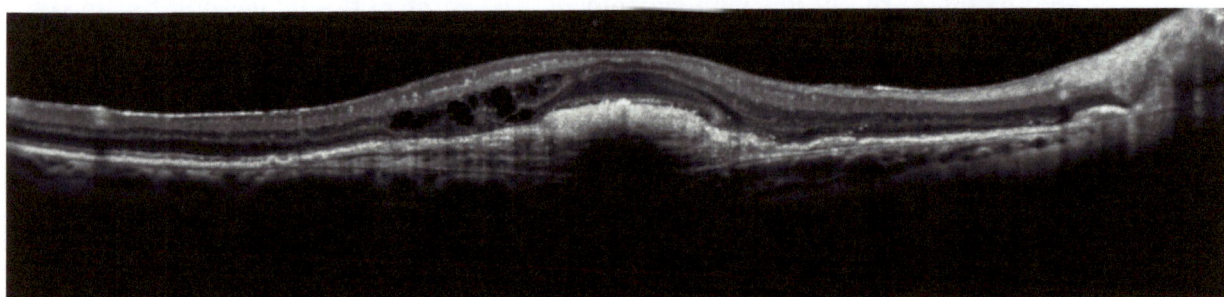

A large subretinal lesion is found in the center of the image. There is high internal reflectivity throughout the lesion and it appears to be sub-RPE. The high internal reflectivity of this PED suggests that it is largely fibrosis. However, there is intraretinal fluid overlying some parts of the PED consistent with active CNV within the complex.

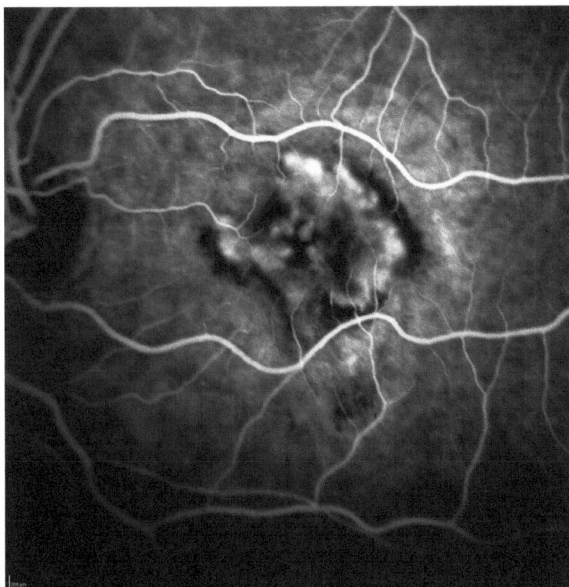

Fluorescein angiogram (above), and OCT (below) of a patient with a classic CNV. The fluorescein angiogram shows a large hyperfluorescent lesion with fairly well defined borders in the mid-phase of the angiogram. There is an outline of hypofluorescent areas surrounding the lesion which suggests the presence of subretinal hemorrhage or fluid. The OCT of the lesion shows a hyperreflective subretinal lesion that is above the RPE and consistent with Type 2 CNV.

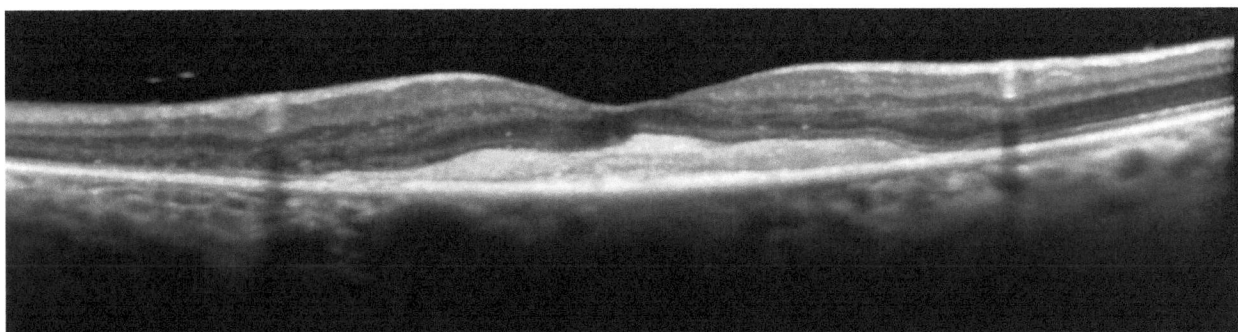

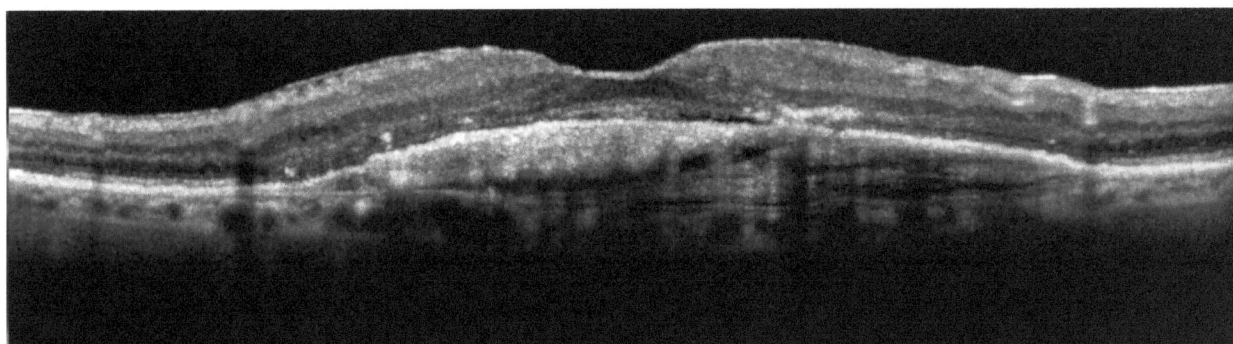

A large PED is observed underneath the retina and is consistent with a fibrovascular lesion. There is a sliver of hyporeflectivity underneath the fovea consistent with subretinal fluid and active CNV complex in the PED.

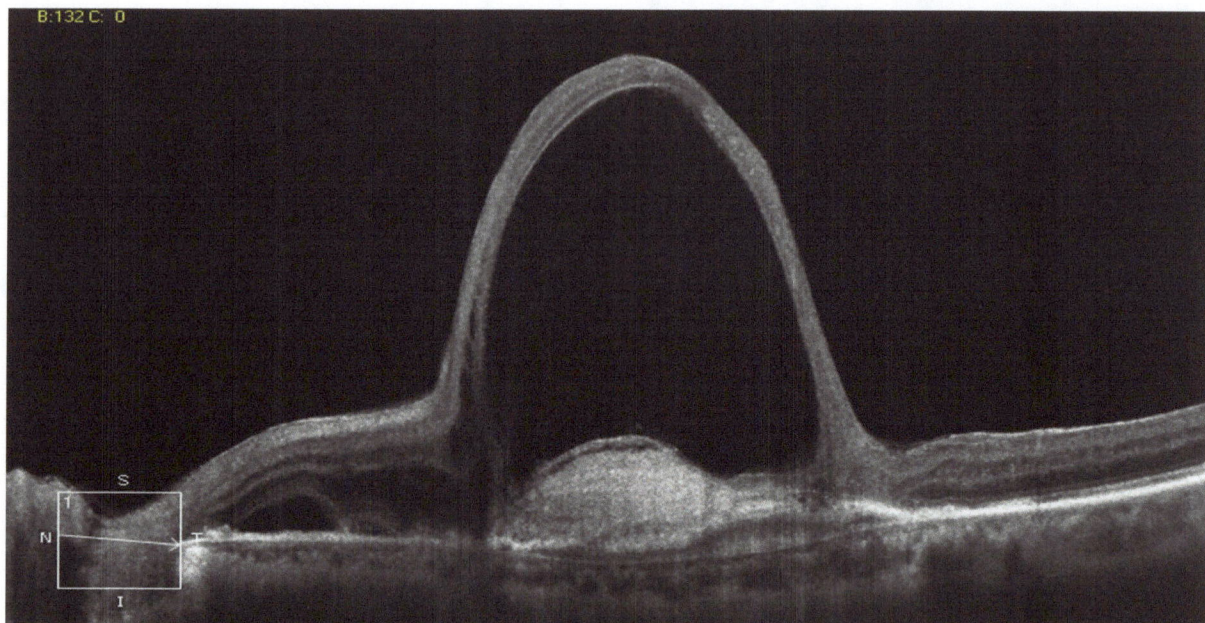

On this OCT B-scan, a very large intraretinal cyst is observed over a hyperreflective lesion with both subretinal and sub-RPE components. The hyperreflectivity of the subretinal lesion is suggestive of a fibrotic scar. The RPE band is broken on the right side of the lesion and the internal contents of the PED demonstrate moderate to high hyperreflectivity. There is subretinal fluid on the far left side of the image. This lesion is consistent with active CNV and the large intraretinal cystoid space and high hyperreflectivity of the subretinal lesion suggest a chronic process.

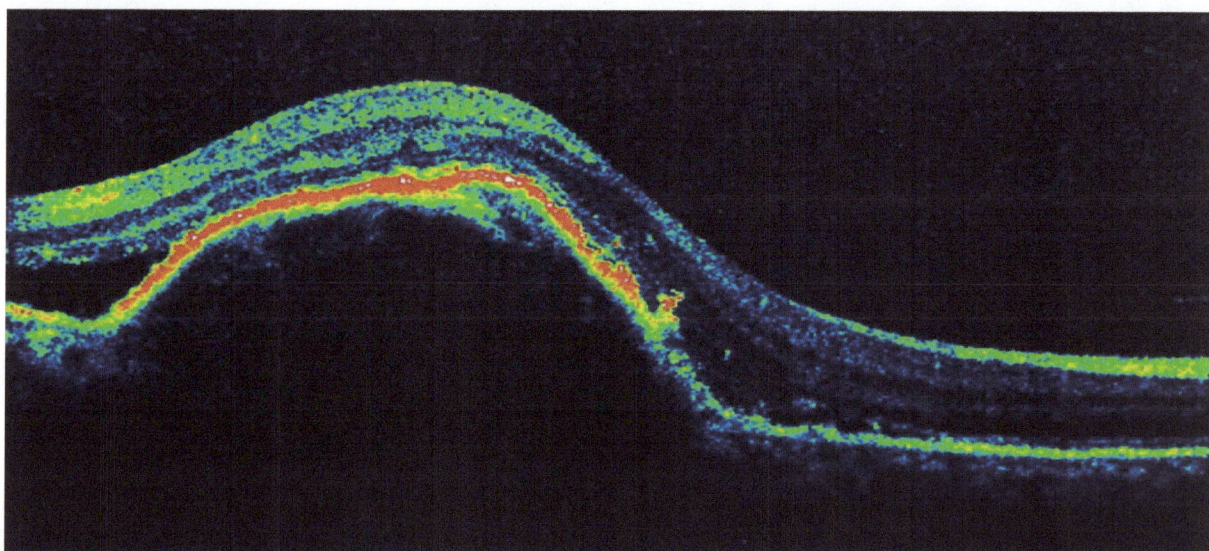

OCT B-scan with a very large PED with sub retinal fluid

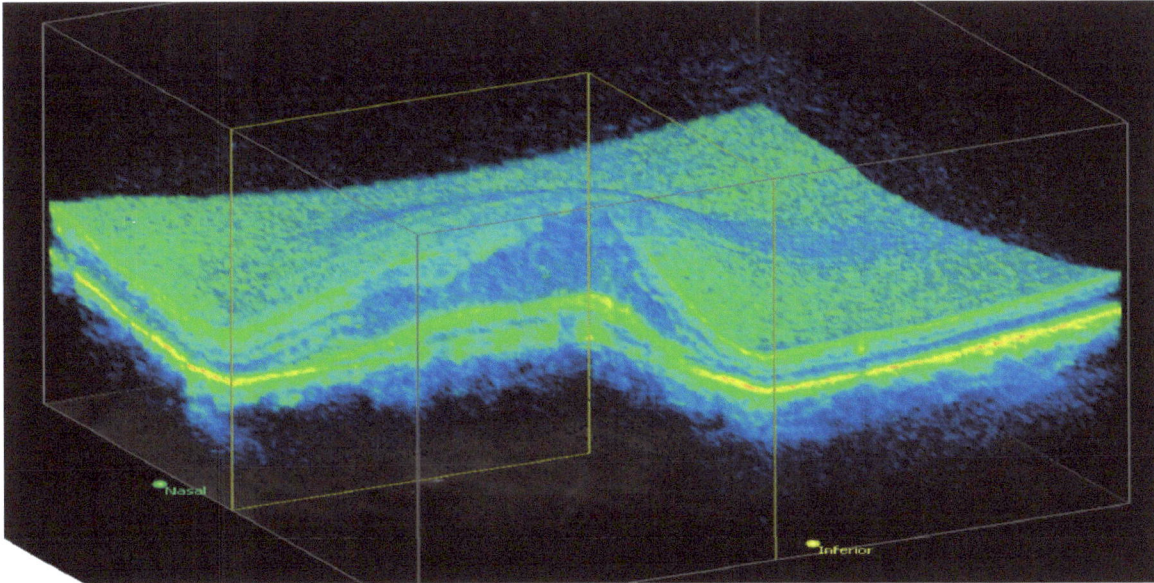

Three-dimensional view of a large pocket of sub retinal fluid

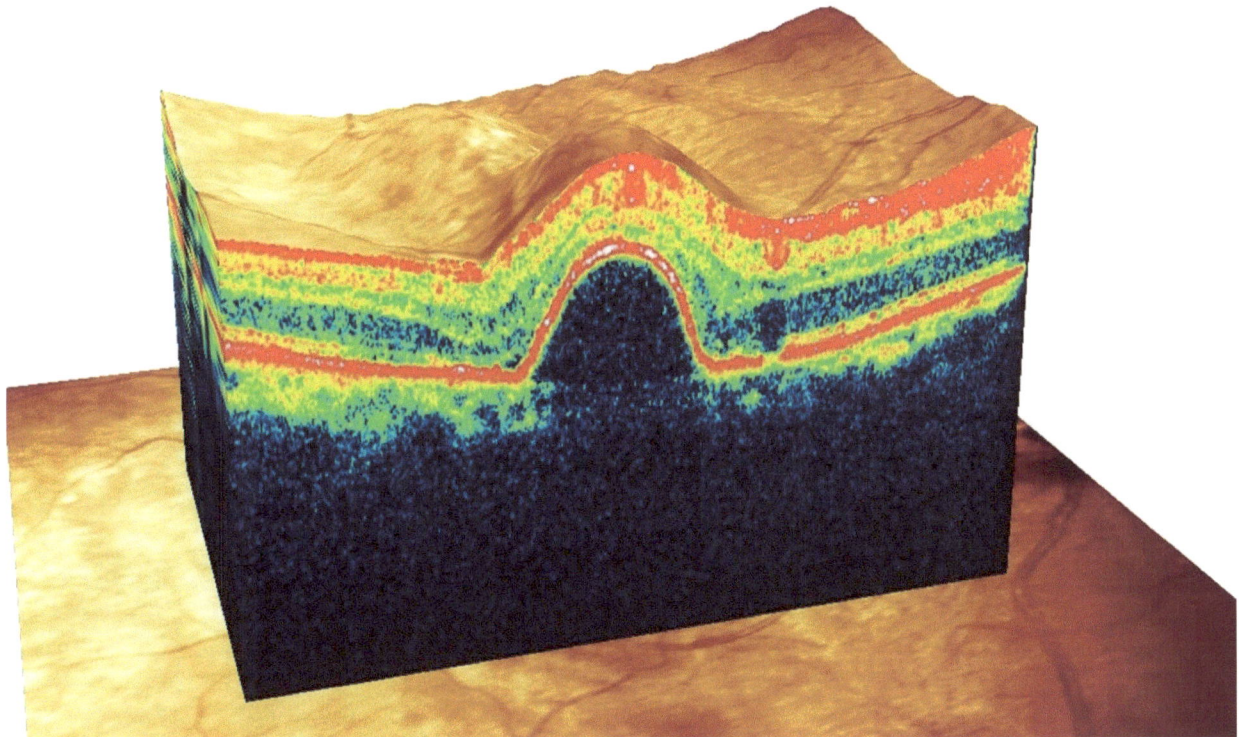

Three dimensional view of a PED

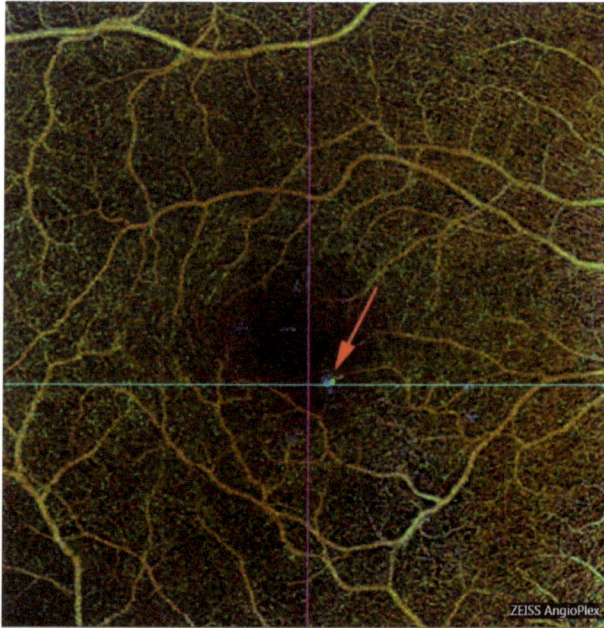

A depth encoded OCTA shows normal retinal vasculature and an area of vascularization in the avascular retinal layers (blue) that is consistent with CNV. The corresponding line scan is shown in the figure below.

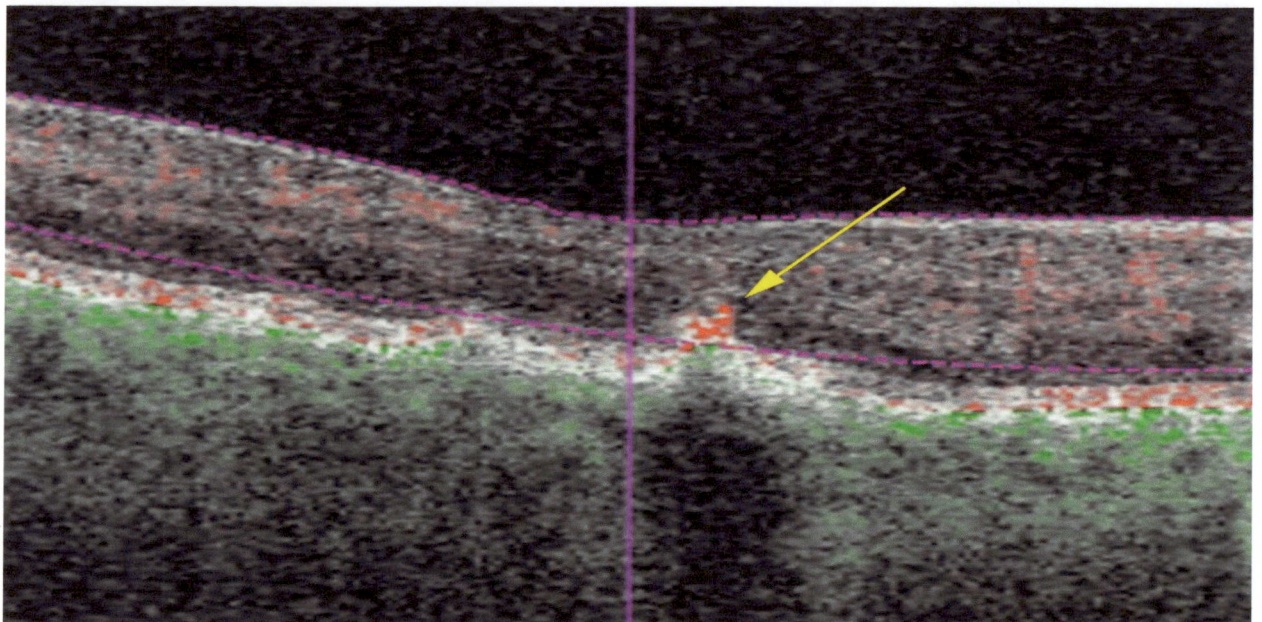

The corresponding area of neovascularization on the blue line scan in the OCTA above. The software assigns retinal vascular flow as red and choroidal vascular flow as green, according to the layer that the flow was detected. In this case, neovascularization at the apex of the elevated RPE is pushed into the normally avascular retinal region, and is highlighted by the yellow arrow. Note that the PED shadows the underlying choroidal vasculature.

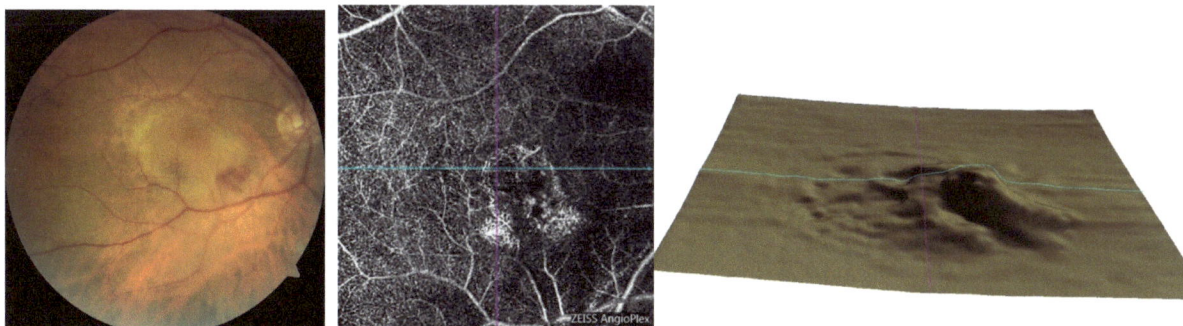

Color fundus image with a large subretinal lesion and intraretinal hemorrhage. The corresponding OCTA showing a large neovascular complex inferior and nasal to the fovea. The RPE slab of the OCT shows a clear elevation of the RPE corresponding to the same region as the neovascular complex.

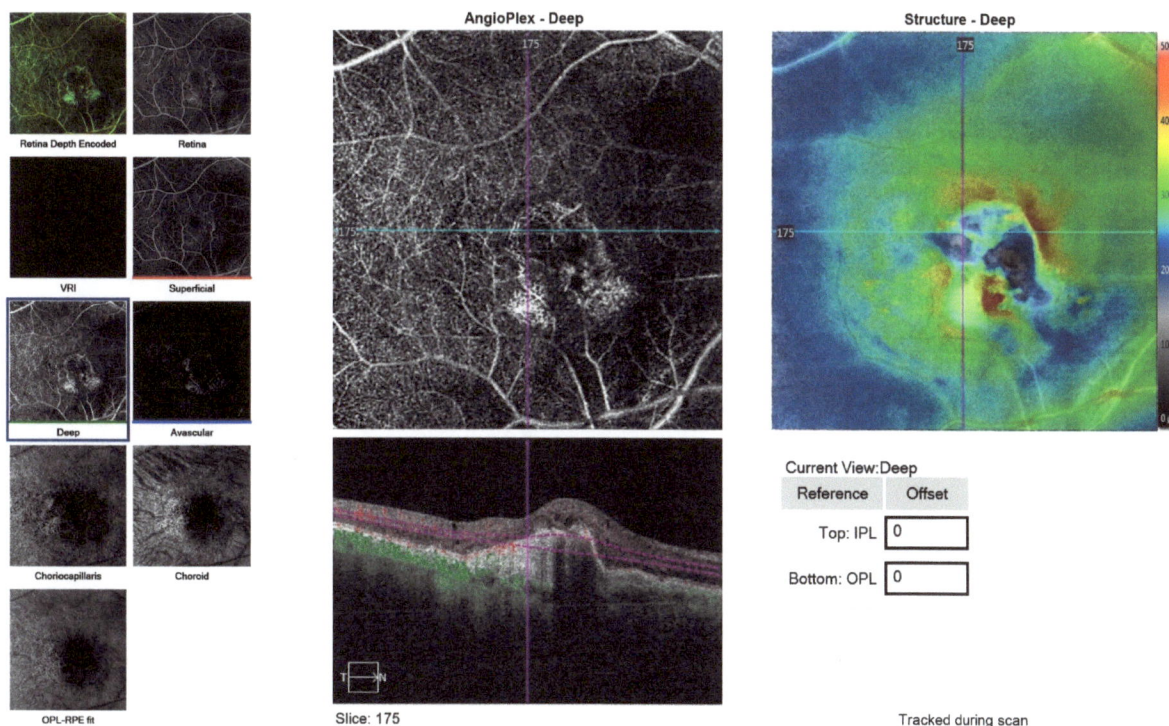

The OCTA report of the same lesion as shown in the last panel. The small panels on the left show the retinal vascularization within each of the preselected layers on the commercial software. These layers are: superficial retina, deep retina, and avascular retina. There are also OCTA slabs for the choriocapillaris, choroid, vitreoretinal interface (VRI), and a depth encoded, pseudo-colored image. The large image in the center shows the deep retinal layer slab as well as the corresponding OCT line B-scan with the segmentation lines that highlight the retinal layer which defines the OCTA slab above it (deep retinal layer).

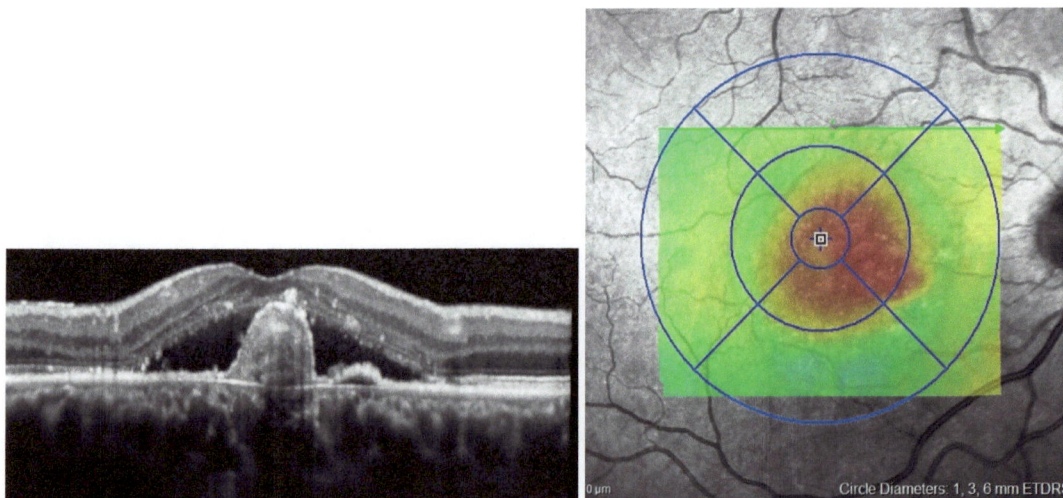

OCT line B-scan shows a large PED with high internal hyperreflectivity directly underneath the fovea and a smaller PED with hyporeflectivity immediately to the right. There is a large amount of overlying subretinal fluid. The volumetric OCT illustrates that the retina is elevated in the region of the PED and sub-retinal fluid.

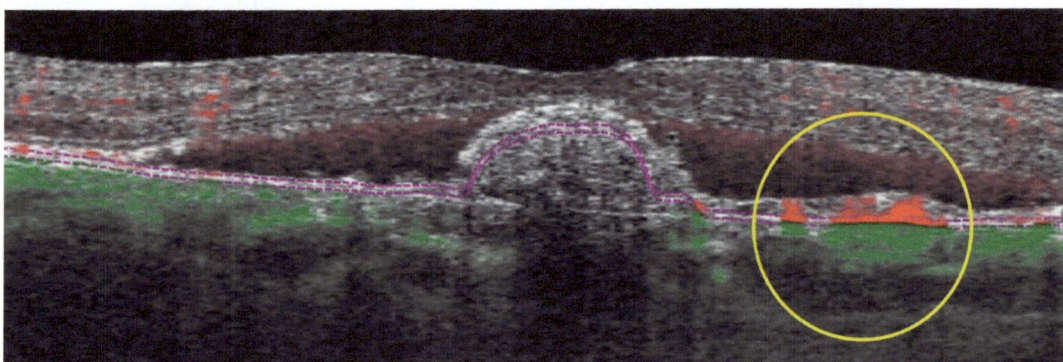

The OCTA B-scan of the same region shows that there is flow signal in the smaller hyporeflective PED consistent with CNV. The larger hyperreflective PED has no flow signal and is consistent with fibrosis.

Retinal Angiomatous Proliferation (RAP)

RAP is also referred to as "Type 3 Neovascularization." The term RAP describes a distinct form of neovascularization that meets one or more of the following criteria: arises out of the deep retinal capillary plexus, invades the retina from an underlying type 1 CNV or invades the retina from breaks in Bruch's membrane. The pathophysiology of this disease is controversial and origin of the anomalous vessels has been debated. The reader is referred to Ryan's Retina or other textbooks of retinal disease for a detailed discussion.

On color fundus imaging, the findings may be subtle. Often there may be focal hemorrhage and edema associated with the site of the vascular lesion. Fluorescein angiography shows findings consistent with either a fibrovascular PED or occult CNV. There is a third category of FA findings termed Late Leakage of Undetermined Significance (LLUS), which is also associated with RAP lesions sometimes. Although FA findings are abnormal in RAP lesions, the details of the vascular lesion are not commonly visualized using FA.

High-speed digital video Indocyanine Green Angiography (ICG), is the main method by which the vascular RAP lesion can be visualized. In prototypical cases the intraretinal anastomosis can be directly visualized on ICG in the very early frames. OCT typically shows the RAP lesion within the center or apex of the PED in cases where a PED is present. This is in contrast to the typical notched appearance of serous PEDs in which the CNV is located at the margins of the PED. In many cases, OCT findings may not be diagnostic.

OCTA provides a potentially powerful method of visualizing RAP lesions because of the depth resolved images that can be produced. In theory, RAP lesions should be visible on OCTA images as the lesion progressed through the retinal layers and some of the examples below highlight this. In evaluating RAP lesions on OCTA care must be taken to identify projection artifacts that may mimic deep retinal vessels.

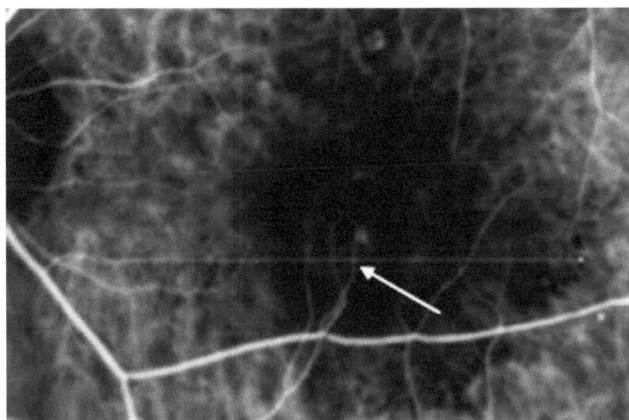

ICG angiogram of RAP lesion with intraretinal anastomosis (arrow)

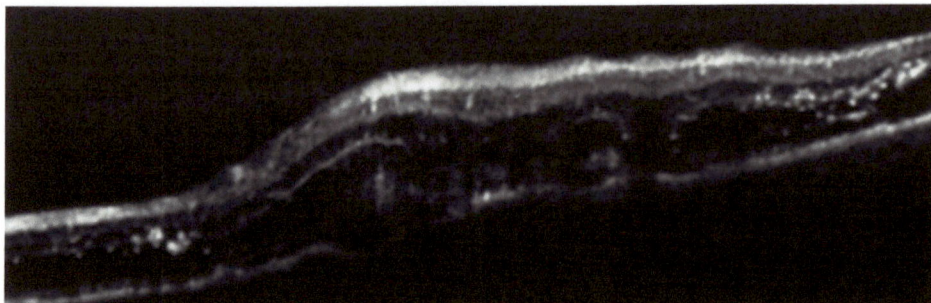

Corresponding B-scan. Although the exact location of the intraretinal vessels are not clear on OCT, the abnormalities in the deep retinal layers suggests the location of the RAP lesion in this case is in the middle third of the OCT scan.

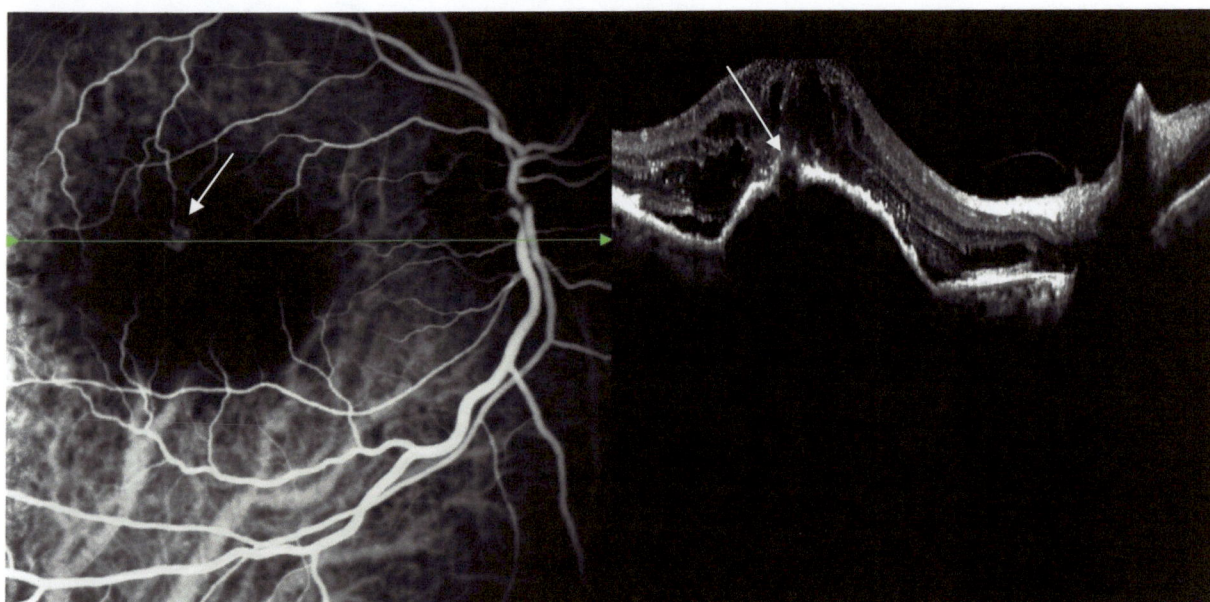

ICG Angiography directed OCT reveals a break in RPE at the apex of the PED corresponding with the retinal vessel illustrated on angiography. Note the location of the RPE break is at or near the apex of the PED.

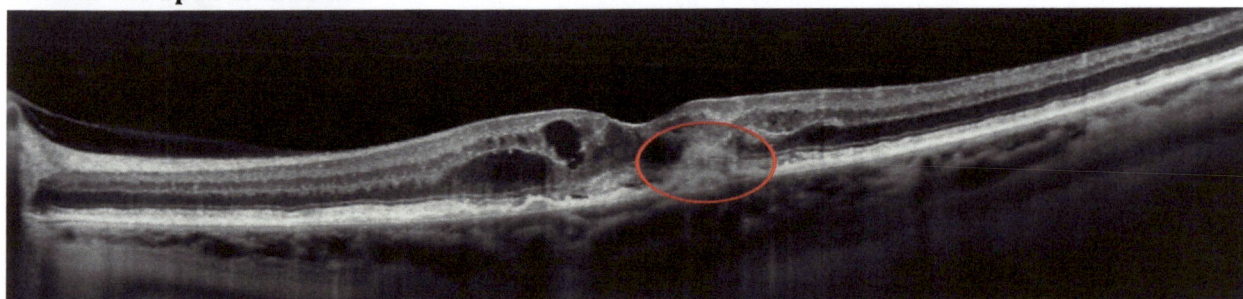

EDI OCT of a RAP lesion. The likely location of the RAP vessel circled in red although ICG angiography would be needed to confirm this.

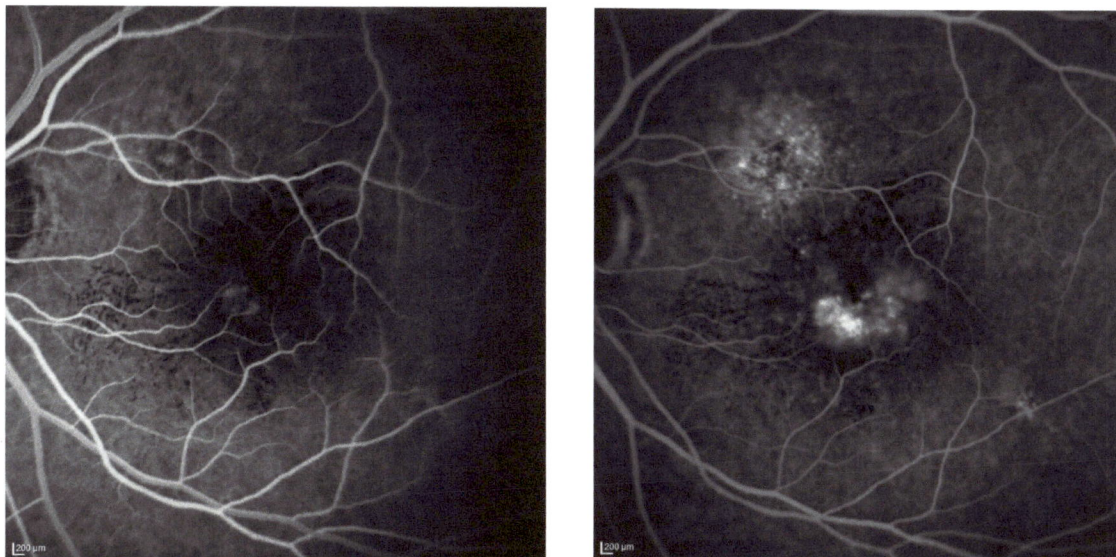

Early phase fluorescein angiogram shows a region of abnormal early staining that suggests an intraretinal anastomosis. There are numerous drusen that are hypofluorescent in this early phase image. Late phase fluorescein angiogram shows a larger region that appears consistent with Late Leakage of Undetermined Significance (LLUS).

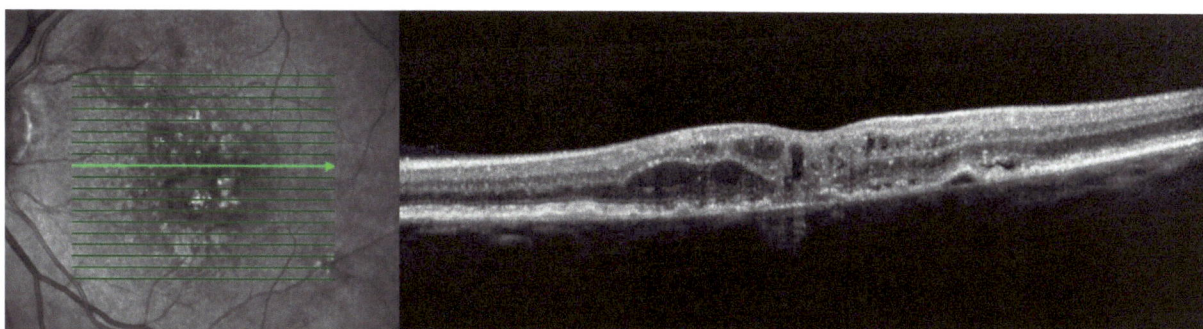

The OCT B-scan shows surrounding intraretinal cystoid spaces consistent with macular edema and small RPE elevations consistent with both serous PEDs (right side of image) and drusen (left side of image). The exact location of the RAP lesion is difficult to identify on OCT.

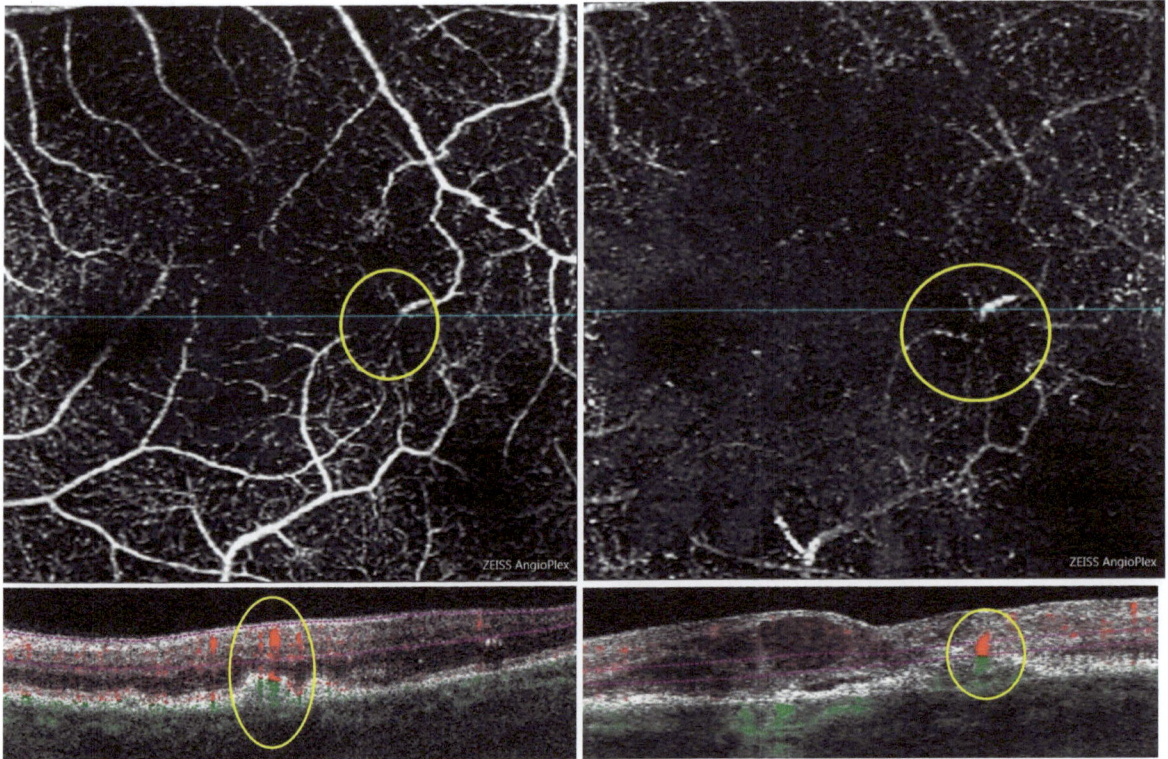

A **B**

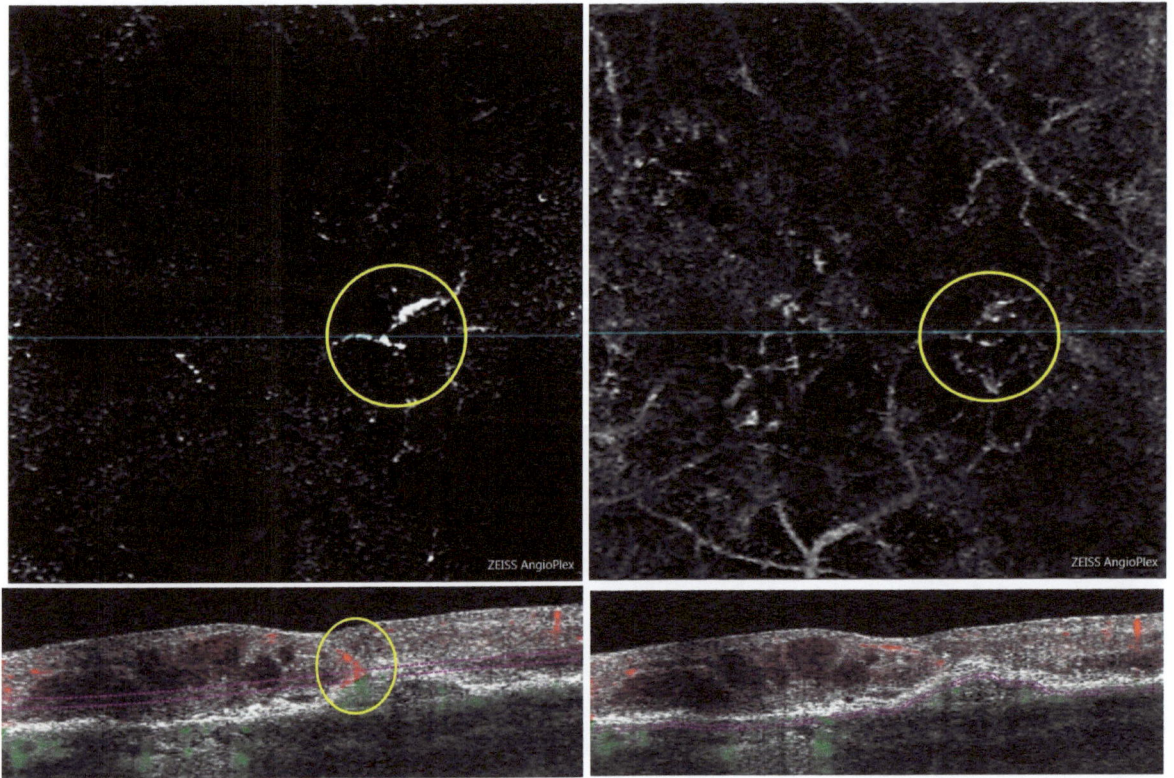

C **D**

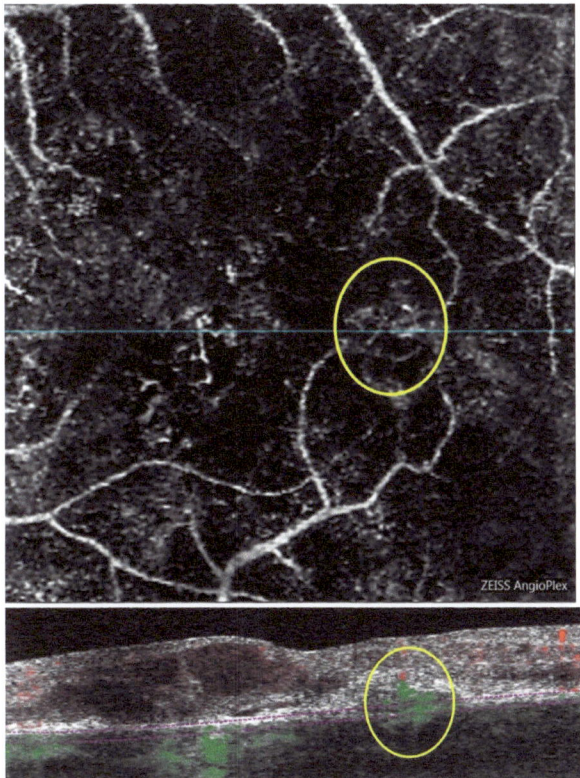

E

OCT Angiogram of the superficial retinal layer **(A)** shows an area where superficial retinal vessels seem to abruptly disappear. The deep retinal layer **(B)** shows continuation of the superficial retinal vessels in this plane. It is difficult to determine if these signals are truly deeper vessels or projection artifacts. The corresponding B-scan shows perfusion in the superficial, deep and sub-RPE layers. The avascular retinal layer **(C)** seems to show an anastomosis between the two retinal vessels at the level of the elevated RPE. This would be a potential site for the RAP lesion to communicate with the choroid. The choriocapillaris layer **(D)** shows abnormal perfusion in the region of the previously noted anastomosis as does the choroid layer **(E)**. Overall this site seems highly suspicious for RAP with anastomosis between retinal and choroidal vessels.

Another case example:

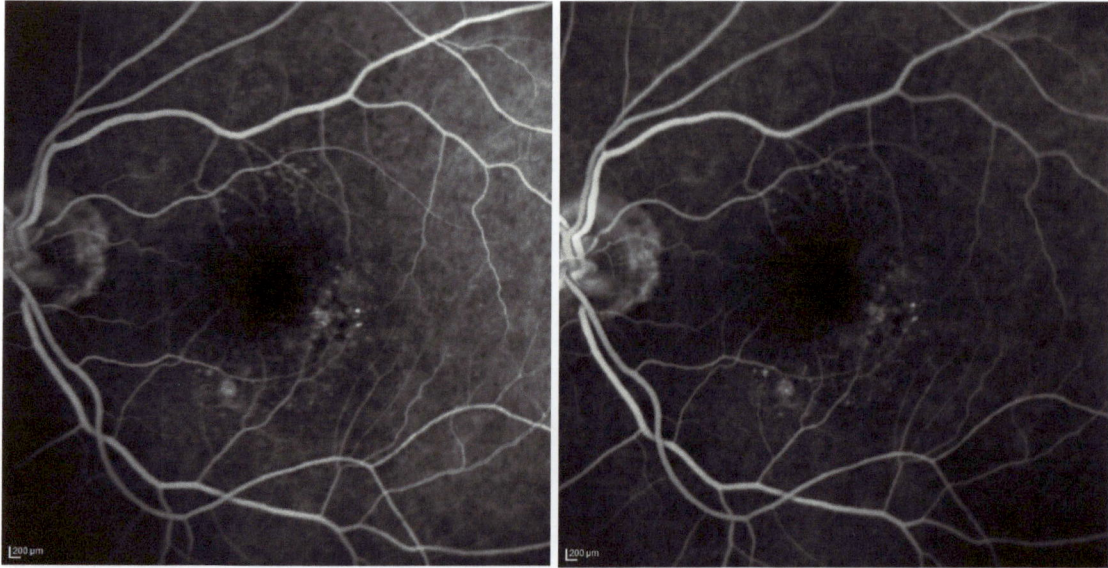

Mid-phase fluorescein angiogram (left) shows an area in the temporal and superior retina with small pinpoint hyperfluorescent lesions and staining of the retinal tissue. These findings are consistent with Late Leakage of Undetermined Significance (LLUS). Late phase FA (right) confirms the same finding.

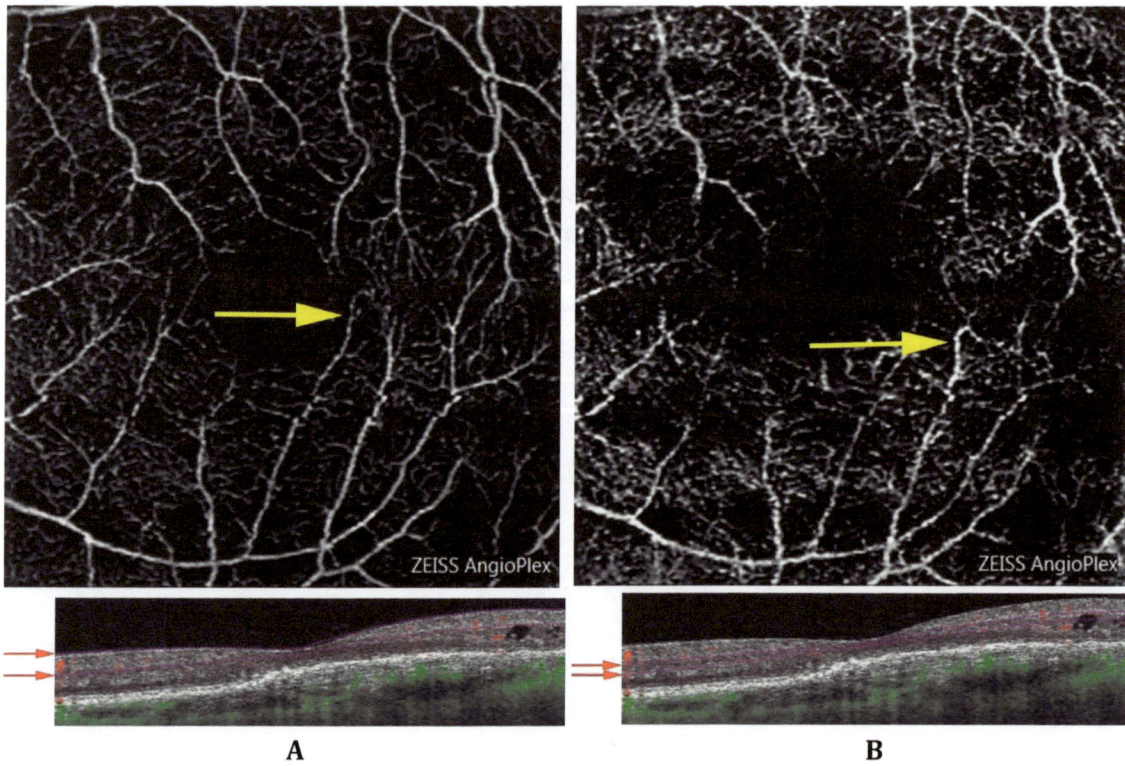

A   B

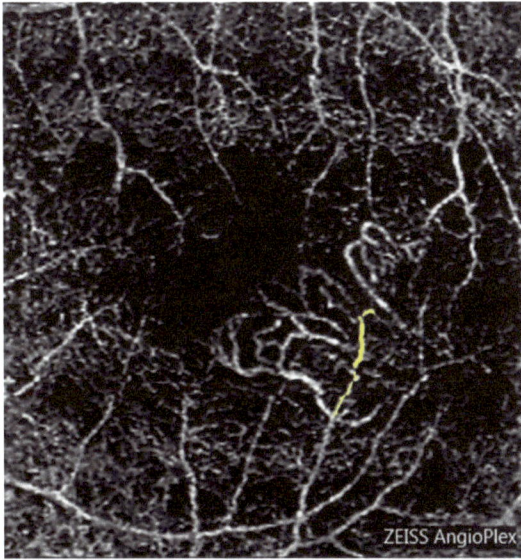
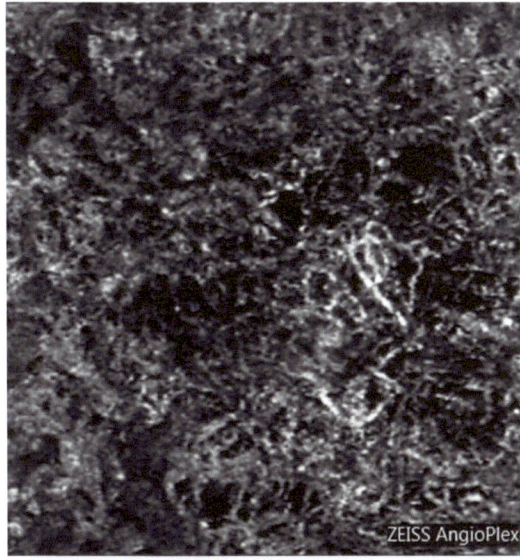

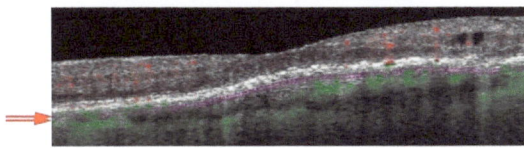
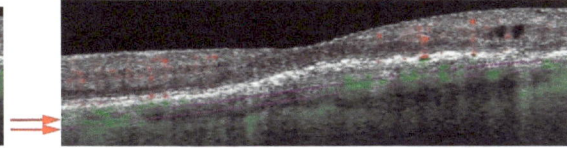

C

D

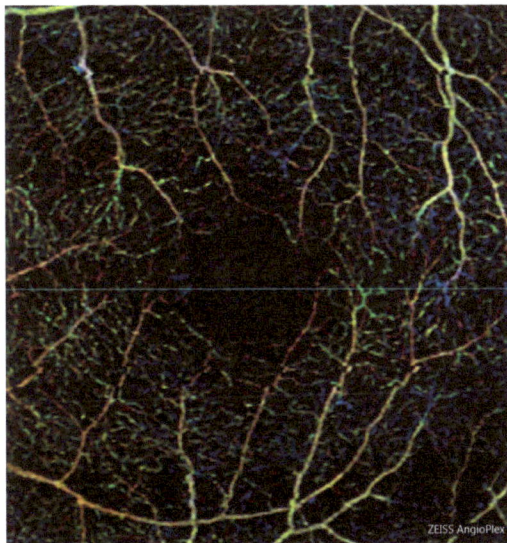
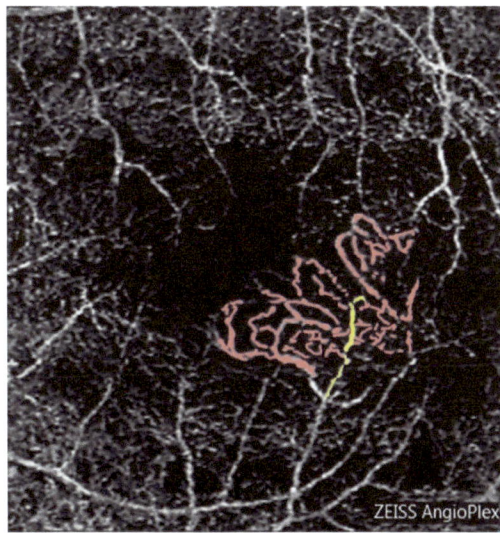

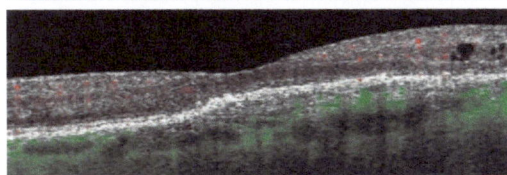
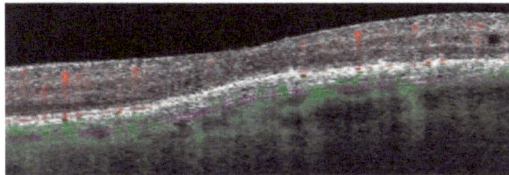

E

F

Likely RAP vessel (*yellow arrow*) on OCTA is evident on different layers. Superficial retinal layer **(A)** shows a vessel making an unusual turn and appearing to anastomose with the adjacent vessel on its immediate right. Deep retinal layer **(B)** shows the anastomoses more clearly with the receiving vessel appearing slightly more dilated and prominent than the neighboring vessels in that area. The associated B-scans show perfusion signal in the region of the anastomosis and intraretinal cystoid spaces consistent with macular edema. Choriocapillaris layer **(C)** (vessel highlighted in yellow) shows the projection artifact of the retinal anastomosis as well as the dilated choroidal vessels in that region that are likely feeding or emptying the RAP lesion. Choroidal layer **(D)** confirms earlier findings. The B-scans show a large but shallow PED with high internal reflectivity and associated perfusion (green) suggesting a CNV in the region where choroidal vessels are prominent on the en face images. Depth encoded OCTA with corresponding B-scan **(E)**. Deeper level of choriocapillaris with corresponding B-scan **(F)** with RAP vessel (in yellow) and neovascular membrane (in red). In this case, projection artifacts were left to illustrate the retinal vessel source of the lesion.

Another case example:

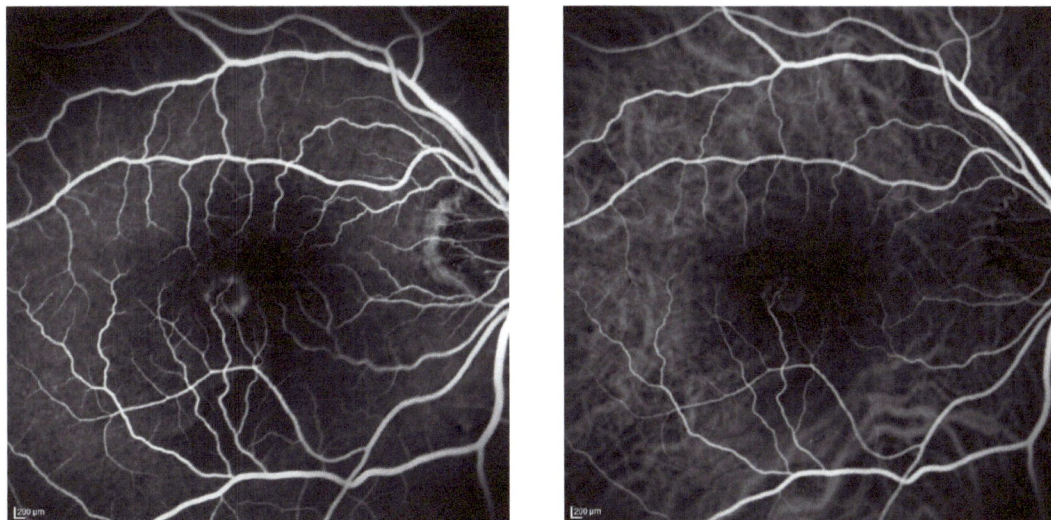

Mid phase fluorescein angiogram (left) shows an area of circular staining surrounding a retinal vessel just temporal to the fovea. Early to mid phase ICG (right) shows the retinal vessel more clearly and no clear choroidal anastomosis is visible. OCTA images (next page) confirm the location of the anastomotic retinal vessel (yellow) in the superficial (A), deep (B) and choriocapillaris (C) layers. The enlarged draining retinal vessel is most prominent in the deep layer. The corresponding B-scans show an elevated RPE with moderate to high internal reflectivity and perfusion signal (green) that suggests CNV. There are a few pockets of intraretinal fluid apparent as well.

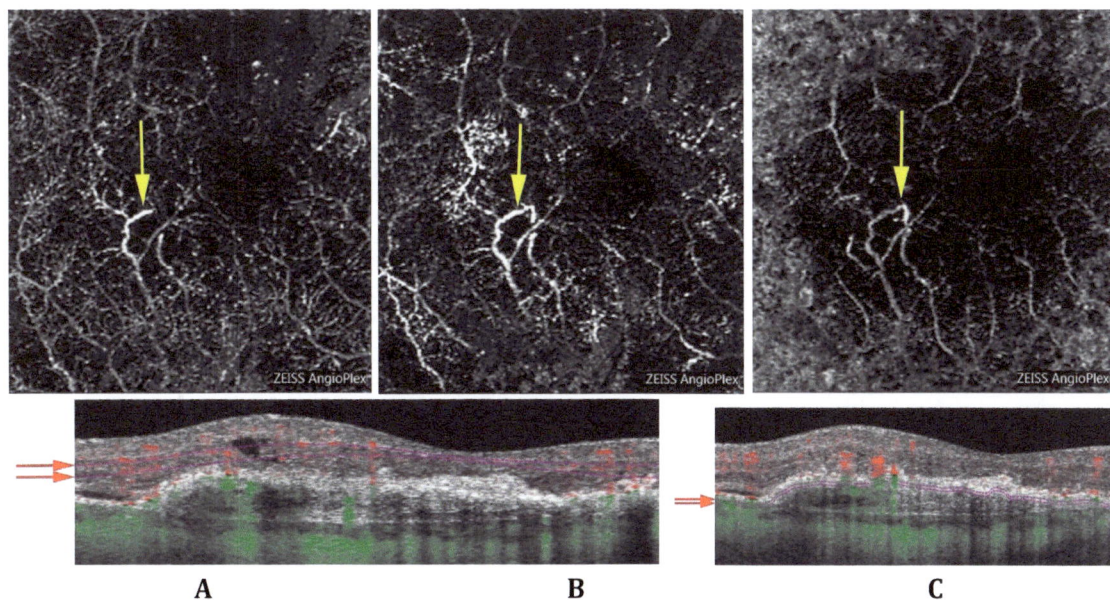

A   B   C

OCTA shows the anastomosis of the retinal and choroidal circulations in this lesion.
Superficial retinal layer OCTA **(A)** and deep retinal layer OCTA **(B)** with corresponding B-scan.
Choriocapillaris OCTA with corresponding B-scan **(C)**.

Polypoidal Choroidal Vasculopathy (PCV)

PCV is an exudative macular disorder that mimics many of the findings in AMD and CSR. In general, these three disorders can appear very similar especially in chronic cases and the clinical diagnosis may be challenging. Characterizing PCV as a subset of AMD or as an entirely separate entity is still under debate. PCV lesions may be considered as a form of Type 1 (sub-RPE) choroidal neovascularization.

PCV is more common among people from African ancestry or from the Asian subcontinent and usually requires ICG for accurate diagnosis. Key anatomic findings include orange-red subretinal nodules, intraretinal hemorrhage, PED, and subretinal fluid.

Fluorescein angiography may show polyp type hyperfluorescent nodules early in the angiogram that leak in the late phase but because fluorescein dye leaks out of the fenestrated choriocapillaris vessels the polyps are often obscured on FA.

ICG angiography is the standard imaging modality for PCV, as the larger molecule dye will create a hypofluorescent halo around the polyps in the early phase of the angiogram and will highlight the polyps in the later phases (~6 min). The presence of orange-red lesions on examination that correspond to hyperfluorescent lesions in the choroid on ICG is a key finding in PCV. ICG may also show a branching network of inner choroidal vessels.

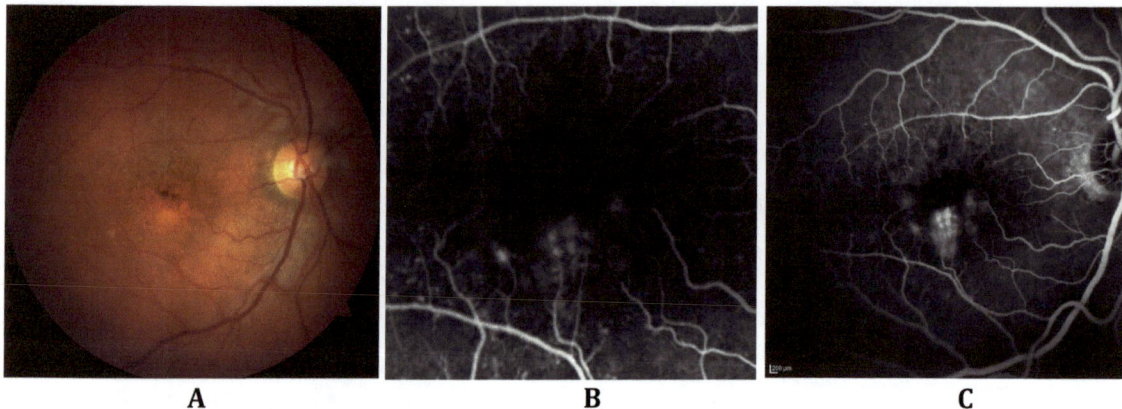

A **B** **C**

Color fundus image (**A**). Magnified mid-phase fluorescein angiogram (**B**) shows several hyperfluorescent lesions inferior to the fovea that appear in same region as the orange lesion on the color image. Late phase fluorescein angiogram (**C**) shows the polyp-like lesions more clearly.

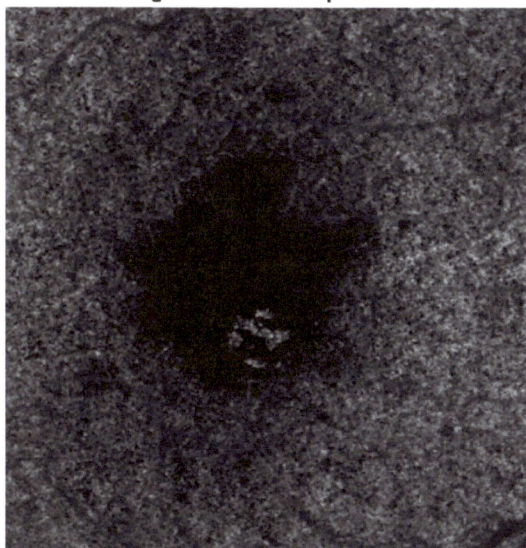
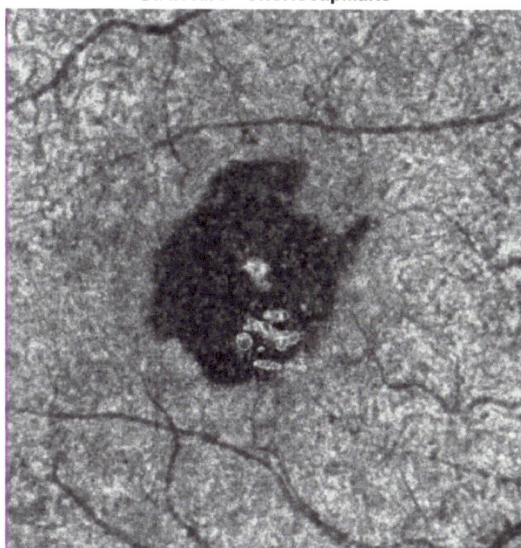

6x6 mm choriocapillaris layer OCTA (left) with corresponding IR en face image (right).

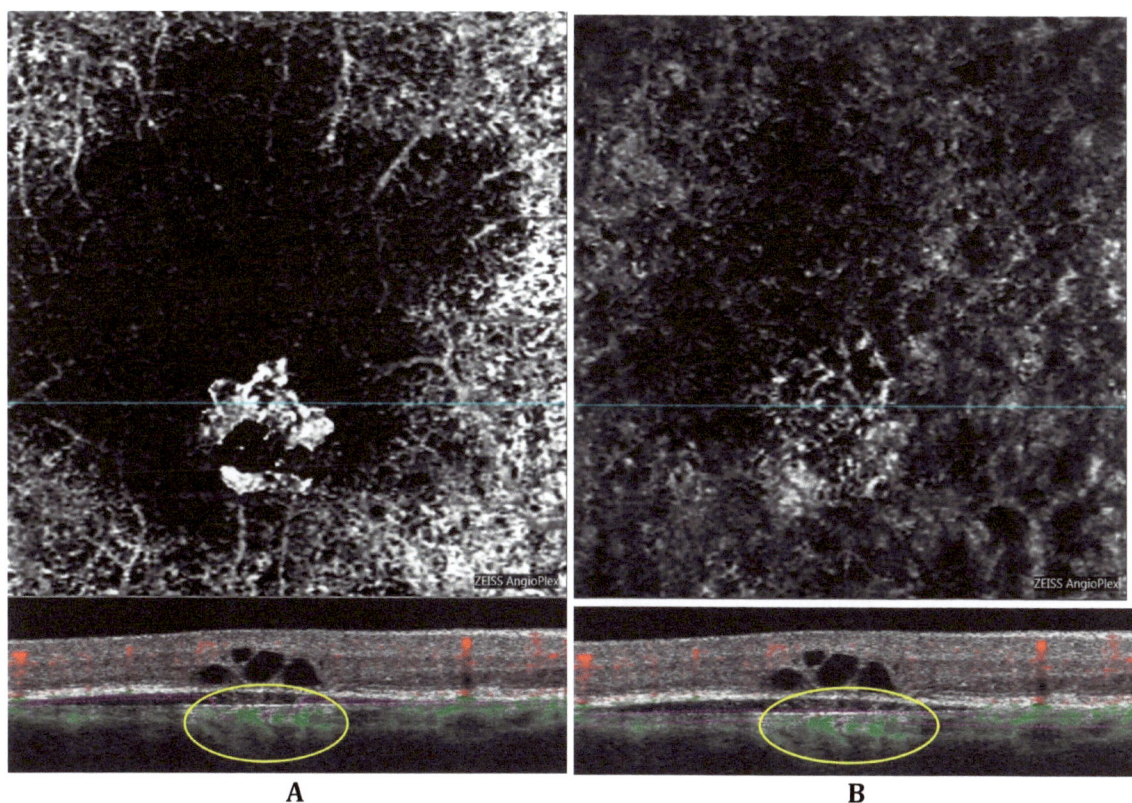

A   B

The choriocapillaris OCTA with corresponding B-scan **(A)** shows increased flow from focal lesions in the area of decreased flow. Polyps in PCV may alter the flow patterns in the surrounding choriocapillaris as is shown in the en face image or this may reflect an artifact of the overlying retinal changes and shallow PED in this case. The en face choriocapillaris OCTA image shows an area of abnormal flow corresponding to the polyps. The choroidal layer OCTA **(B)** shows the abnormal perfusion patterns in the area surrounding the polyps.

164

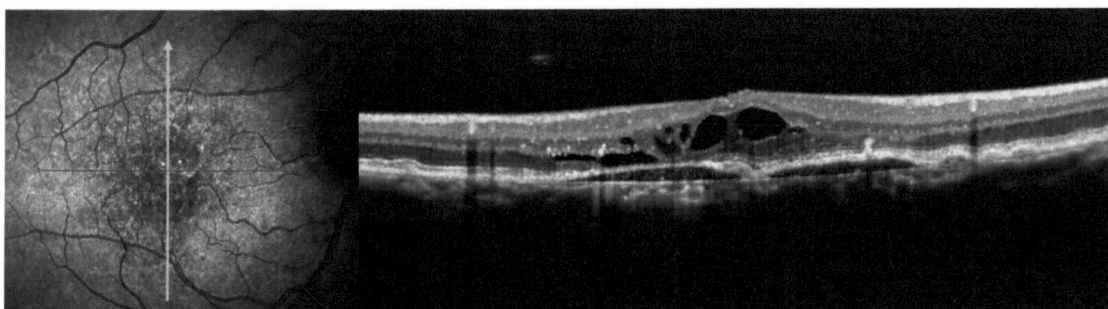

B-scan OCT shows intraretinal cystoid spaces over the shallow PED with internal hyporeflectivity corresponding to serous PED.

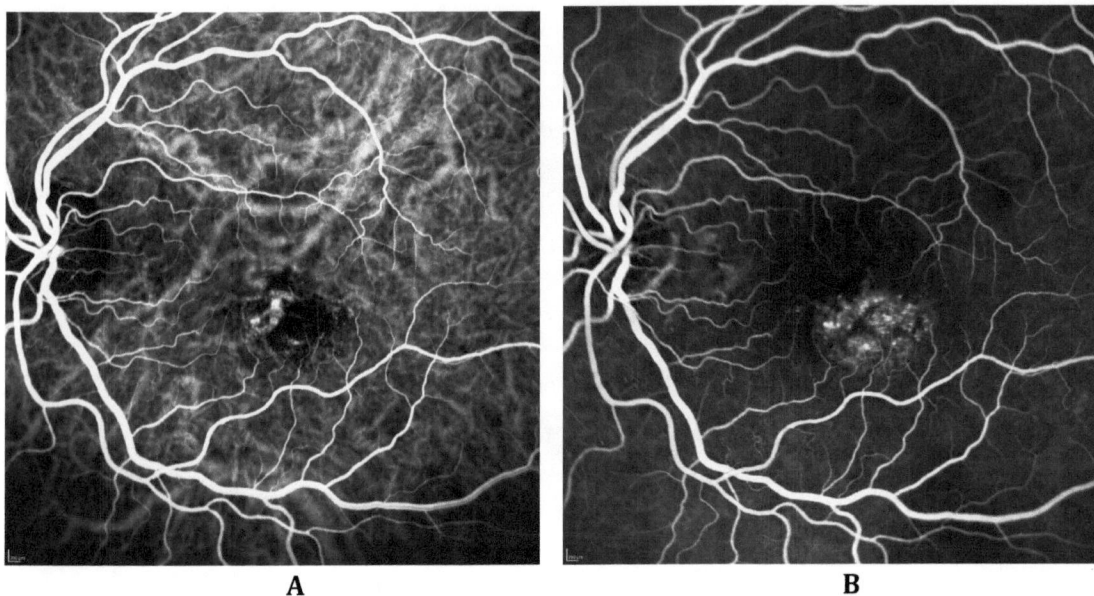

A

B

Mid phase ICG angiogram **(A)** of PCV with 2-3 clearly defined polyps in the area of choroidal hypoperfusion. Mid phase fluorescein angiogram **(B)** of PCV shows overlying hyperfluorescent pinpoint changes and late staining.

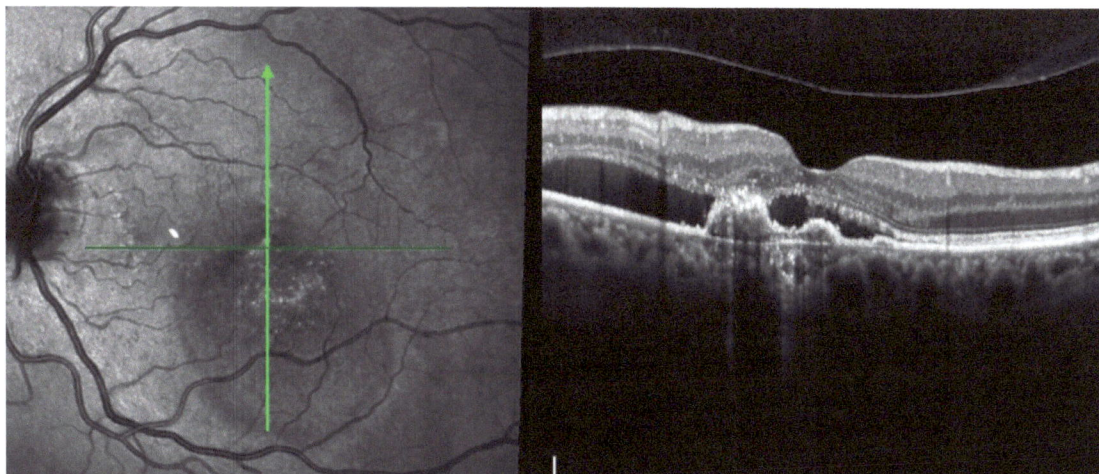

Vertical B scan OCT through lesion shows subretinal fluid and multilobulated PED with hyporeflective internal contents suggesting of a serous PED.

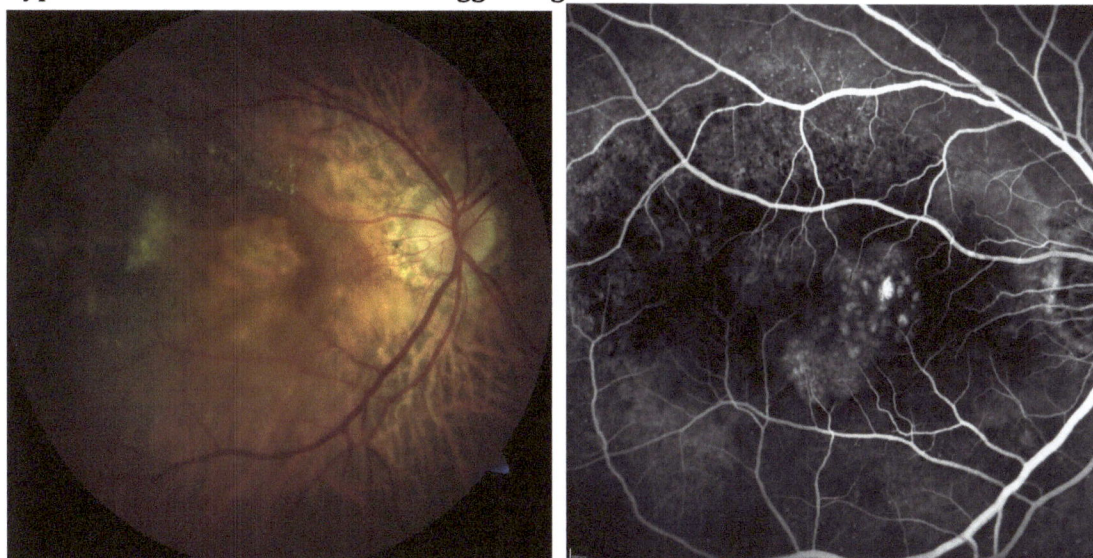

Color fundus image demonstrates subretinal fluid and yellow-gold deposits consistent with resolving lipoproteinaceous material associated with IRF or SRF. There is an area of GA in the center of the macula. The mid-phase FA shows several polyp type lesions in the nasal macula and diffuse areas of hypoperfusion throughout the macula.

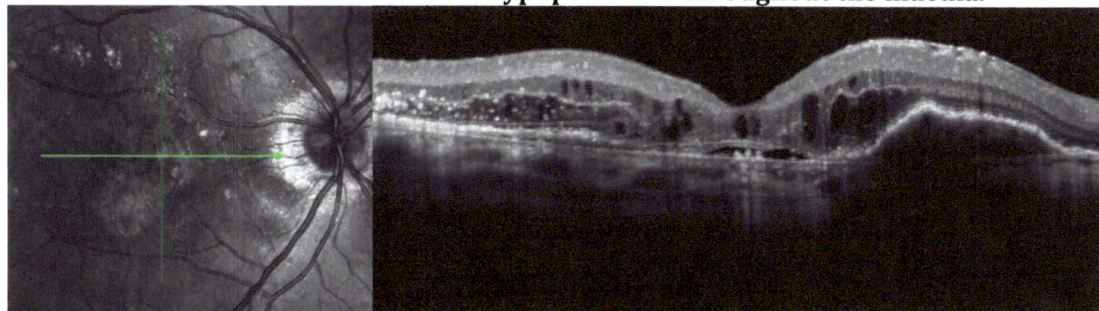

Horizontal B-scan OCT of same patient as above shows multiple intraretinal cystoid spaces. There is sub-retinal fluid directly underneath the fovea, and a large PED with hyporeflective internal contents consistent with a serous PED. The numerous pin-point hyperreflective spots likely correspond to hard exudates in the color image above.

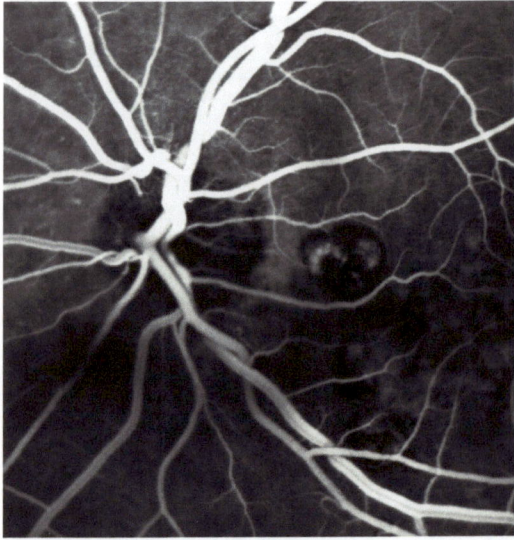

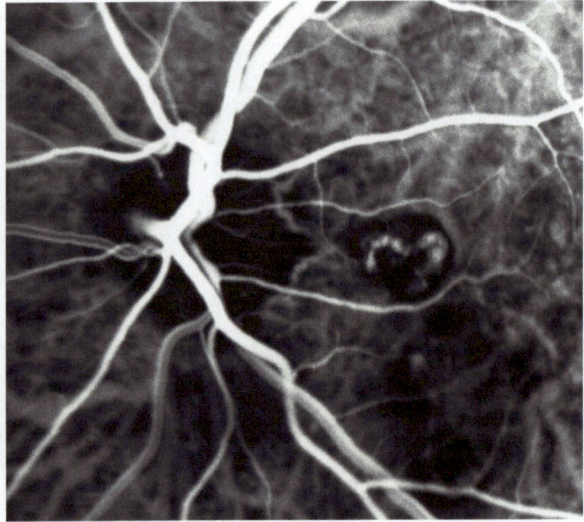

A

B

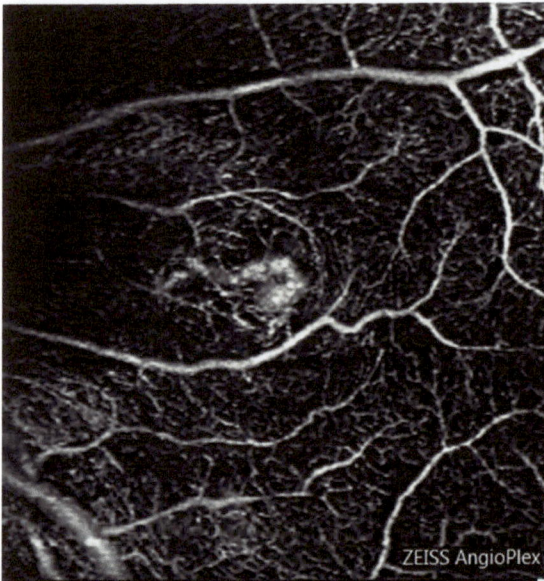

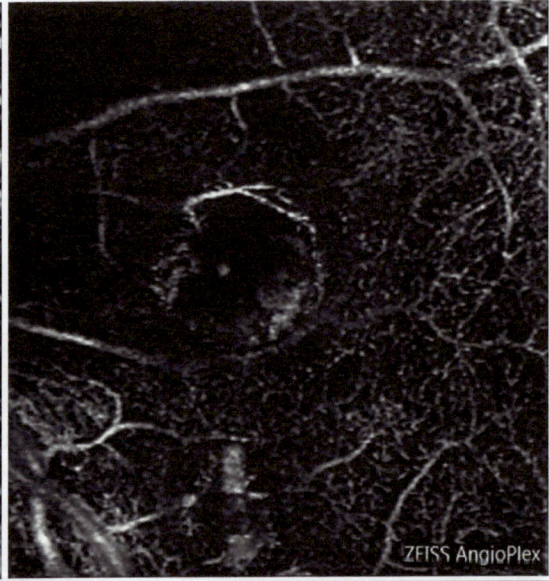

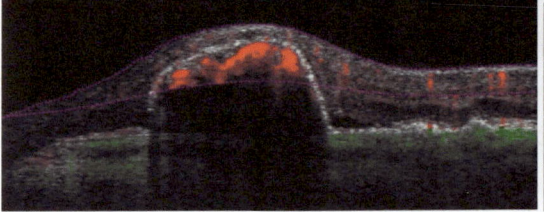

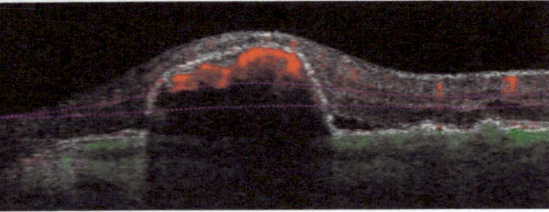

C

D

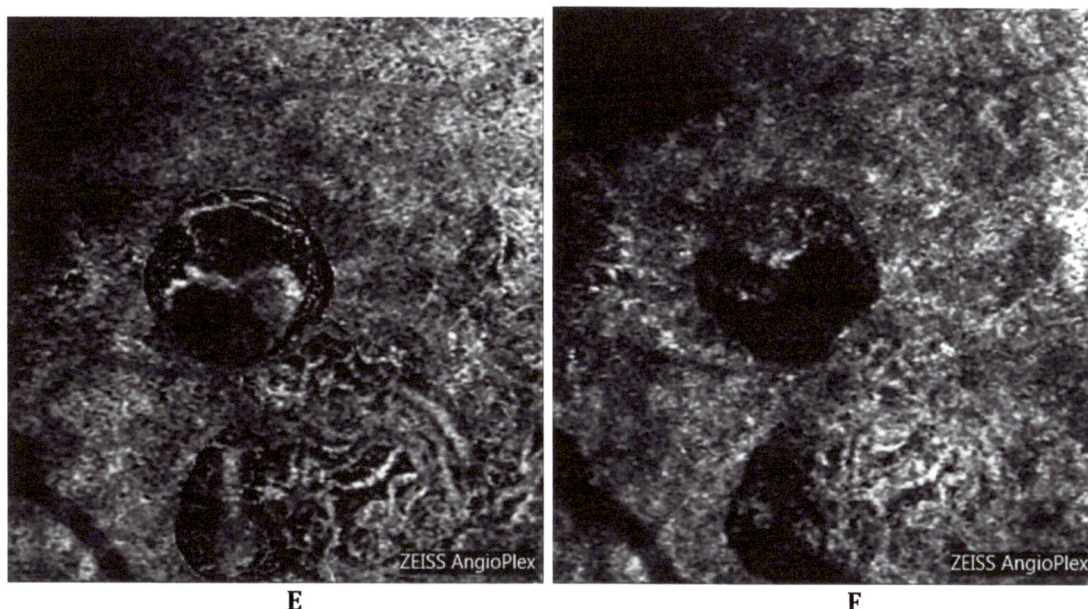

E   F

Mid phase fluorescein angiogram **(A)** shows several pockets of hypoperfusion with polyp like lesions in the nasal macula. The corresponding ICG **(B)** confirms the polyp like lesions and associated choroidal hypoperfusion. The OCTA of the superficial retina **(C)** shows the polyp like lesion with perfusion signal. In this case, the elevated PED has been artifactually displaced into the superficial retinal layer of the OCTA as is well demonstrated in the corresponding B-scan. Notice the nodular lesion with perfusion signal from the PED. There is a small amount of SRF adjacent to the PED. This is a great example that it is necessary to evaluate B-scans corresponding to unusual retinal changes in the en face OCTA in order to accurately identify the lesion. OCTA of the deep retinal layer **(D)** does not demonstrate lack of flow due to artifactual elevation of the deep retinal layer out of the plane. Choriocapillaris **(E)** and choroidal **(F)** level OCTA show focal regions of hypoperfusion surrounding the polyps.

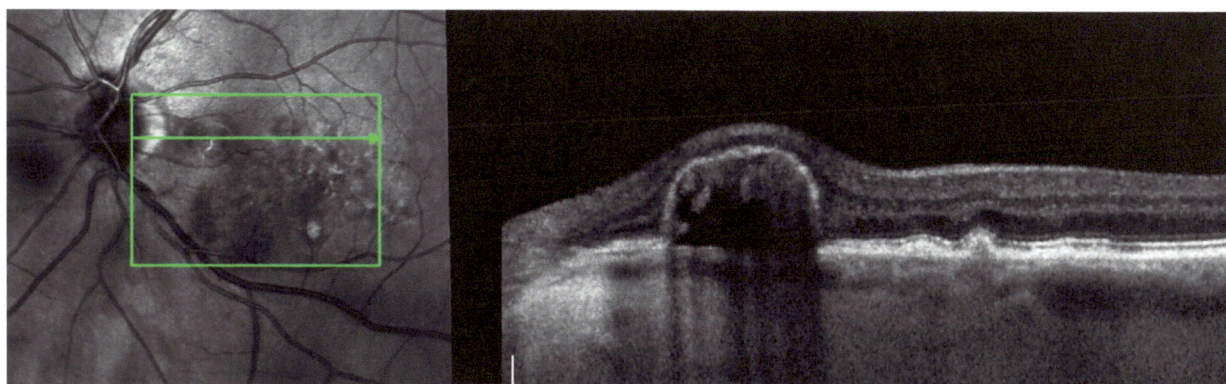

Horizontal B-scan OCT of the case above, illustrating dense polyp structures below the level of RPE (in the PED) that cast shadows onto deeper structures.

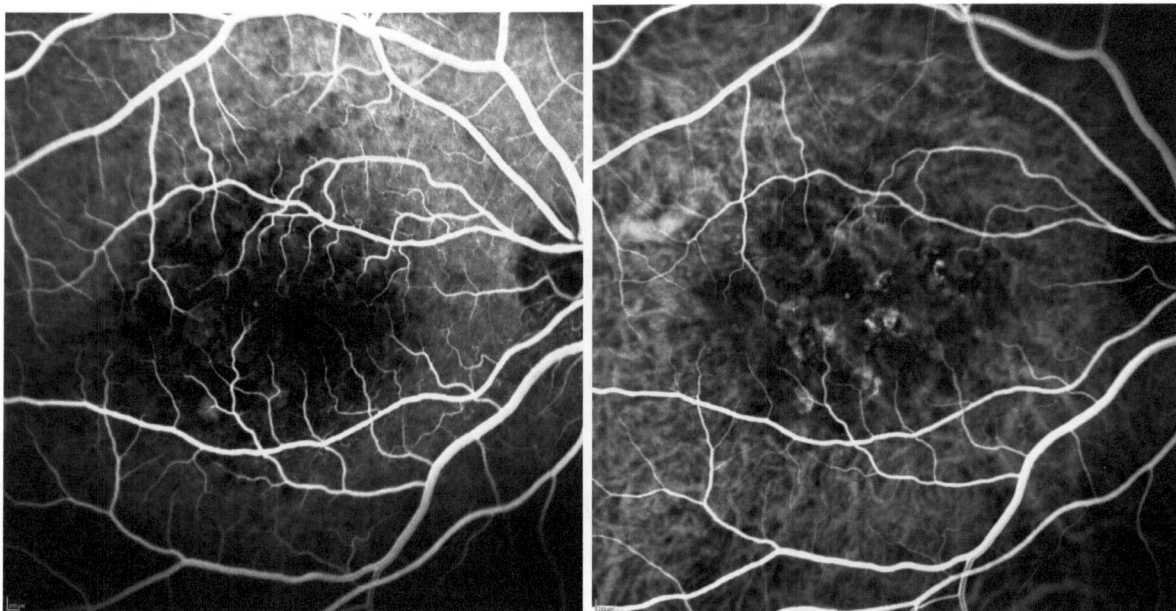

Early phase FA (left) shows numerous areas of RPE changes with mild staining throughout the macula. Early phase ICG (right) shows corresponding areas of hypoperfusion and some polyp like structures with hyperfluorescence.

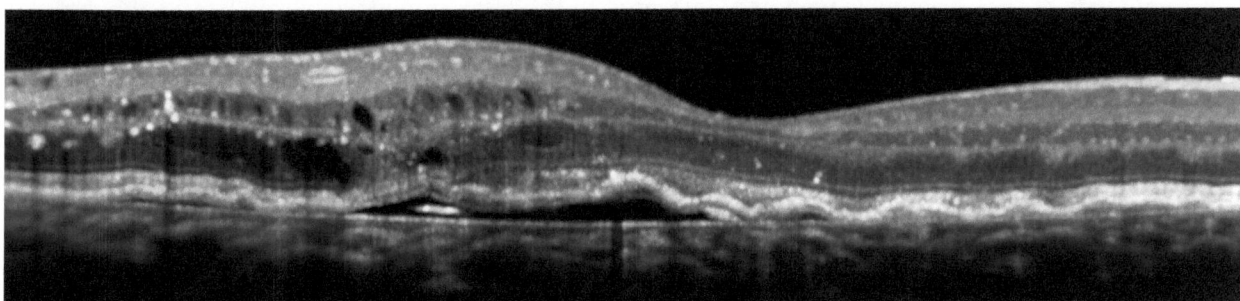

Horizontal B-scan OCT of PCV shows shallow PED with hyporeflective internal contents consistent with serous PED. There are several cystoid pockets within the retina.

Central Serous Chorioretinopathy (CSCR)

CSCR is a chorioretinal disease that is classically characterized by a neurosensory retinal detachment with or without a retinal pigment epithelial detachment. Although sometimes termed retinopathy, it is more appropriately designated a choroidopathy or chorioretinopathy. The typical CSCR patient is between 20 and 50 years old, and it affects men more than women. CSCR has also been associated with increased stress and systemic steroid use. With appropriate precautions, CSCR is usually self-limiting, and tends to clear within weeks or months. Most patients with an acute or single episode recover vision but recurrent episodes can lead to severe vision loss.

On OCT, CSCR presents with a single or multiple fluid pockets in the subretinal space. Areas with a "stalactite" appearance of the overlying neurosensory retina likely represent the accumulation of photoreceptor outer segments. This may occur because the underlying RPE is not present to phagocytose the photoreceptor debris as occurs in the normal retinal anatomy. Undulations in the RPE are common but not necessarily always present. Recurrent and chronic CSCR can result in RPE loss and CNV. Enhanced depth imaging of CSCR cases typically demonstrates a thickened choroid.

OCT angiography can be extremely useful in detecting CNV associated with CSCR and in differentiating CSCR with age related macular degeneration in some cases.

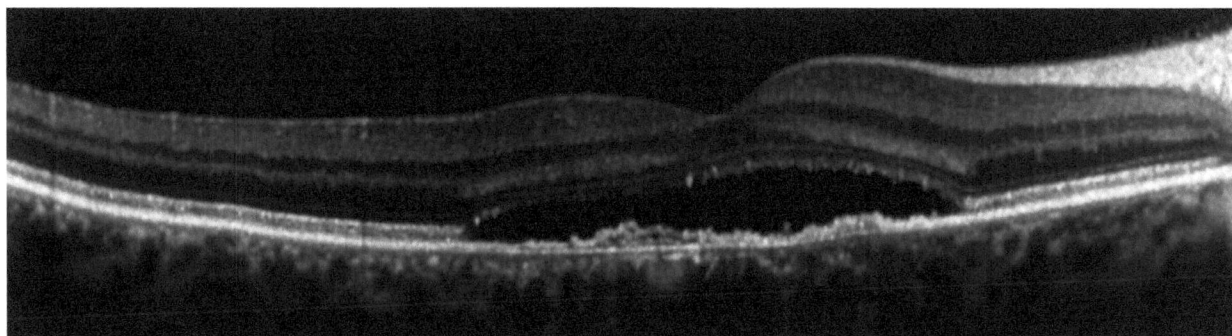

OCT line B-scan of the fovea in CSCR. Note the subretinal fluid, stalactite appearance of the photoreceptor outer segments in the area of the neurosensory detachment and the RPE undulations.

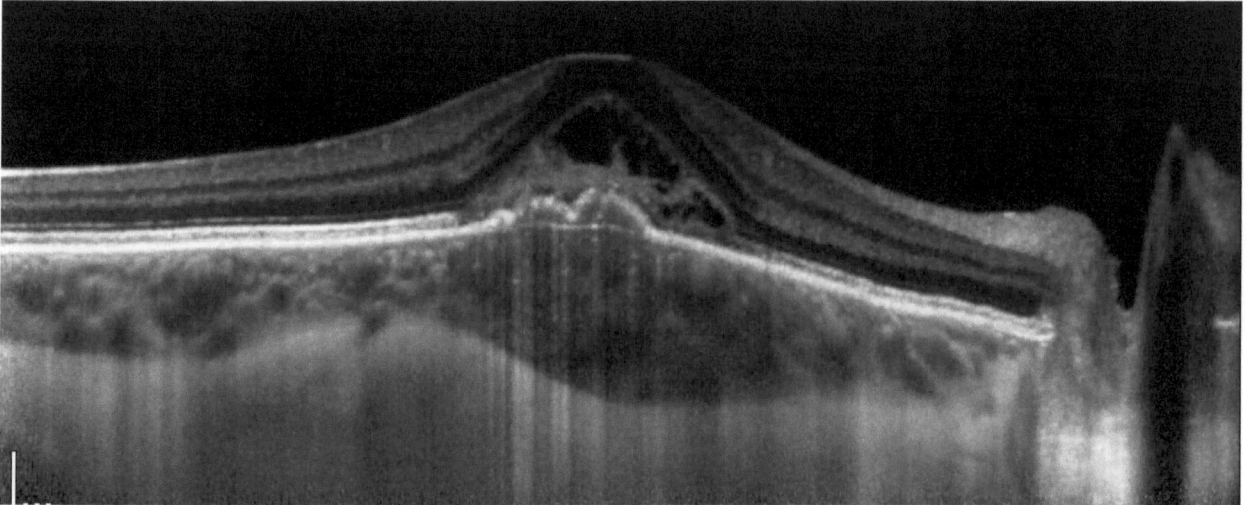

EDI OCT B-scan of a patient with CSCR. There is a neurosensory detachment under the fovea that is blunting the foveal depression. The subretinal fluid has hyperreflective material in it that suggests the fluid has been there for a long period of time, and the underlying RPE has two elevations consistent with pigment epithelial detachments directly underneath the fovea. Note the thickened choroid that is most prominent in the area underneath the neurosensory detachment.

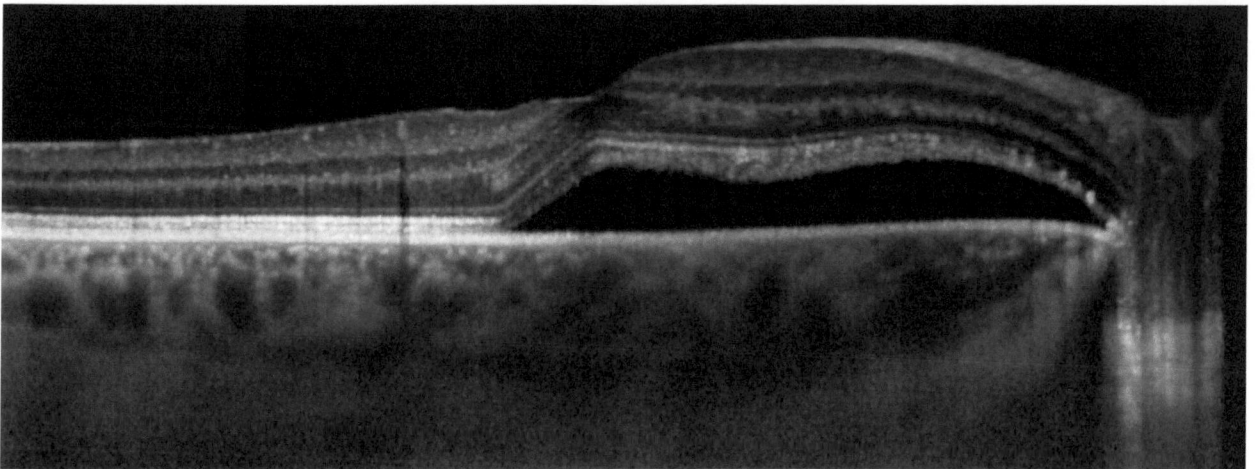

EDI OCT B-scan of a patient with CSCR. There is a neurosensory detachment under the fovea extending to the edge of the nerve. Note the abnormally long photoreceptor outer segments that are forming a continuous contour in this case (rather than the stalactite configuration of the last image). No pigment epithelial detachment is evident on this scan. The choroid appears thicker than usual. Manual choroidal measurements in the case of CSCR may be useful to follow the progression or regression of the disease.

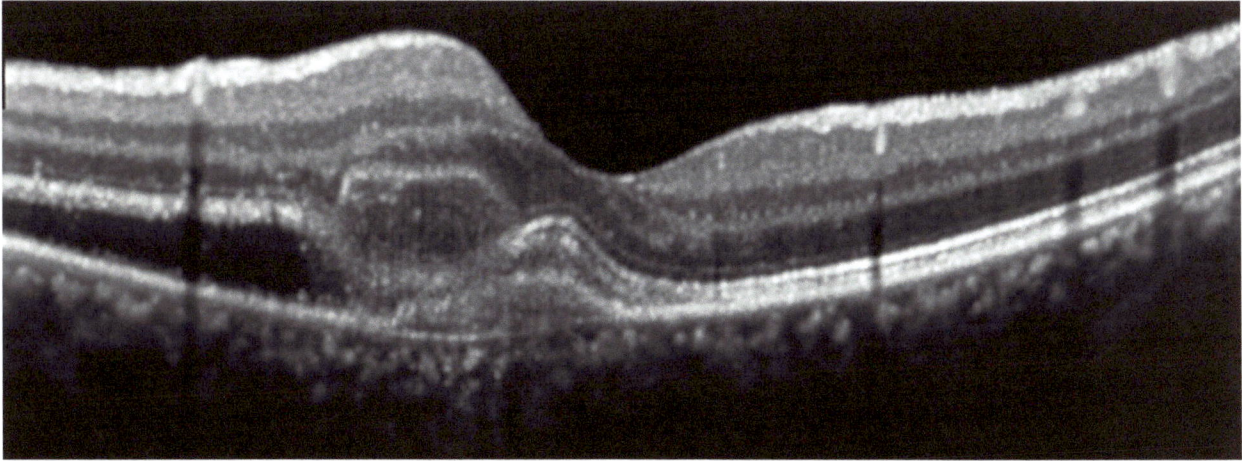

B-scan OCT of a patient with CSCR. There is subretinal fluid in the far left of the image as well as some adjacent areas of retinal thickening that suggest intraretinal edema. Intraretinal edema is not characteristic of CSCR but may be present in some cases. There is elevation of the retina and RPE below the fovea in this case. The combination of the irregular RPE elevation as well as intraretinal thickening in this case is concerning for CNV in the setting of chronic CSCR.

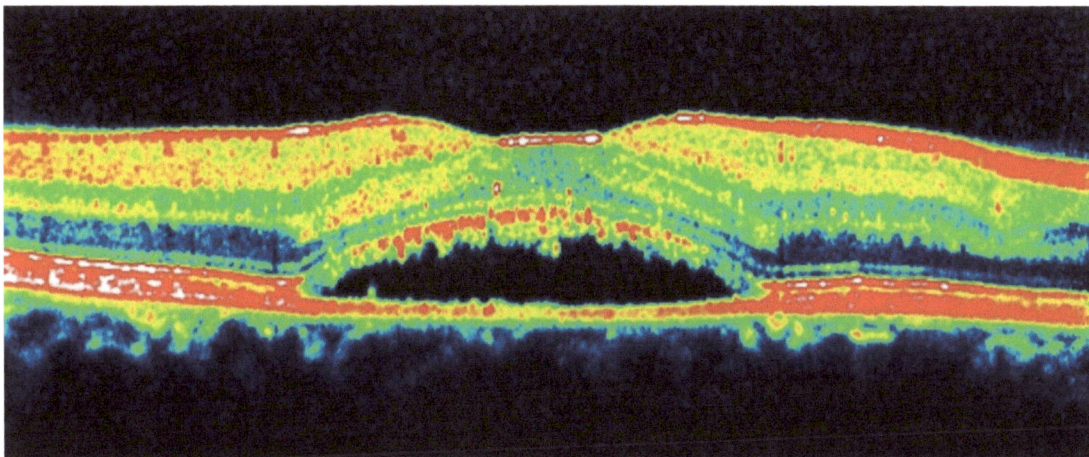

Typical "stalactite" formation at the roof of the neurosensory detachment

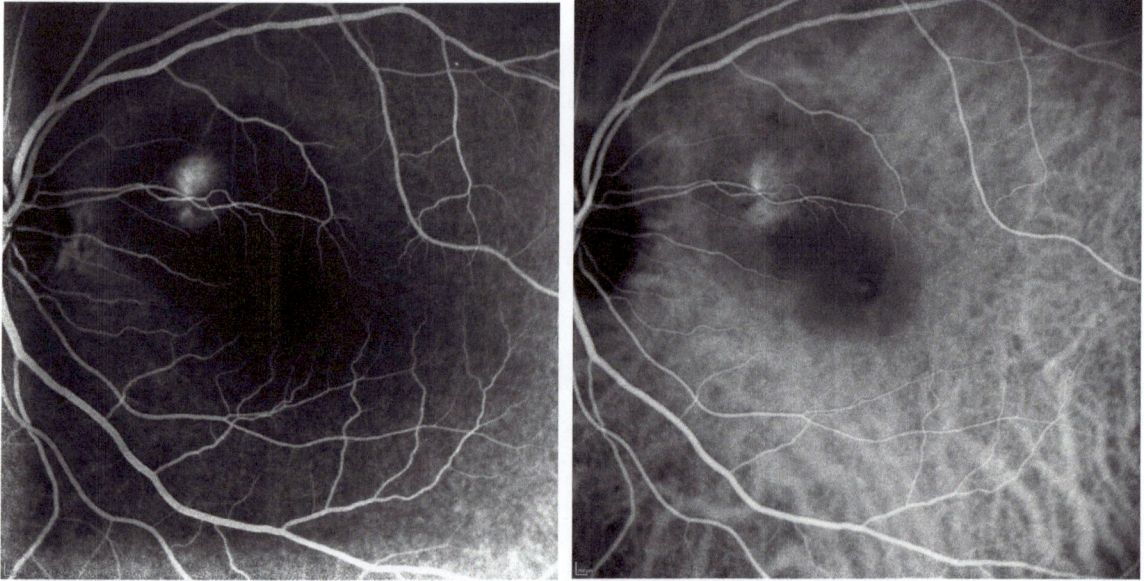

Fluorescein angiogram (left) shows an expansile dot pattern of leakage in this case of CSCR. Note the surrounding hypofluorescence, which is consistent with a ring of subretinal fluid and neurosensory detachment. ICG angiogram (right) shows a hotspot corresponding to the region of the expansile dot on fluorescein angiography. The ICG hypofluorescence is similarly attenuated here by the subretinal fluid in the neurosensory detachment. The OCT B-scan and volume map of CSCR is provided below as well.

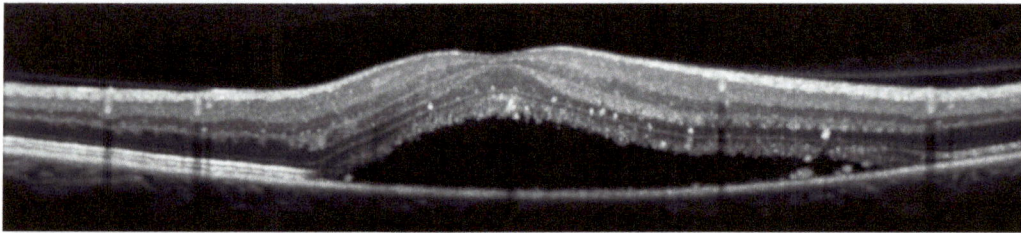

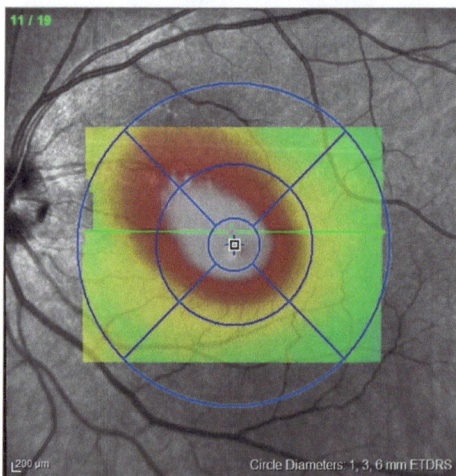

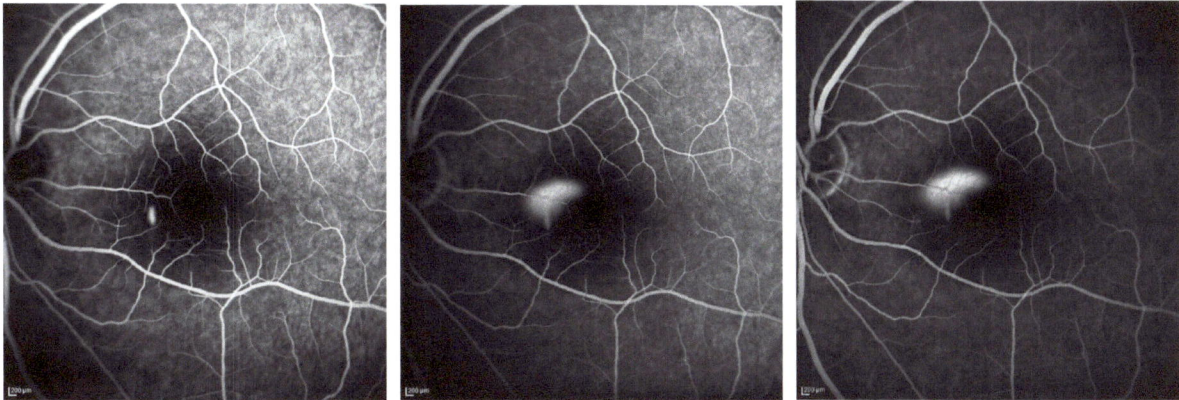

Early (left), mid (middle) and late (right) phase fluorescein angiogram of CSCR with classic "smokestack" appearance.

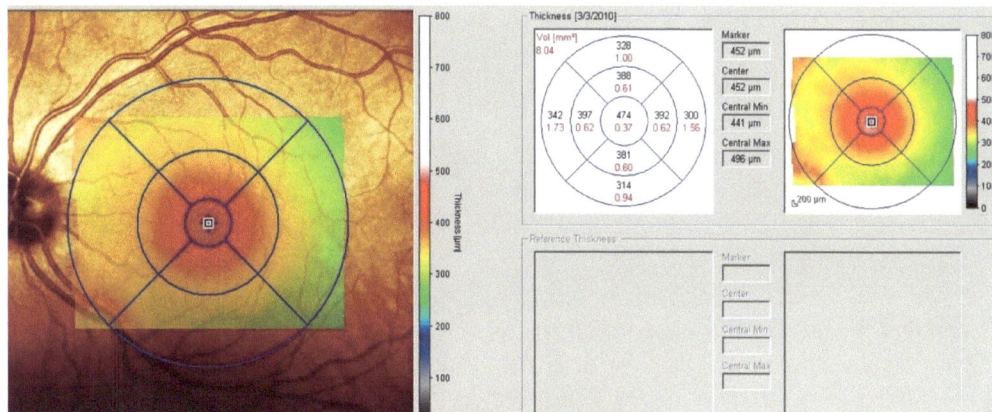

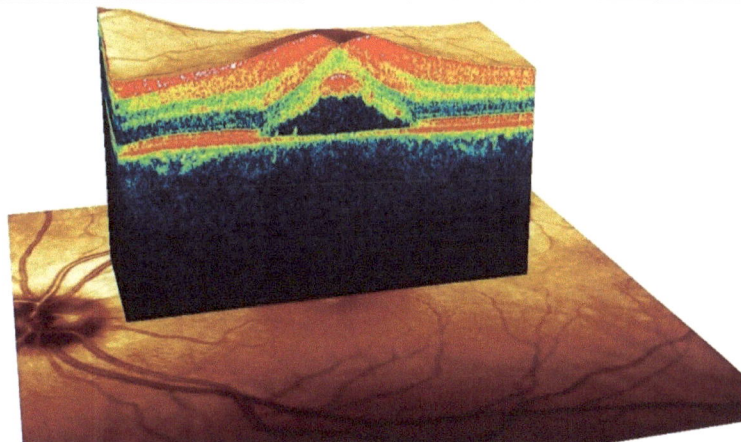

Volumetric OCT (top) and 3D cube OCT (bottom) of CSR

Case 1: *Epiretinal Membrane*

Clinical Summary

77-year-old white male presents with metamorphopsia and general decreased vision OS progressing over a 6-month period. Visual acuity is 20/200 in the symptomatic eye.

Image Summary

A. Color Fundus: Shows vessel tortuosity within the macula, a grey sheen overlying the macula and distorted macular anatomy.

B. Fluorescein angiography: Late phase image reveals severe distortion of macular vessels and leakage in the foveal and parafoveal region. There are also a few microaneurysms in the periphery.

C. OCT Angiography: **C1**: Shows predominantly superficial retinal perfusion (red) on the depth-encoded image. **C2**: Full depth retina composite OCTA. **C3**: B-scan near the fovea shows attenuated flow where the presumptive fovea would be. In this case and others, epiretinal membranes often distort and elevate parts of the retina into more superficial scan planes thereby artifactually increasing the superficial perfusion and decreasing the deep retinal perfusion. Despite this, it is evident that overall capillary flow is attenuated around the fovea. **C4a-c**: Monochromatic composite OCTA with corresponding B-scan from superior, mid and inferior retina shows more prominent flow in the superficial retinal layer throughout.

D. OCT: A vertical B-scan through the fovea shows a hyperreflective retinal surface consistent with an ERM. Cystoid spaces are also apparent throughout the retina and the retina is diffusely thickened, and the foveal contour is completely blunted.

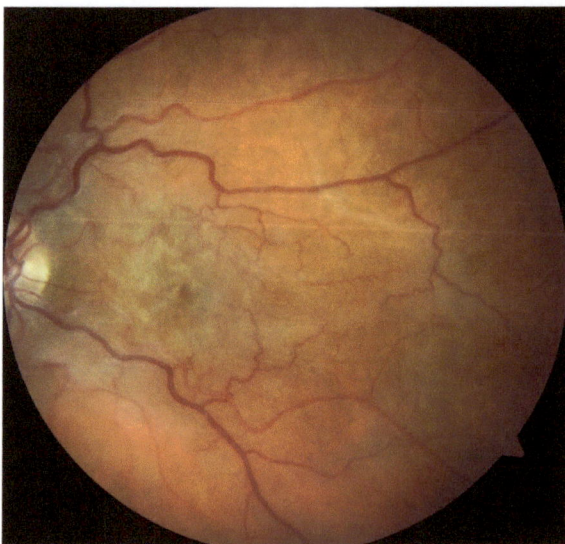

A

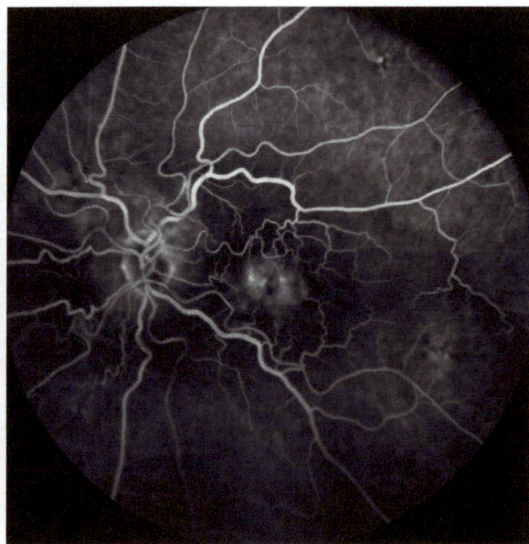

B

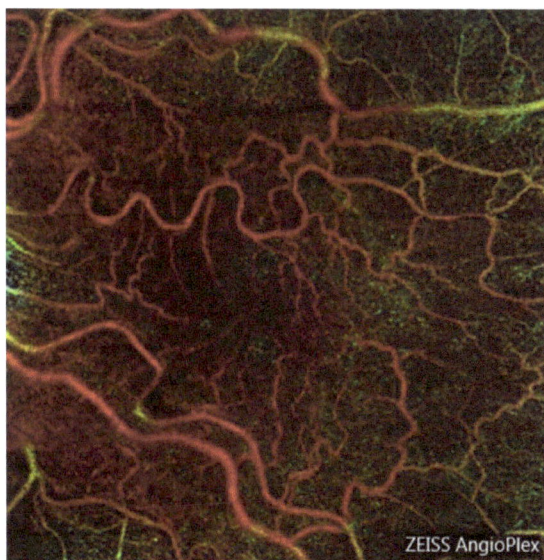

C1

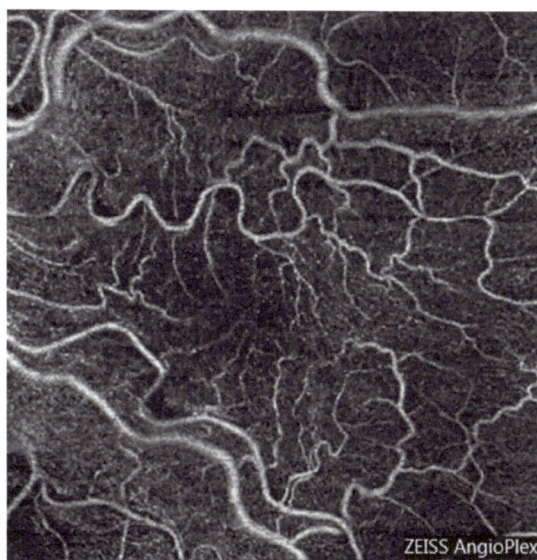

C2

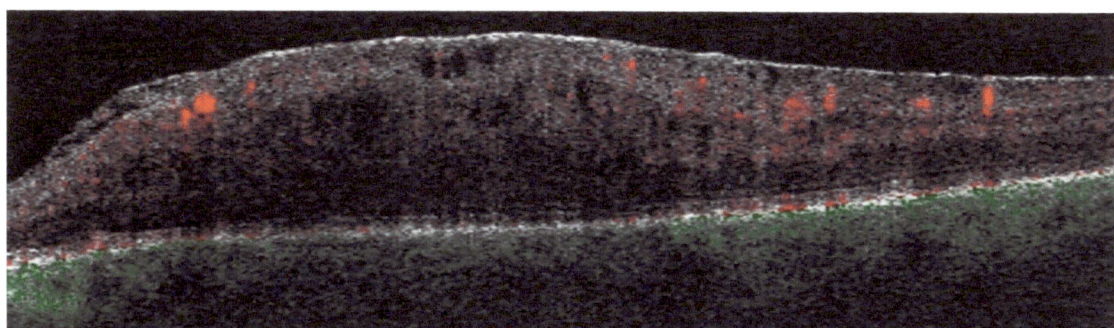

C3

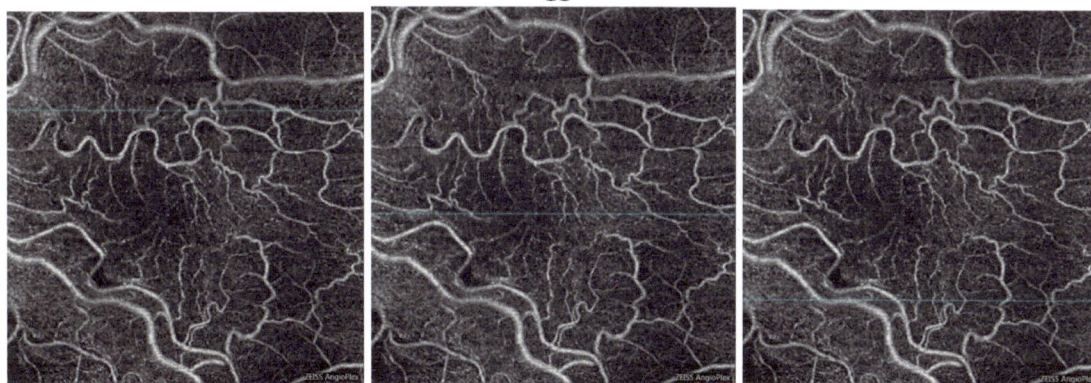

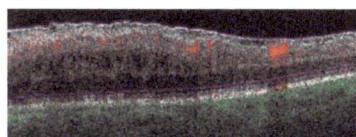

C4a

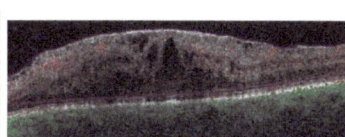

C4b

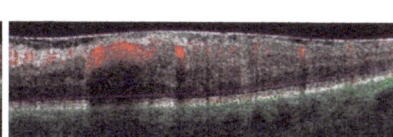

C4c

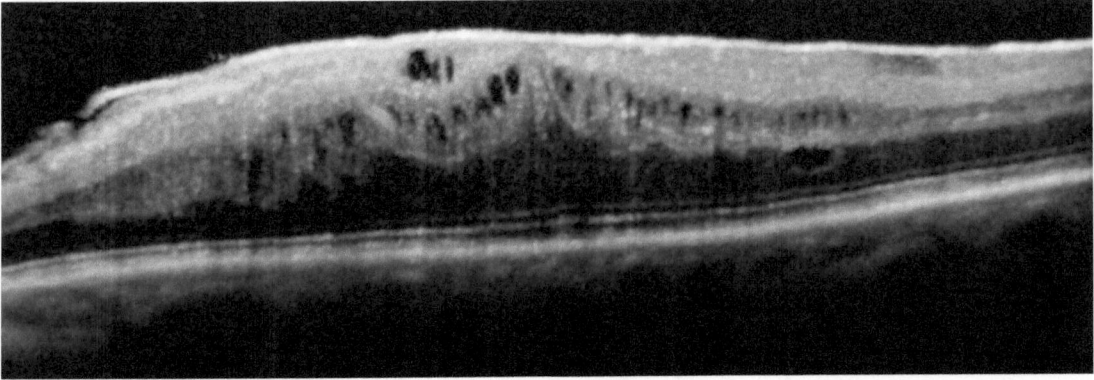

D

Intraretinal Diseases

- Cystoid Macular Edema

- Diabetic Macular Edema

- Non-proliferative Diabetic Retinopathy

- Proliferative Diabetic Retinopathy

- Branch Retinal Vein Occlusion

- Central Retinal Vein Occlusion

- Branch Retinal Artery Occlusion

- Central Retinal Artery Occlusion

Case 2: *Cystoid Macular Edema*

Clinical Summary:

75-year-old white female presents with complaints of decrease in vision one week after cataract surgery OD. Visual acuity is 20/200 OD. History of drusen OU, pre-cataract vision 20/100 OD.

Image Summary

A. Color Fundus: Shows RPE changes in the macula as well as some yellow deposits consistent with drusen. There appears to be a yellow-green sheen to the macula suggesting subretinal pathology.

B. Fluorescein Angiography: Late phase image shows diffuse leakage and staining with poorly defined borders throughout the macula consistent with an occult choroidal neovascular lesion. Numerous cystoid spaces are evident.

C. OCT Angiography: C1: Full thickness retina composite OCTA with corresponding B-scan shows attenuated perfusion that is more severe in the right side of the image. **C2**: Depth encoded OCTA with corresponding B-scan illustrates the macula edema with raised (red) superficial retinal vessels. **C3**: Retina composite en face intensity image shows numerous large hypo-intense regions consistent with cystoid spaces. Several horizontal black lines in the superior half of the image are movement artifacts.

D. OCT: D1: Volume representation of the macula shows prominent thickening. **D2**: Line B-scan shows a bright hyperreflective line anterior to the retina that is consistent with vitreomacular adhesion. There is a large amount of intraretinal cystoid spaces consistent with macular edema. There is a large, shallow lesion consisting of a PED with an overlying area of hyperreflectivity in the center suggestive of CNV or fibrosis.

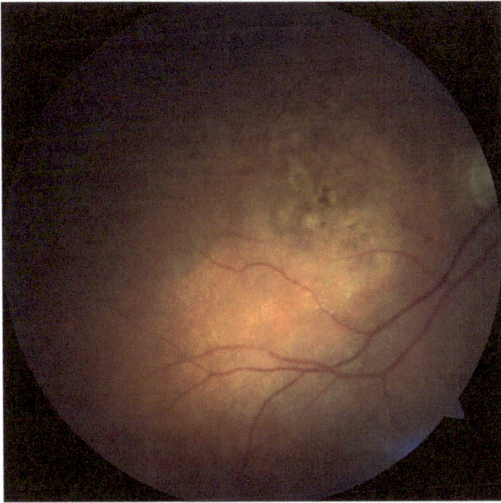

A

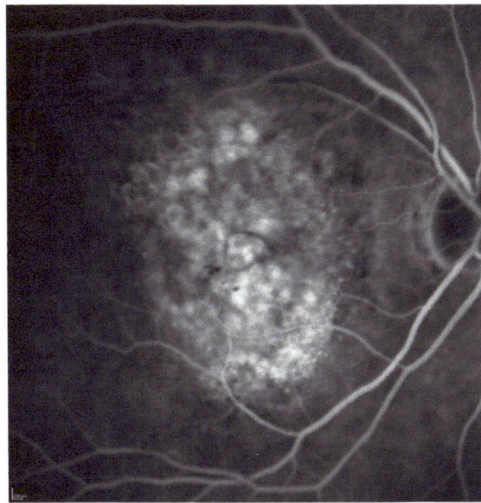

B

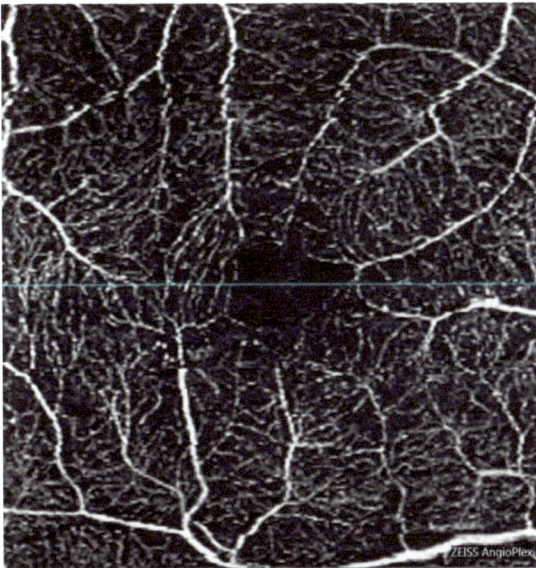

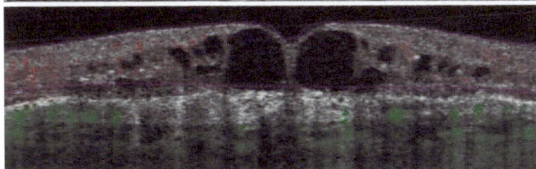

C1

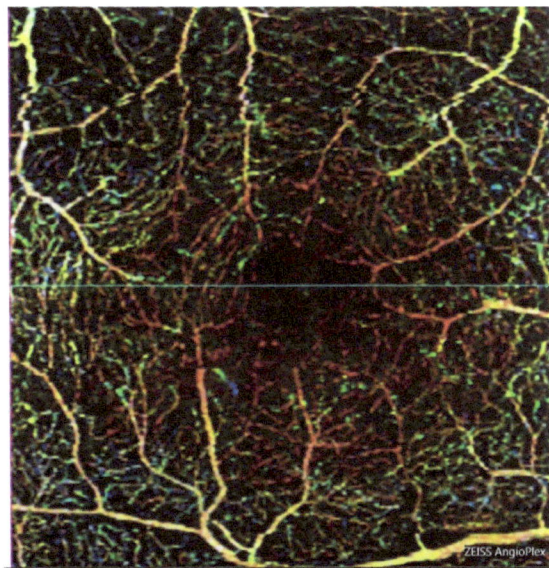

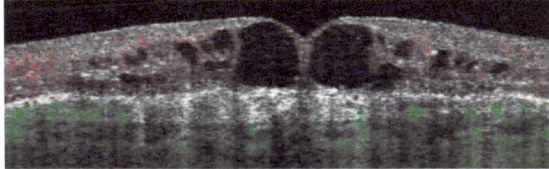

C2

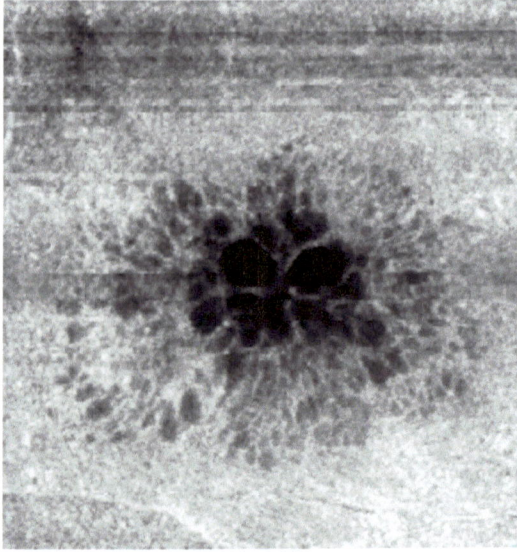

C3

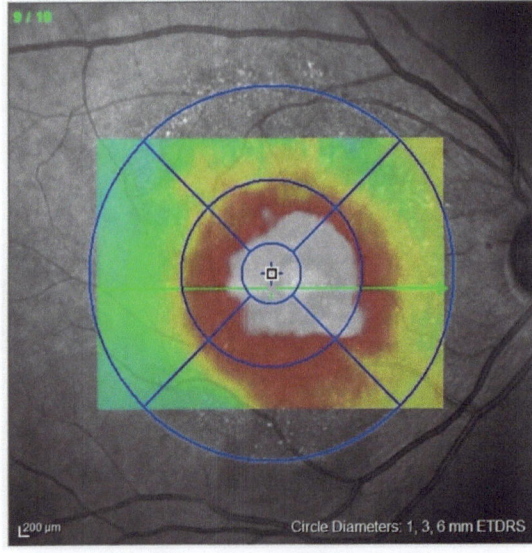

D1

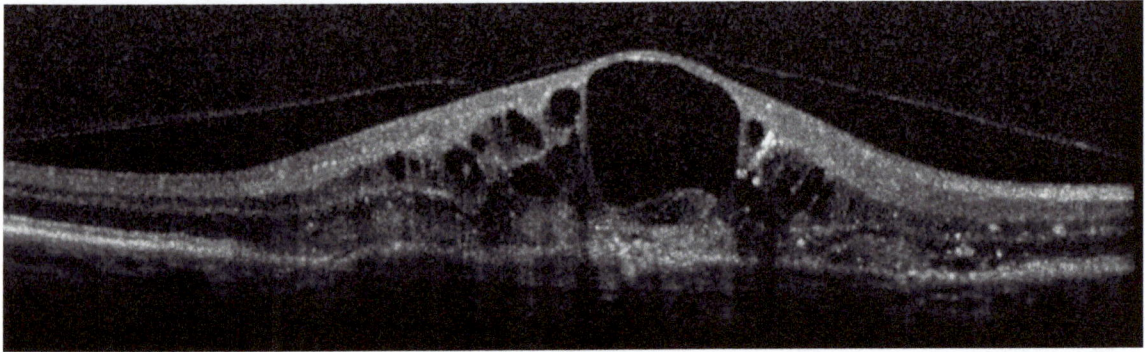

D2

Case 3: *Cystoid Macular Edema*

Clinical Summary:

60-year-old white male presents 2-months post cataract surgery and complains of gradual blurriness OS x 1 month. Post-operative vision OS is 20/60 and pre-op cataract vision 20/100.

Image Summary

A. Color Fundus: Shows limited detail due to posterior capsule opacity.

B. En face: Full thickness en face intensity image shows decreased reflectivity from numerous cystoid spaces arranged in a petaloid pattern slightly temporal to the fovea.

C. OCT Angiography: C1: Depth encoded image shows an area of impaired perfusion slightly temporal and inferior to the fovea. The impairment in perfusion appears to be largely limited to the deep retinal layer (green) since there is notable perfusion in the superficial layer (red) in the region of the defect. **C2**: Deep retinal plexus layer OCTA with corresponding B-scan and OCTA segmentation lines demonstrating the deep retinal layer. The red in the B-scan represents perfusion signal. In this case, the presence of the cystoid spaces has displaced the retina superiorly and this may have artifactually decreased the perfusion signal from the deep retinal layer. Notice that there is still perfusion along the boundary of the outer plexiform layer that is displaced slightly superior to the segmentation lines.

D. OCT: D1: Line B-scan shows areas of hyperreflectivity along the surface of the retina suggestive of an ERM that may be contributing to the retinal thickening as well. The foveal contour is significantly blunted, and there are several cystoid spaces temporal to the fovea. These correspond in location to the area of decreased perfusion on OCTA. **D2**: Volumetric OCT shows thickening involving the central subfields.

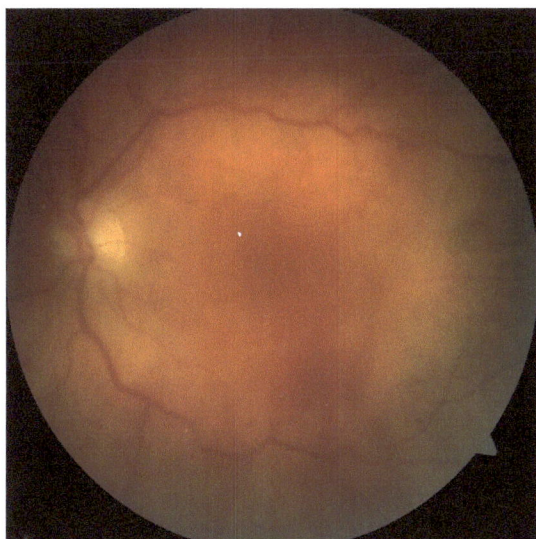

A

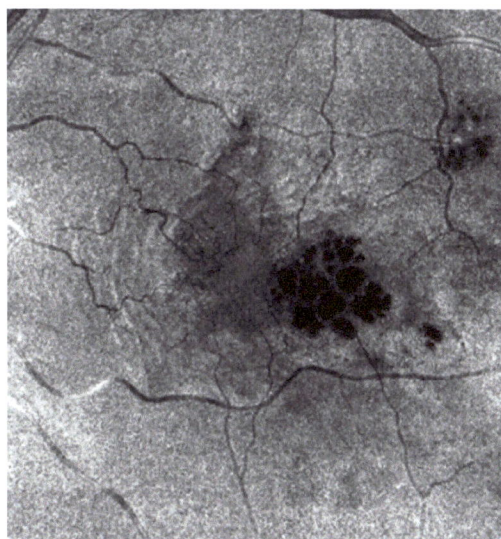

B

182

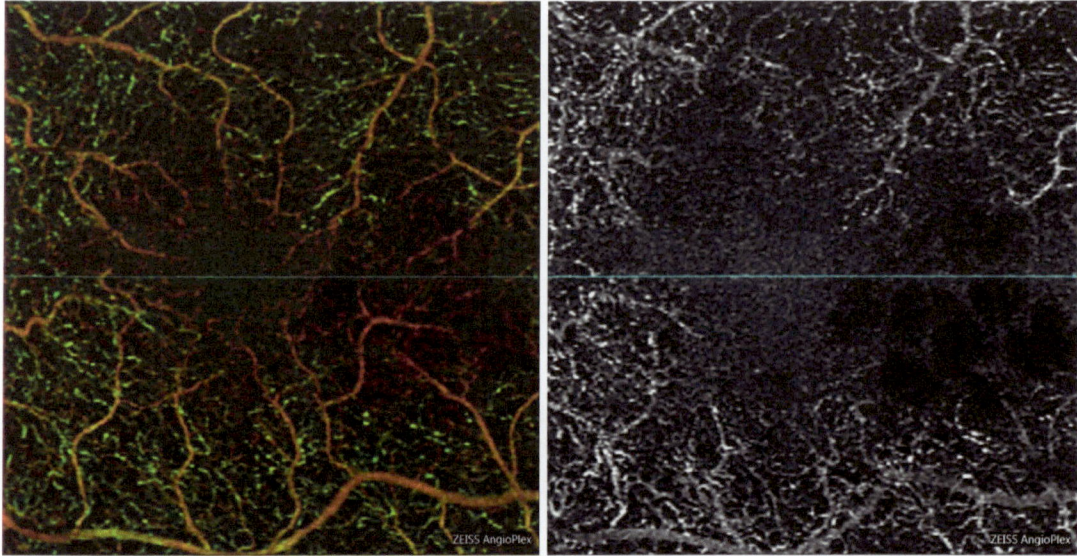

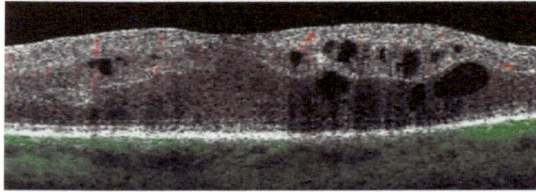

C1

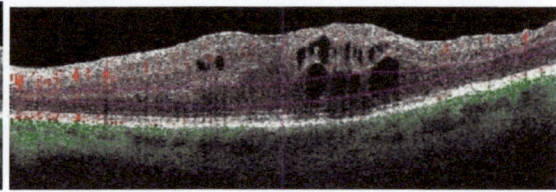

C2

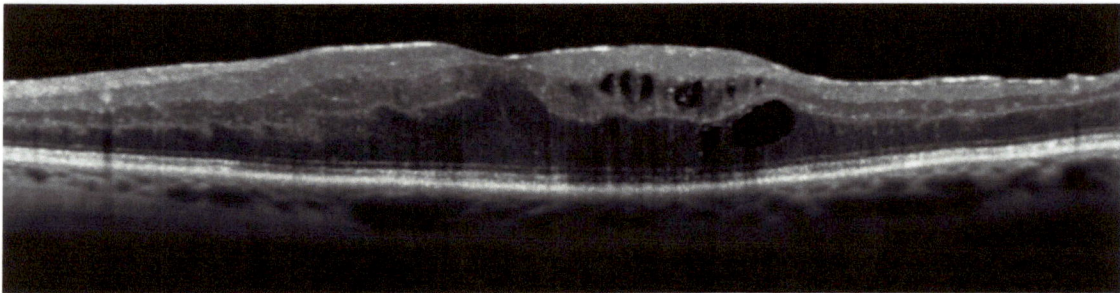

D1

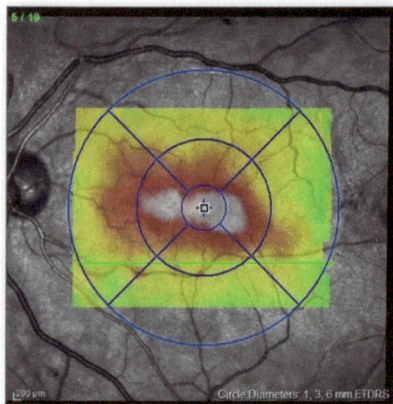

D2

Case 4: *Cystoid Macular Edema*

Clinical Summary

65-year-old white female with complaints of gradual decrease in vision OD x 3 months with metamorphopsia. Vision OD is 20/60.

Image Summary

A. Color Fundus: Shows fine yellow deposits consistent with fine drusen. There is a small choroidal nevus along the temporal aspect of the inferior arcade.

B. Fluorescein Angiography: Late phase image shows hyperfluorescence in a petaloid pattern that is concentrated around the fovea.

C. OCT Angiography: C1: Full thickness retinal composite OCTA image shows an abnormal foveal avascular zone. There are several focal enlargements of the capillaries that are consistent with microaneurysms. **C2**: The full thickness en face intensity image shows the decreased reflectivity from the cystoid spaces. The horizontal motion artifacts are obvious on this image.

D. OCT: D1: B-scan with segmentation of the full retinal thickness and perfusion signal shown in red. Note that the cystoid spaces displace the surrounding retina and the flow signal. **D2**: Line B-scan shows hyperreflective white band along retinal surface consistent with an ERM. There are several large hyporeflective intraretinal spaces consistent with macular edema.

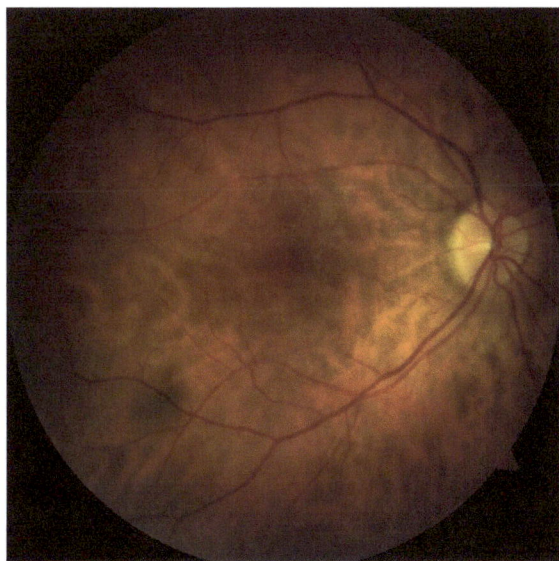

A

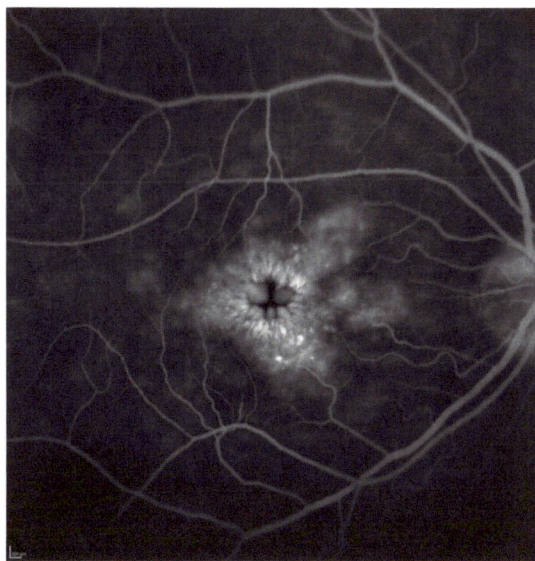

B

184

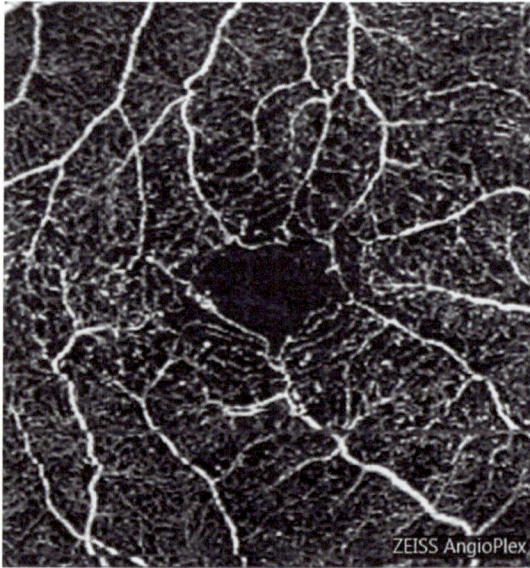

C1

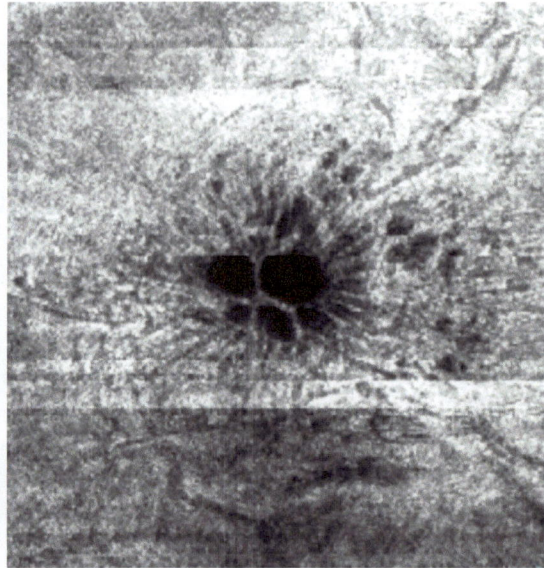

C2

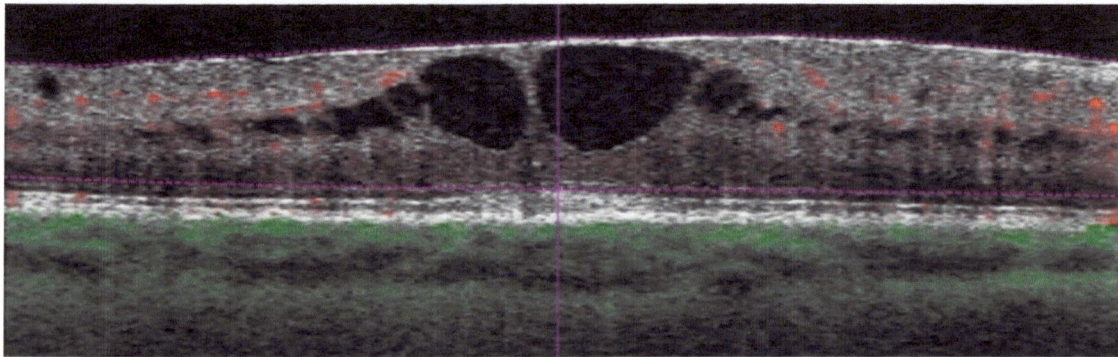

D1

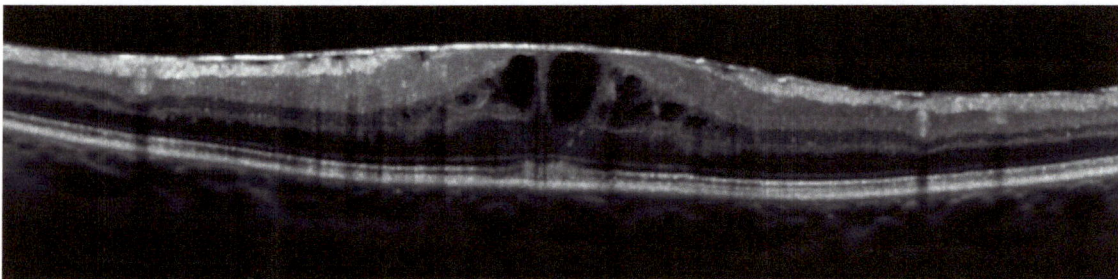

D2

Case 5: *Cystoid Macular Edema*

Clinical Summary

73-year-old white male, post cataract surgery OS, complains of gradual decrease in vision OS, starting 1-month post op. Vision is 20/70 OS.

Image Summary

A. Color Fundus: Shows a blunted foveal reflex.

B. Fluorescein Angiography: B1: Late venous phase image shows early leakage surrounding the fovea. **B2**: Late phase image shows hyperfluorescence from the optic disc as well as significantly increased fluorescence from the central macula. There are also numerous other pinpoint foci of hyperfluorescence.

C. OCT Angiography: C1: Full thickness retinal composite OCTA image shows mild distortion of the foveal avascular ring and modest attenuation of perfusion signal surrounding the fovea. **C2**: Depth encoded OCTA shows the same findings more clearly. **C3**: Full thickness en face intensity image shows numerous large and small hyporeflective regions consistent with intraretinal cystoid spaces. **C4**: B-scan from full thickness OCTA with attenuated perfusion immediately surrounding the fovea.

D. OCT: D1: Line B-scan shows a few areas of mildly increased reflectivity along the retinal surface consistent with an ERM. The foveal contour is inverted and there are several large hyporeflective cystoid spaces within the macula. There is also subretinal fluid immediately underneath the fovea. **D2**: Volumetric OCT shows significant increase in retinal thickness.

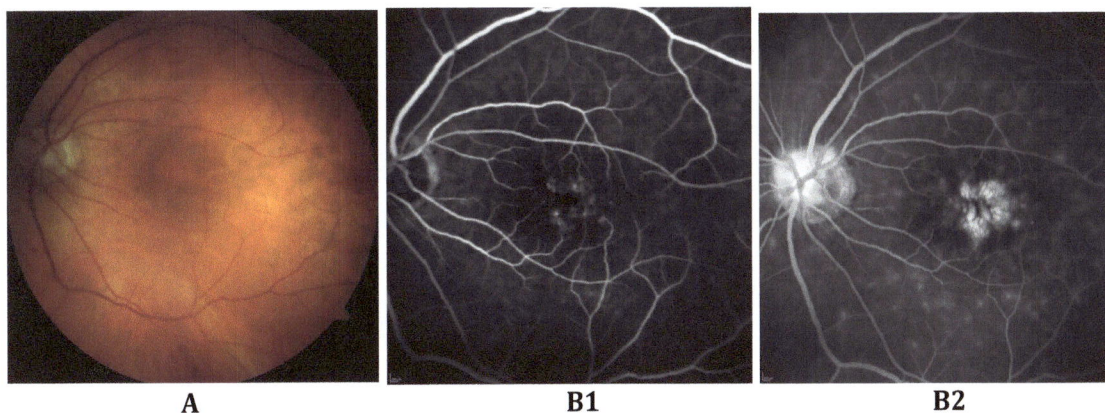

A   B1   B2

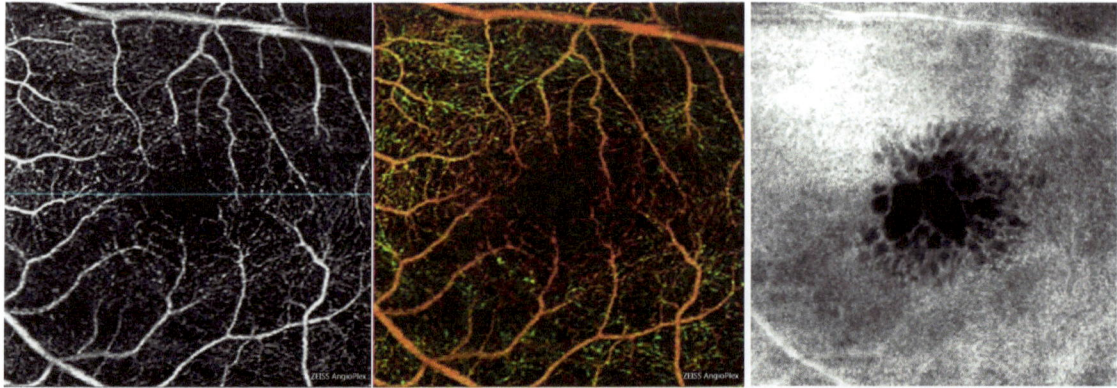

C1 **C2** **C3**

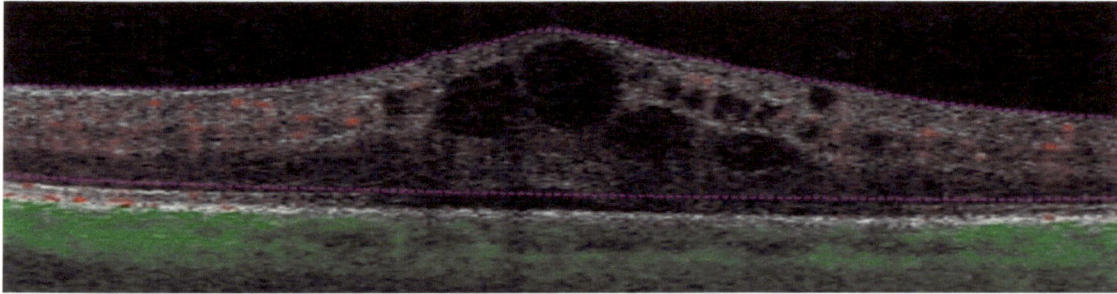

C4

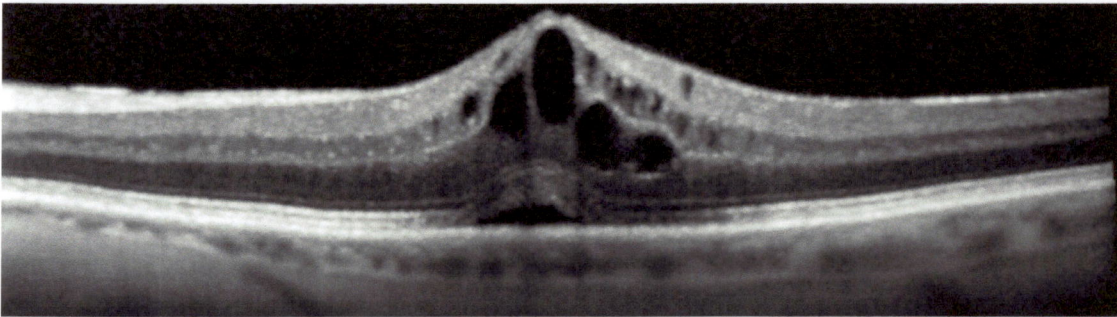

D1

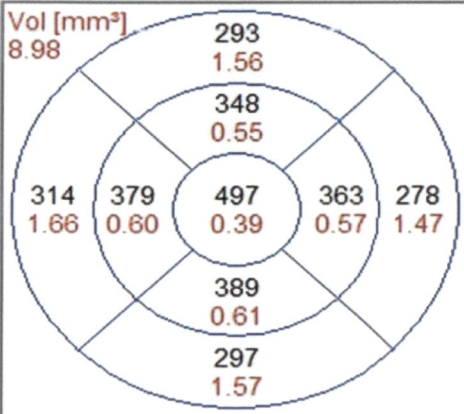
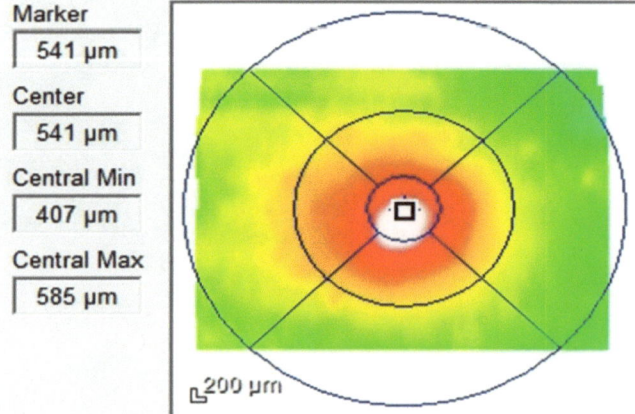

D2

Case 6: *Diabetic Macular Edema*

Clinical Summary

62-year-old white male with history of NIDDM x 15 years. Complains of blurry vision OS x 1+ year. Vision is 20/100 OS.

Image Summary

A. Color Fundus: Shows moderate to severe amounts of yellow deposits consistent with hard exudates threatening the fovea. There are several dot-blot hemorrhages. These findings suggest at least severe non-proliferative diabetic retinopathy and likely clinically significant macular edema.

B. Fluorescein Angiography: B1: Mid-phase fluorescein angiogram shows numerous areas of blockage consistent with the hard exudates and hemorrhages in the color image. There appear to be areas of impaired flow most prominent temporal to the fovea. **B2**: Late phase fluorescein angiogram shows numerous microaneurysms and diffuse hyperfluorescence consistent with diabetic macular edema. Several regions of impaired perfusion are evident inferotemporal to the fovea.

C. OCT Angiography: C1: Depth encoded OCTA with corresponding B-scan clearly shows the impaired perfusion in the deep retinal layer inferotemporal to the fovea. **C2**: Full thickness retina composite OCTA with corresponding B-scan.

D. OCT: D1: Horizontal B-scan OCT illustrates the area of edema temporal to the fovea. There are hyporeflective cystic spaces along with hyperreflective areas consistent with hard exudate. **D2**: Volumetric OCT illustrates the extent of the edema centrally and inferotemporal.

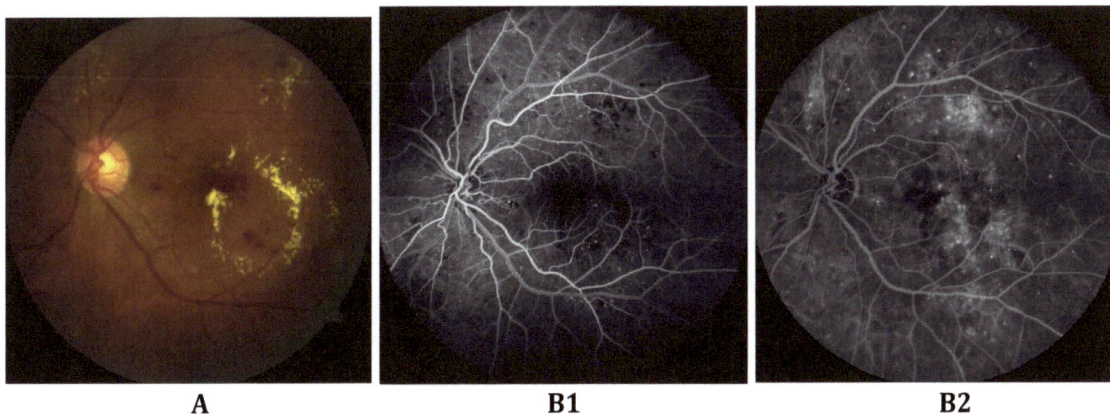

| A | B1 | B2 |

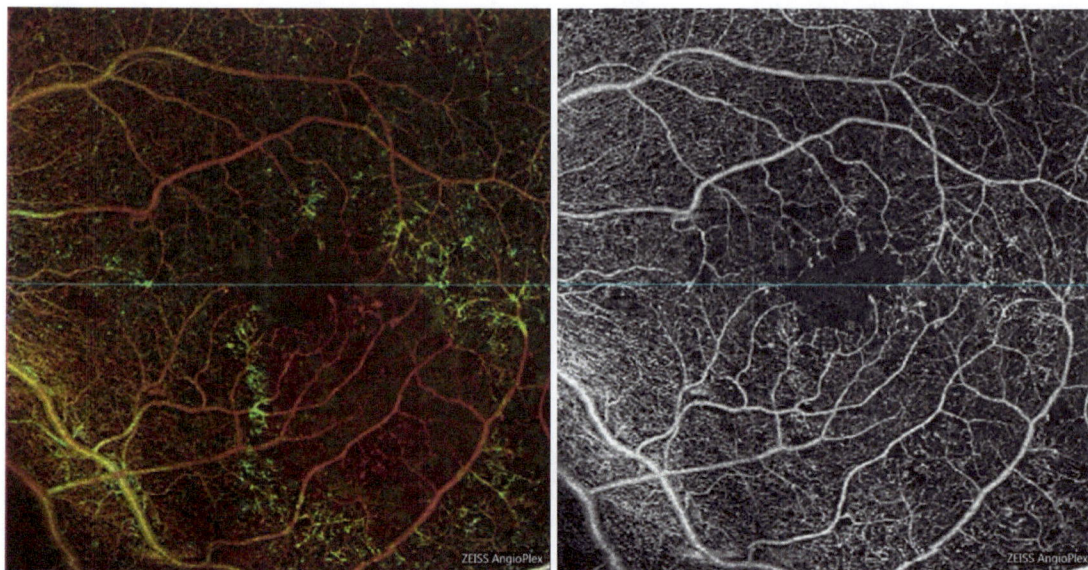

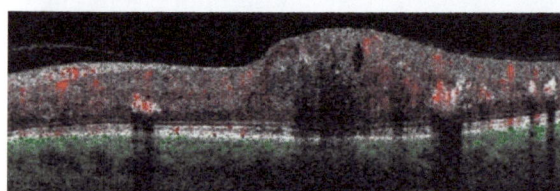
C1

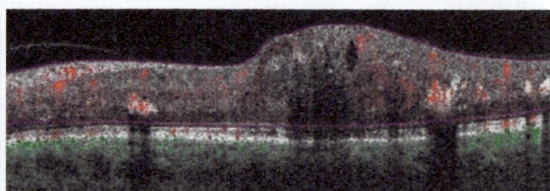
C2

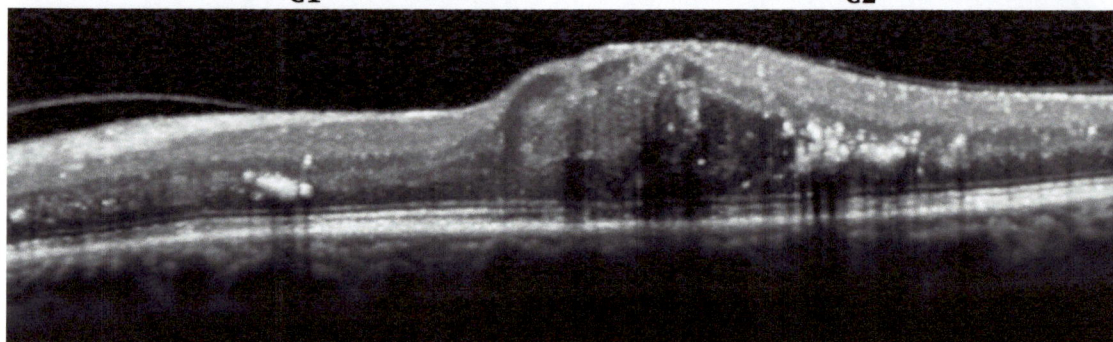
D1

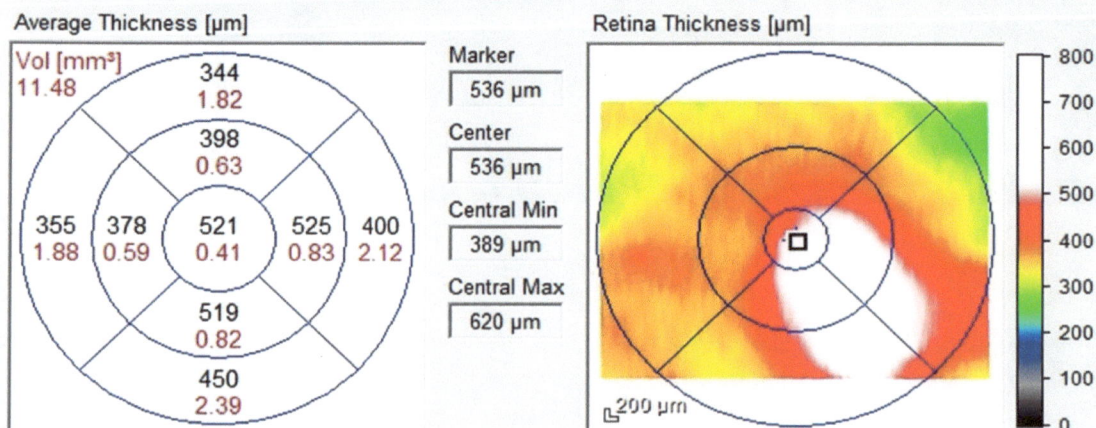
D2

Case 7: *Diabetic Macular Edema*

Clinical Summary

58-year-old white female presents with a history of non-proliferative diabetic retinopathy and complaints of general blurriness OU. Visual acuity is 20/80 OU. The patient has a history of insulin dependent diabetes mellitus for 15 years.

Image Summary

A. Color Fundus: Shows moderate to severe amounts of yellow deposits consistent with hard exudates threatening the fovea. There are several dot-blot hemorrhages. These findings suggest at least severe non-proliferative diabetic retinopathy and likely clinically significant macular edema.

B. Fluorescein Angiography: B1: Mid-phase fluorescein angiogram shows numerous areas of blockage consistent with the hard exudates and hemorrhages in the color image. There appear to be areas of impaired flow most prominent temporal to the fovea. **B2**: Late phase fluorescein angiogram shows numerous microaneurysms and diffuse hyperfluorescence corresponding to diabetic macular edema. Several regions of impaired perfusion are evident inferotemporal to the fovea.

C. OCT Angiography: C1: Superficial retinal layer OCTA shows focal areas of impaired perfusion in the temporal macula and also scattered throughout the macula. **C2**: Deep retinal layer OCTA shows more severe abnormalities in perfusion in the temporal macula and numerous foci of intense flow signal that are likely microaneurysms. **C3**: Depth encoded OCTA shows the combined image demonstrating the attenuated perfusion and numerous microaneurysmal lesions. The B-scans show that some of the microaneurysmal lesions have perfusion.

D. En face: D1: Superficial retina intensity en face and **D2**: Deep retinal layer intensity en face images show minimal artifacts and numerous hyper and hyporeflective regions. In this case the hyporeflective regions are likely cystoid spaces, while the hyperreflective regions are hard exudates.

E. OCT: E1: B-scan shows prominent intraretinal fluid in the outer retina associated with hard exudate. The overlying vitreous is attached and the pre-macular bursa is evident. **E2**: Volumetric OCT demonstrates thickened retina from edema that extends temporally.

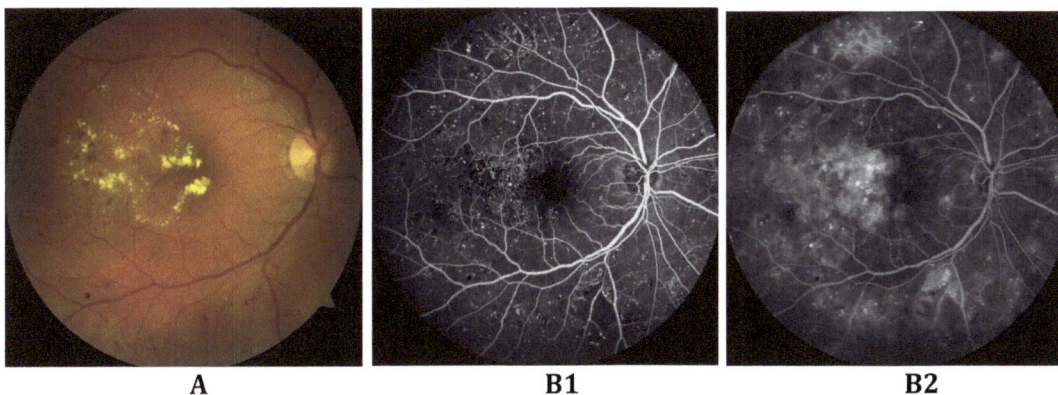

A   B1   B2

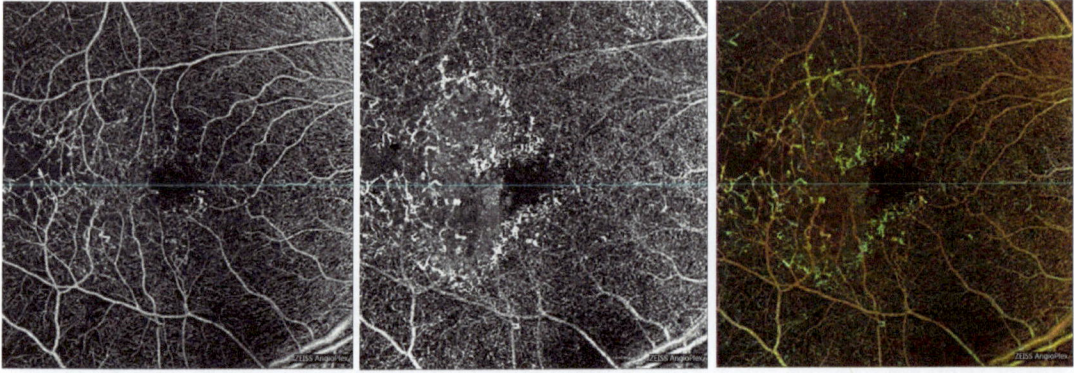

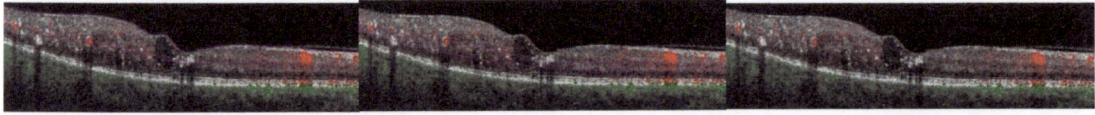

C1 C2 C3

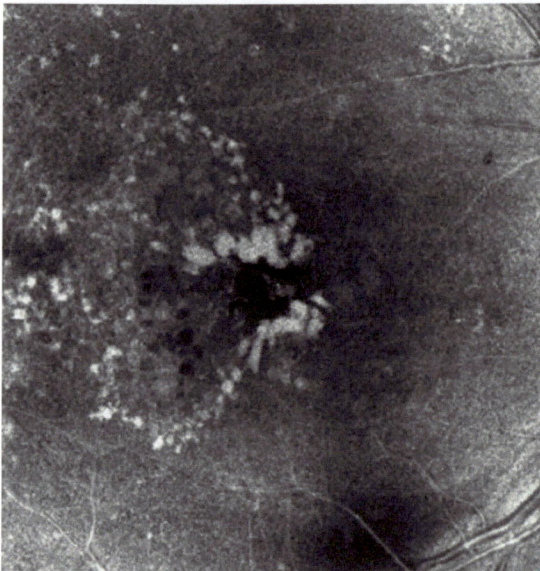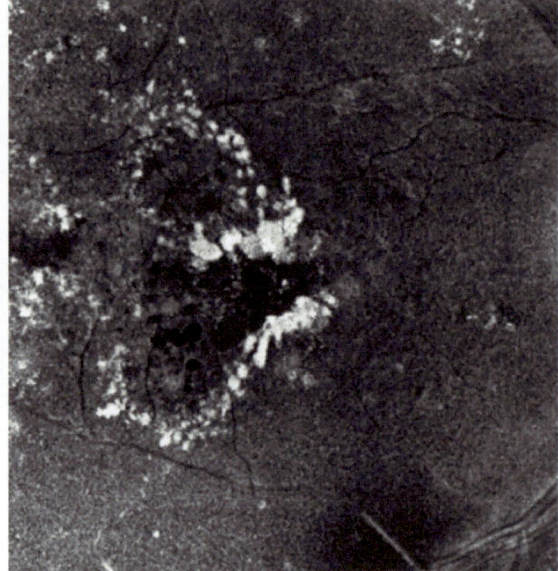

D1 D2

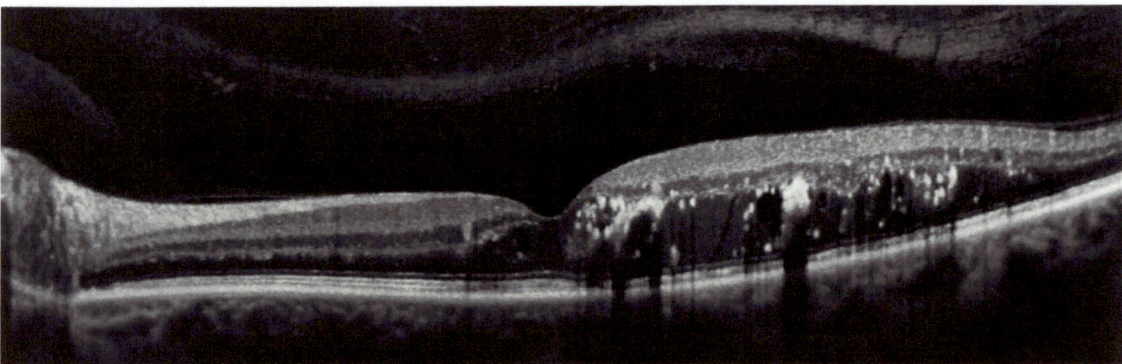

E1

191

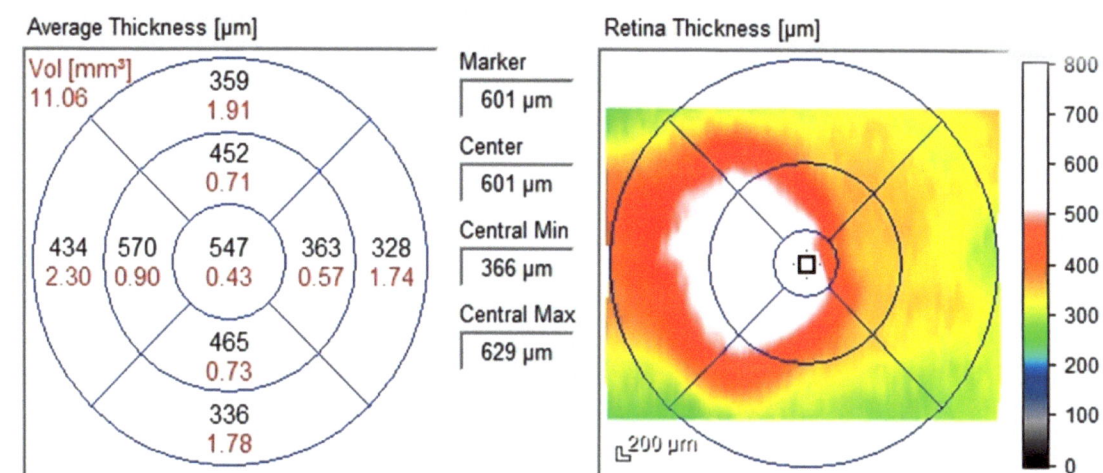

E2

Case 8: *Diabetic Macular Edema*

Clinical Summary

52-year-old African American male with IDDM x 10 years, who presents with complaints of chronic blurry vision OU. Vision OU is 20/70-. We present the right eye findings here.

Image Summary

A. Color Fundus: Shows numerous areas of intraretinal hemorrhages as well as mild amounts of hard exudate immediately inferior to the fovea. The arteries appear attenuated and there are several cotton wool spots throughout the periphery of the image. There are also a few nerve fiber layer hemorrhages along the superior arcade.

B. Fluorescein Angiography: B1: Mid-phase fluorescein angiogram shows numerous areas of impaired perfusion as well as blockage consistent with the intraretinal hemorrhages and cotton wool spots seen on the color image. **B2**: Late fluorescein angiogram shows similar findings without any diabetic macular edema.

C. OCT Angiography: C1: 3mm x 3mm depth encoded OCTA with corresponding B-scan shows impaired flow in the deep retinal layer as well as numerous areas of bright green signal, consistent with intraretinal edema associated with hard exudate. The perfusion in the superficial retinal layer also appears to be attenuated throughout. The B-scan confirms the intraretinal edema associated with hard exudate as well as the overall decrease in perfusion throughout the image. **C2**: 6mm x 6mm depth encoded OCTA with corresponding B-scan with similar findings. **C3**: Deep retinal layer OCTA with corresponding B-scan confirms the location of the intraretinal edema associated with hard exudate. **C4**: Deep retinal layer en face intensity image shows numerous areas of hyporeflectivity corresponding to intraretinal cystoid spaces, as well as numerous areas of hyperreflectivity corresponding to hard exudate.

D. OCT: D1: B-scan shows intra-retinal cystoid spaces associated with hard exudate. **D2**: Volumetric OCT illustrates thickened retina due to diffuse edema.

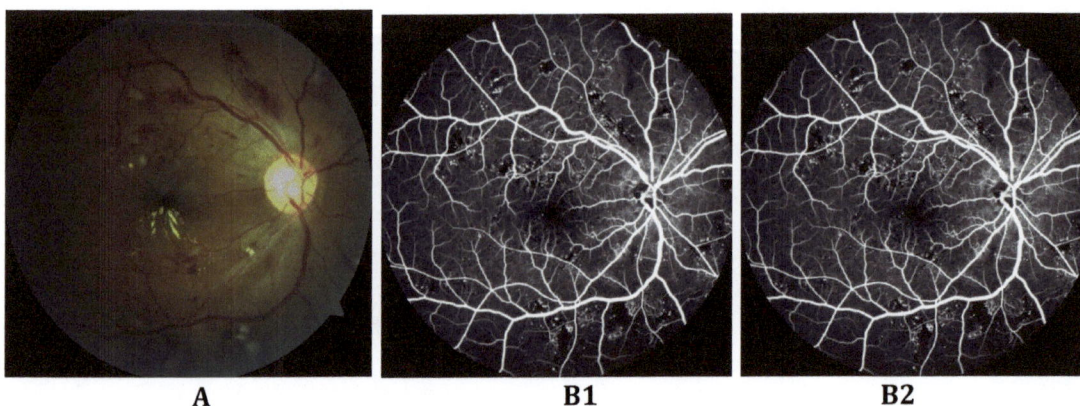

A   B1   B2

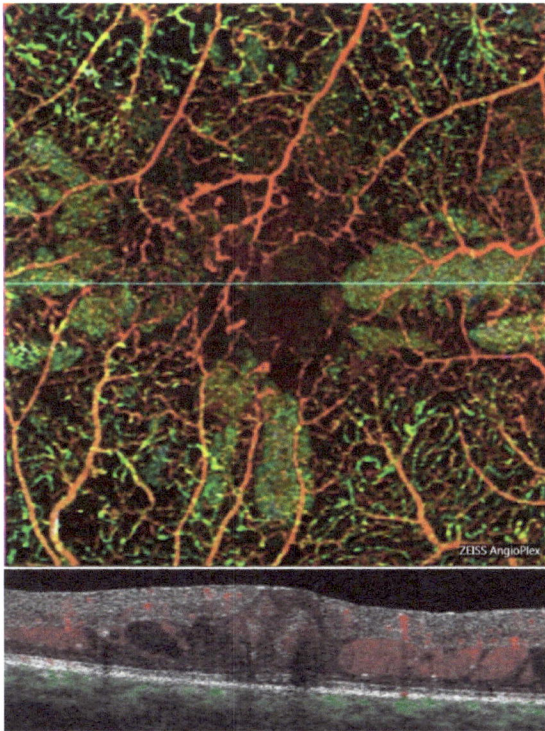
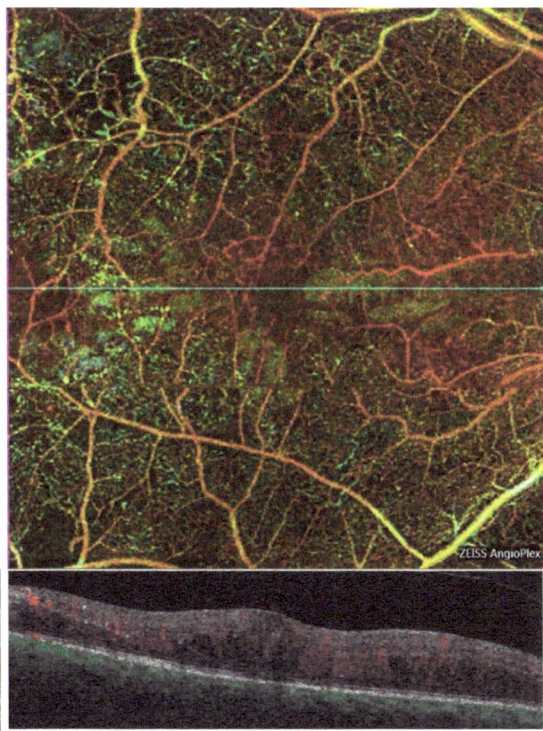

C1　　　　　　　　　**C2**

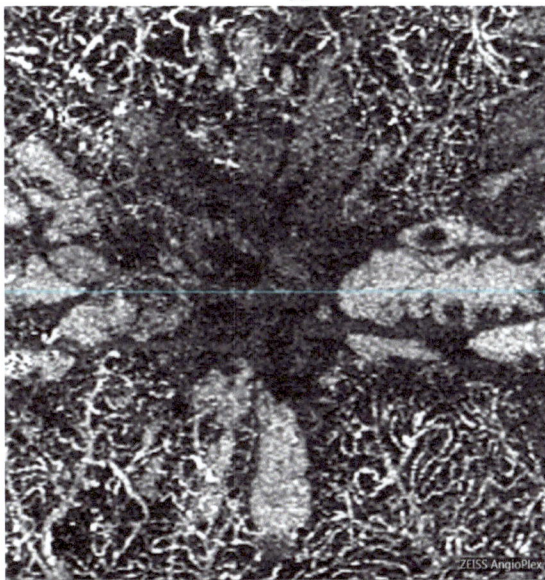
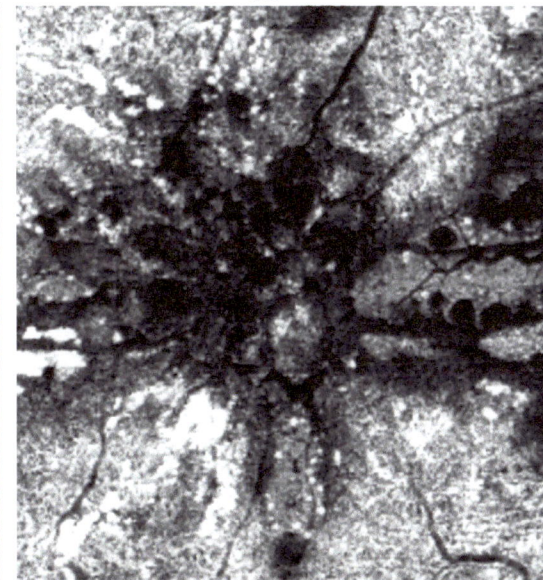

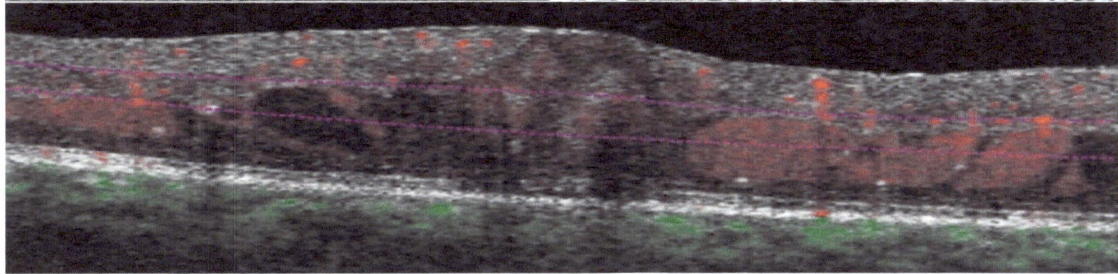

C3　　　　　　　　　**C4**

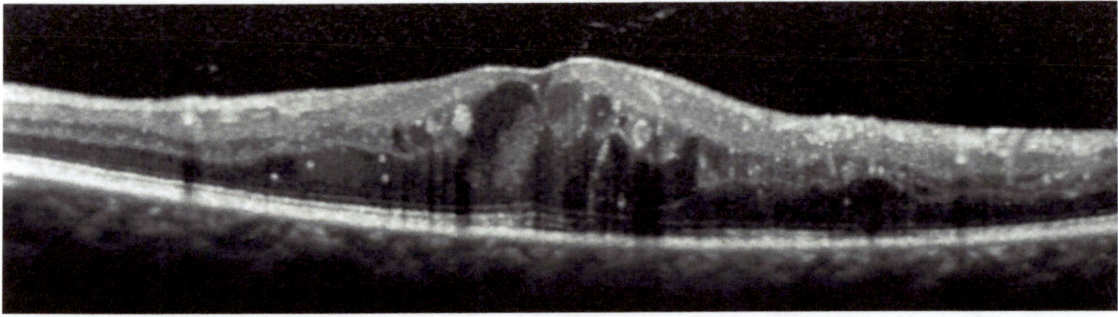

D1

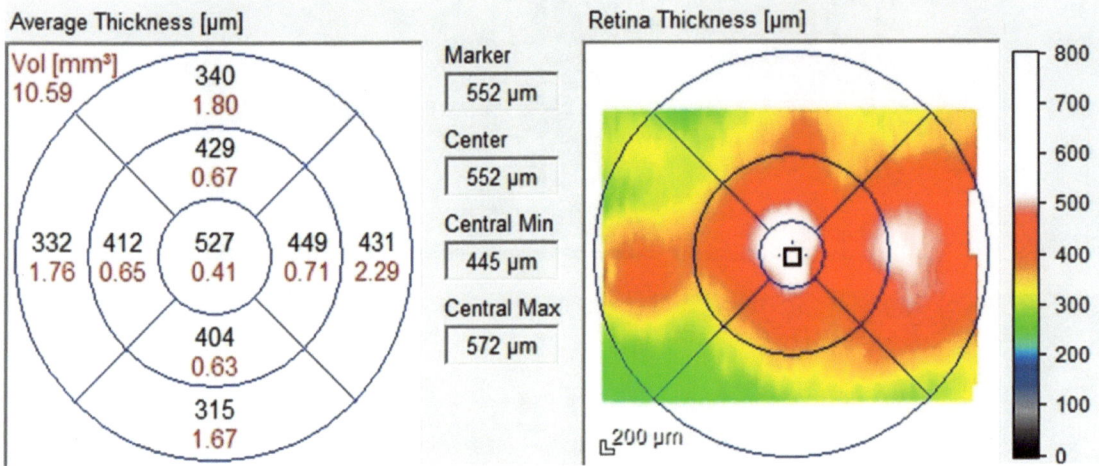

D2

Case 9: *Diabetic Macular Edema*

Clinical Summary

42-year-old white male with history of IDDM x 8 years, who presents with complaints of decrease vision OU x "months". Vision OD is 20/40, OS is 20/30. We present the right eye findings here.

Image Summary

A. Color Fundus: Shows numerous intraretinal hemorrhages and very fine yellow deposits consistent with hard exudate.

B. Fluorescein Angiography: B1: Early phase fluorescein angiogram shows a large area of impaired capillary perfusion in the temporal macula as well as numerous areas of hypofluorescence consistent with blockage from dot-blot hemorrhages. There are numerous areas of scattered impaired perfusion throughout the periphery. **B2**: Late phase fluorescein angiogram shows diffuse leakage consistent with diabetic macular edema involving nearly the entire macula. There are a few focal regions of impaired capillary perfusion or "non-perfusion".

C. OCT Angiography: C1: Depth encoded OCTA with corresponding B-scan shows several areas of impaired retinal perfusion in the periphery of the image. **C2**: Superficial retina layer OCTA with corresponding B-scan shows layer specific impairments in perfusion as well as several dilated capillaries consistent with microaneurysms. The B-scan images show that some of these microaneurysmal lesions have perfusion.

D. OCT: D1: B-scan OCT shows several small pockets of intraretinal fluid consistent with diabetic macular edema. **D2**: Volumetric OCT illustrates retinal thickening parafoveally and extending beyond in a circular pattern.

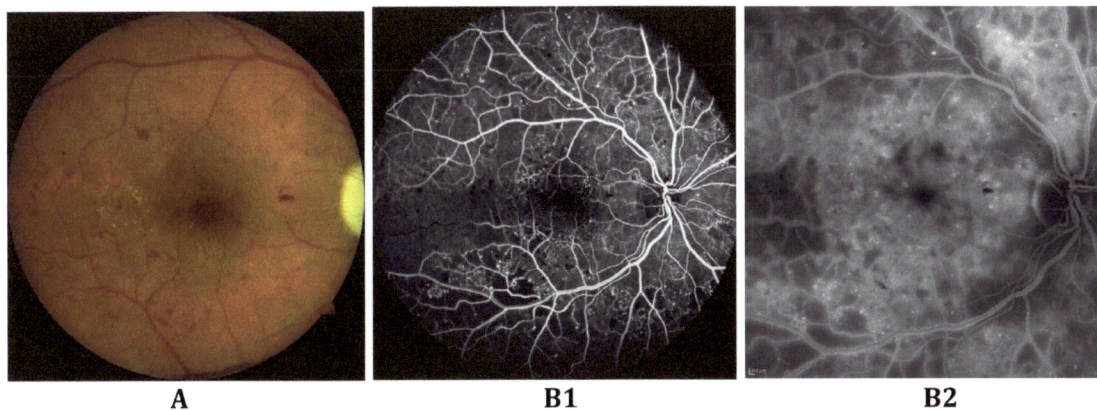

A   B1   B2

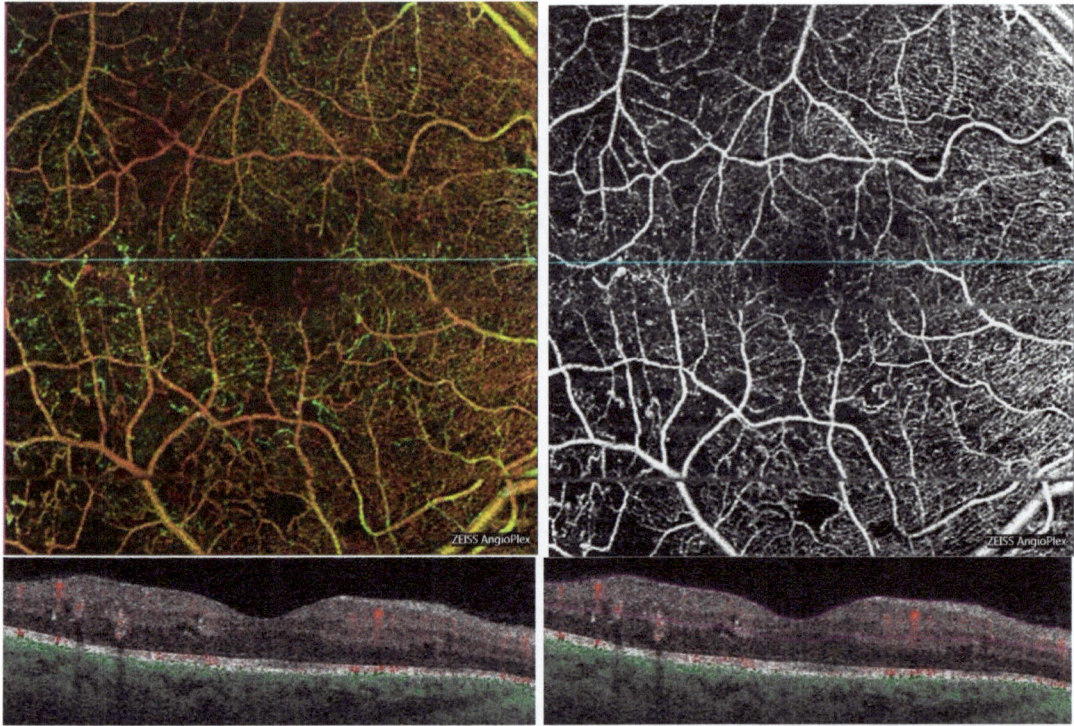

C1 **C2**

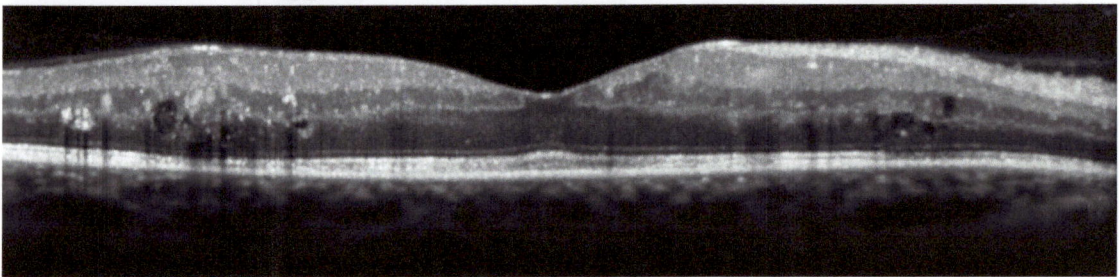

D1

Average Thickness [µm]

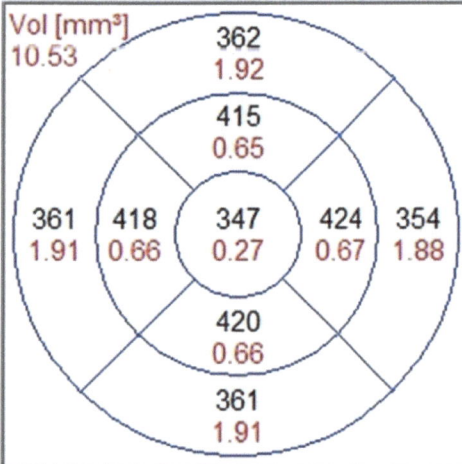

Vol [mm³]
10.53

	362	
	1.92	
	415	
	0.65	
361	418	347	424	354
1.91	0.66	0.27	0.67	1.88
	420	
	0.66	
	361	
	1.91	

Marker
287 µm

Center
287 µm

Central Min
284 µm

Central Max
402 µm

Retina Thickness [µm]

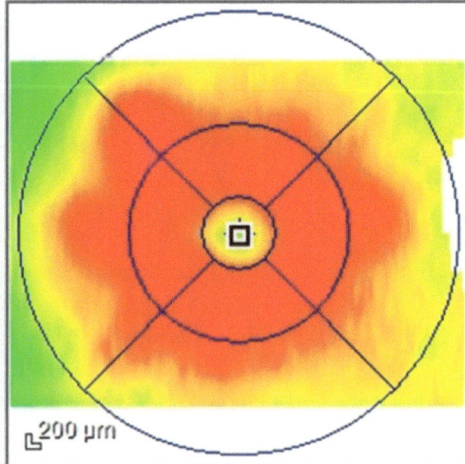

200 µm

D2

Case 10: *Non-Proliferative Diabetic Retinopathy*

Clinical Summary

56-year-old white female with history of NIDDM x 6 years, who presents with complaints of blurred vision OU, gradually worsening x 2 months. Vision is 20/50 OD and 20/70 OS.

Image Summary

A. Color Fundus: A1: Color OD shows dilated veins and attenuated arteries with an ischemic appearance to the retina. The foveal reflex is severely blunted. **A2**: Color OS shows dilated veins and attenuated arteries. There are several intraretinal hemorrhages in the temporal periphery. White or yellow lesions are present in the macula, which are consistent with the old focal scars.

B. Fluorescein Angiography: B1: Early phase fluorescein angiogram OD shows an enlarged foveal avascular zone as well as numerous pinpoint areas of hyperfluorescence consistent with microaneurysms. There are numerous regions of impaired perfusion throughout the periphery of the image. **B2**: Late phase fluorescein angiogram OD shows diffuse areas of late staining consistent with diabetic macular edema throughout most of the macula. There are two large areas of impaired perfusion in the temporal macula. The majority of the nasal half of the macula appears non-perfused as well. **B3**: Early to mid phase fluorescein angiogram OS shows similar findings to the contralateral eye. **B4**: Late phase fluorescein angiogram OS reveal intense late staining associated with the areas that had focal scars on the color image. There are a few areas of late hyperfluorescence in the periphery that maybe consistent with neovascularization.

C. OCT Angiography OD: C1: Depth encoded OCTA with corresponding B-scan shows two or three large areas of impaired perfusion in the periphery of the image. Careful examination also shows numerous areas of focal impaired perfusion in the temporal half of the image as well as the area surrounding the fovea. **C2**: Retina composite OCTA with corresponding B-scan. **C3**: Deep retinal plexus OCTA with corresponding B-scan.

D. OCT Angiography OS: D1: Depth encoded OCTA with corresponding B-scan shows a large area of impaired capillary perfusion in the right side of the image. Notice that there are multiple areas where the perfusion is superficial in the deep lead retinal layers are asymmetric as indicated by the predominance of either red or green perfusion signal. **D2**: Retina composite OCTA with corresponding B-scan and **D3**: Deep retinal plexus OCTA with corresponding B-scan confirm the same findings as the depth encoded OCTA image.

E. OCT: E1: B-scan OCT OD shows several large hypo reflective spaces within the retina consistent with cystoid spaces. **E2**: B-scan OCT OS shows blunting of the retinal banding pattern and numerous hyperreflective dots throughout the retina consistent with hard exudates.

E3: Volumetric OCT OD shows central thickening consistent with the cystic edema on the other imaging modalities. **E4**: Volumetric OCT OS shows thinning of the foveal avascular zone and immediate surrounding tissue with some pockets of thickened retina in the superior and nasal macula.

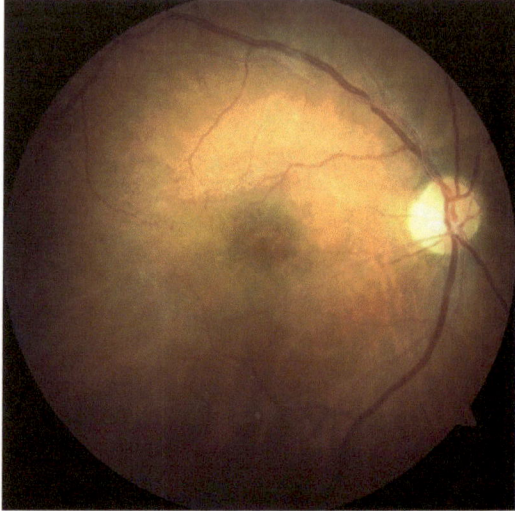

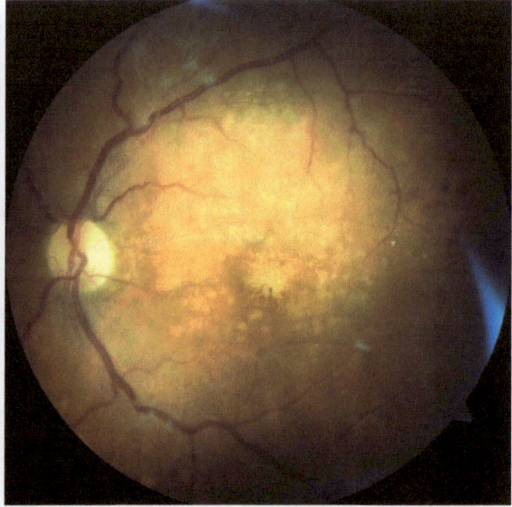

A1   A2

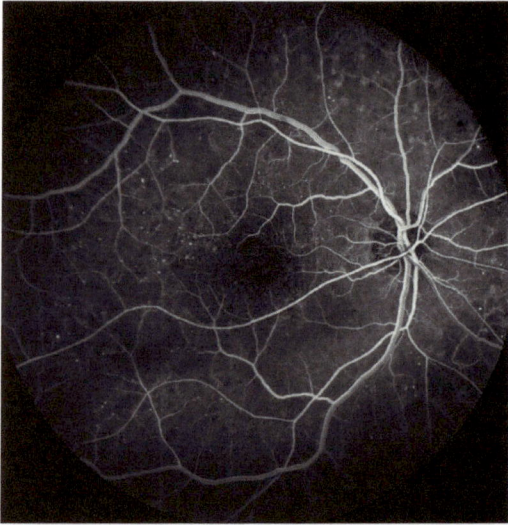

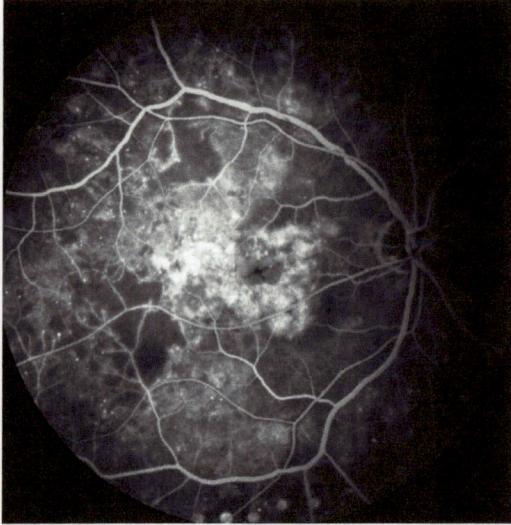

B1   B2

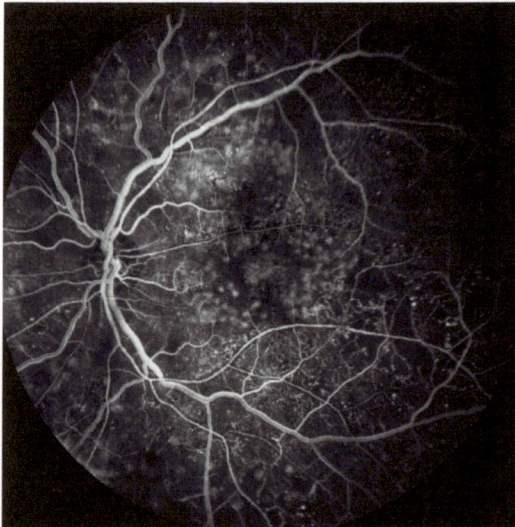

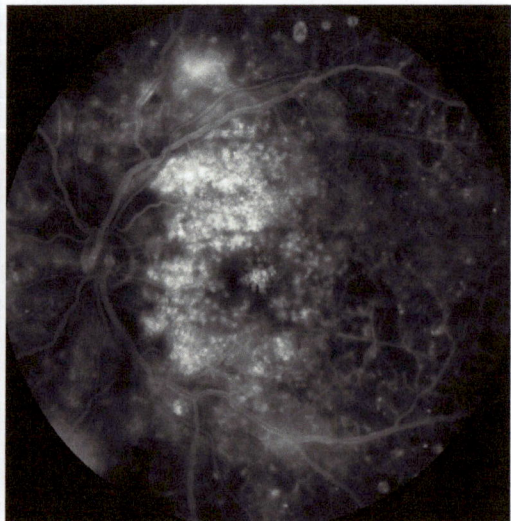

B3   B4

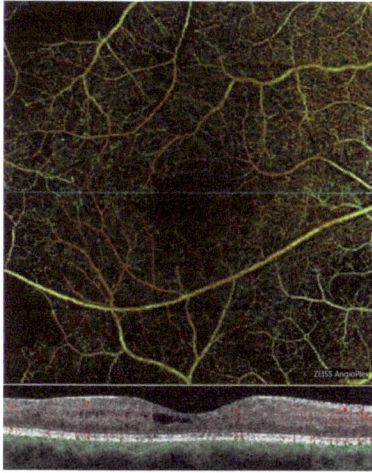
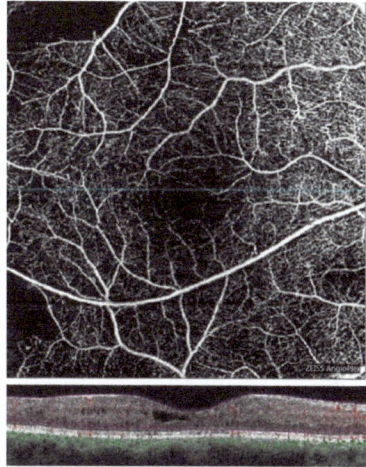
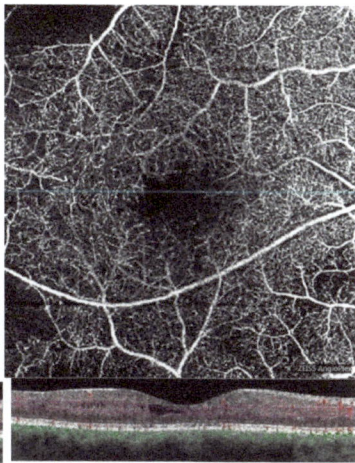

C1   C2   C3

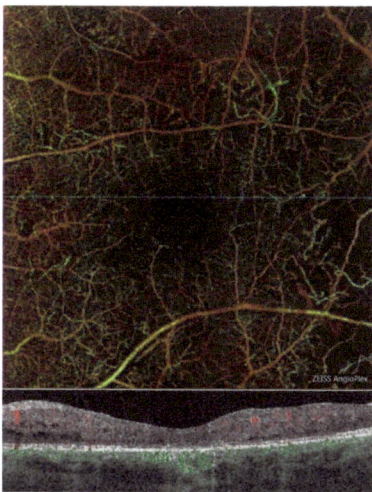
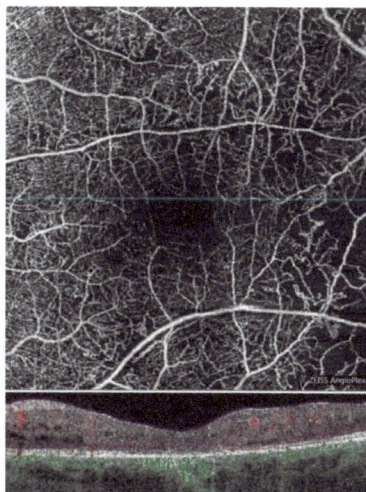
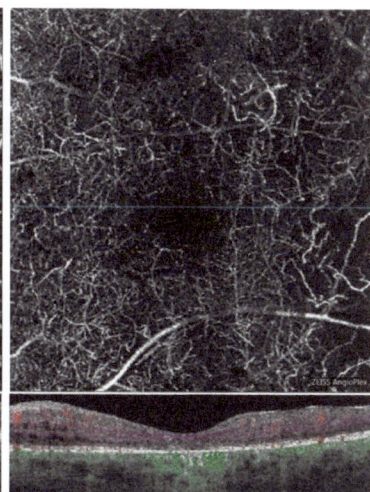

D1   D2   D3

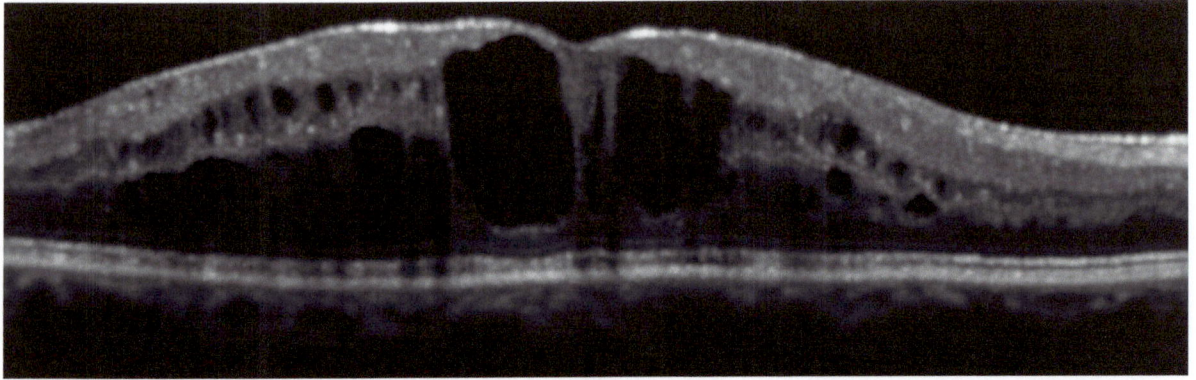

E1

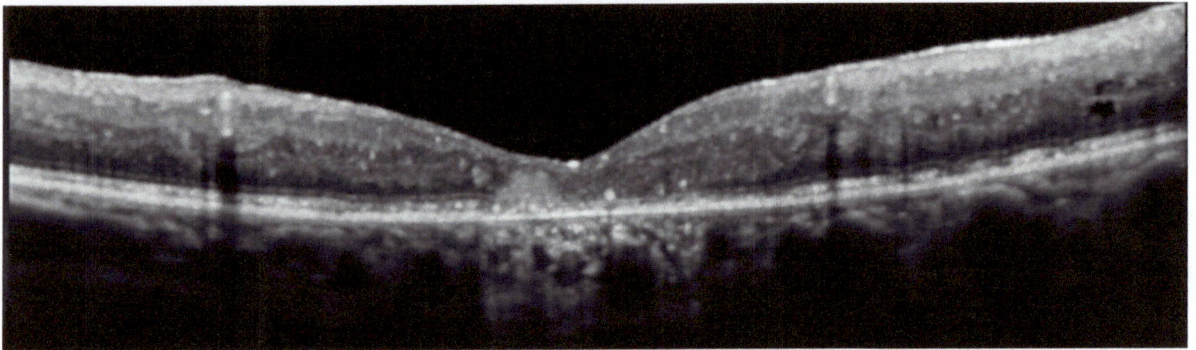

E2

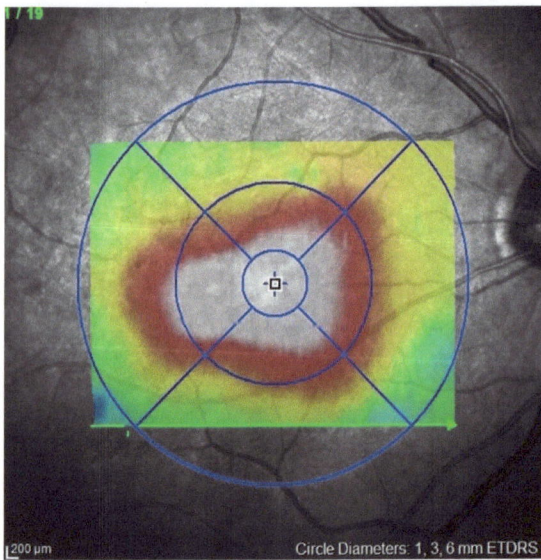

E3

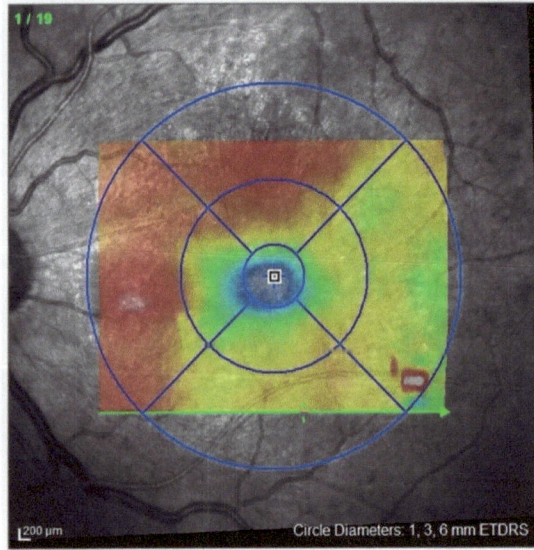

E4

Case 11: *Non-Proliferative Diabetic Retinopathy*

Clinical Summary

66-year-old white male with history of NIDDM x 15 years. referred for diabetic retinal evaluation, with no vision complaints. Vision is 20/40- OS.

Image Summary

A. Color Fundus: Shows several areas with yellow deposits consistent with hard exudates. There are several large microaneurysms that are visible.

B. Fluorescein Angiography: B1: Early to mid phase fluorescein angiogram shows numerous microaneurysms. **B2**: Late phase fluorescein angiogram shows late staining of numerous microaneurysms as well as late hyperfluorescence consistent with neovascularization of the disc.

C. OCT Angiography: C1: Depth encoded OCTA shows focal areas of impaired perfusion throughout the macula. There is asymmetric perfusion in the deep and superficial retinal layers evident by the areas with predominant red signal. The arrow indicates microaneurysms-with corresponding B-scan microaneurysms circled. **C2**: Deep retinal layer OCTA shows large area of impaired perfusion to the left of the fovea.

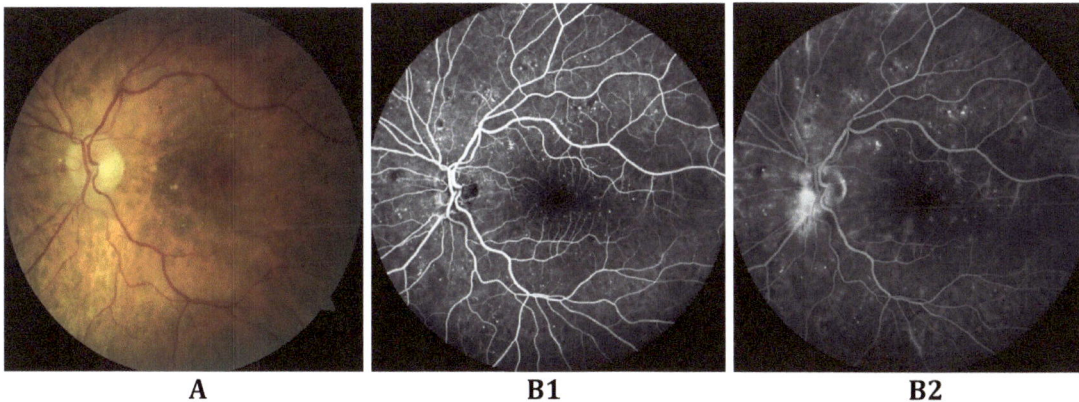

A   B1   B2

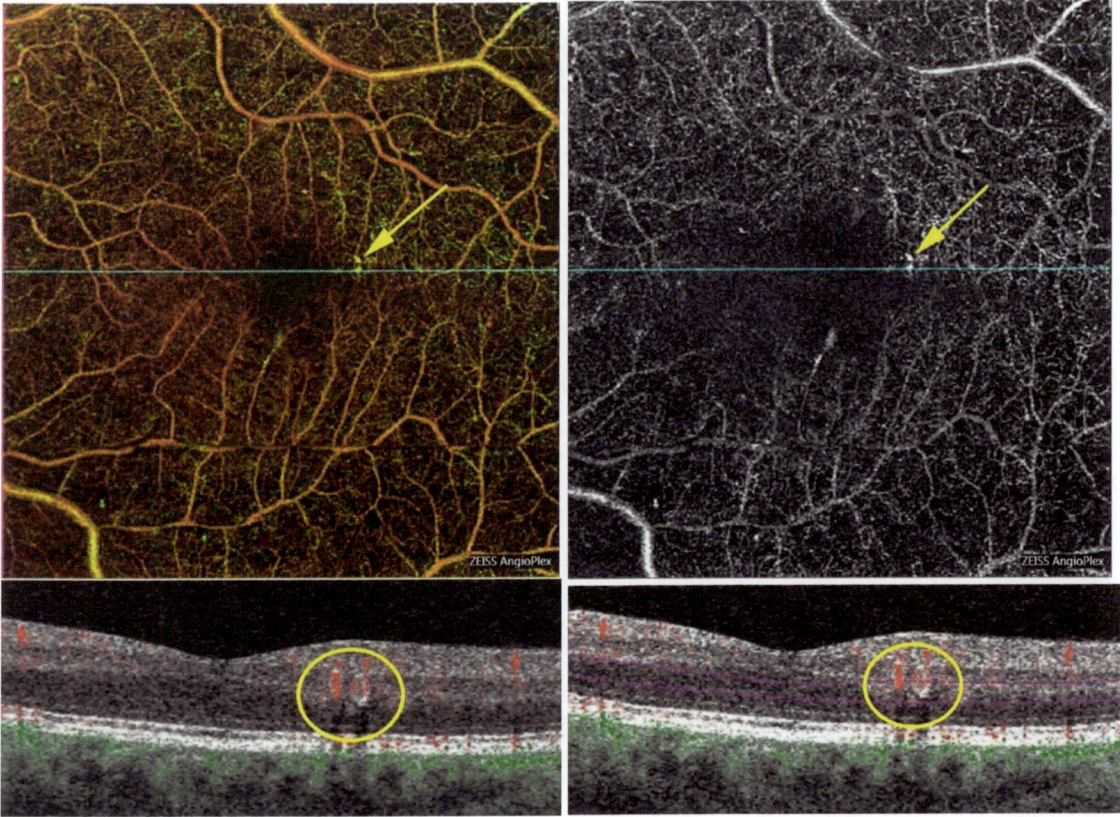

C1   C2

Case 12: *Non-Proliferative Diabetic Retinopathy*

Clinical Summary

53-year-old white male with history of IDDM x 11 years, referred for diabetic retinopathy evaluation. Vision is 20/80- OD and 20/100 OS. We present the right eye findings here. (Proliferative diabetic retinopathy OS case to follow).

Image Summary

A. Color Fundus: Shows several dot-blot hemorrhages. The view is hazy due to a cataract, and there is a blink artifact in the bottom left of the image.

B. Fluorescein Angiography: B1: Mid-phase fluorescein angiogram shows numerous pinpoint areas of hyperfluorescence consistent with microaneurysms. There are large areas of impaired capillary perfusion involving the fovea as well as the temporal half of the image. There is a large shadow to the right of the optic nerve that is consistent with opacity in the vitreous. **B2**: Late phase fluorescein angiogram shows diffuse late hyperfluorescence involving most of the macula consistent with diabetic macular edema.

C. OCT Angiography: C1: Depth encoded OCTA with corresponding B-scan shows large areas of impaired capillary perfusion involving both the superficial and deep retinal layers on the left side of the image. There is also attenuation of the deep retinal layer perfusion surrounding the fovea and immediately inferior to the fovea. **C2**: Full thickness retina composite OCTA with corresponding B-scan better illustrates the impaired capillary perfusion.

D. OCT: D1: B-scan OCT shows numerous large intraretinal hyporeflective lesions consistent with cystoid spaces. The foveal contour is completely blunted. **D2**: Volumetric OCT illustrates central thickening that extends inferiorly, as seen on the depth encoded OCTA.

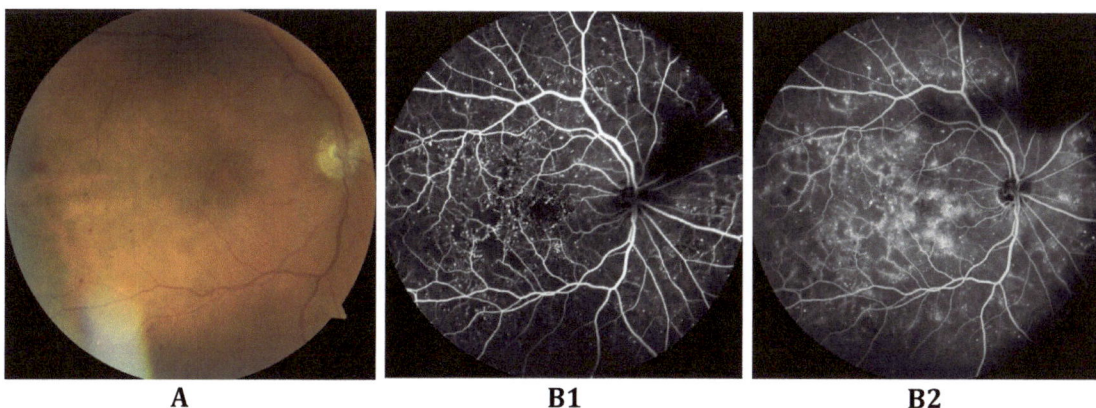

A   B1   B2

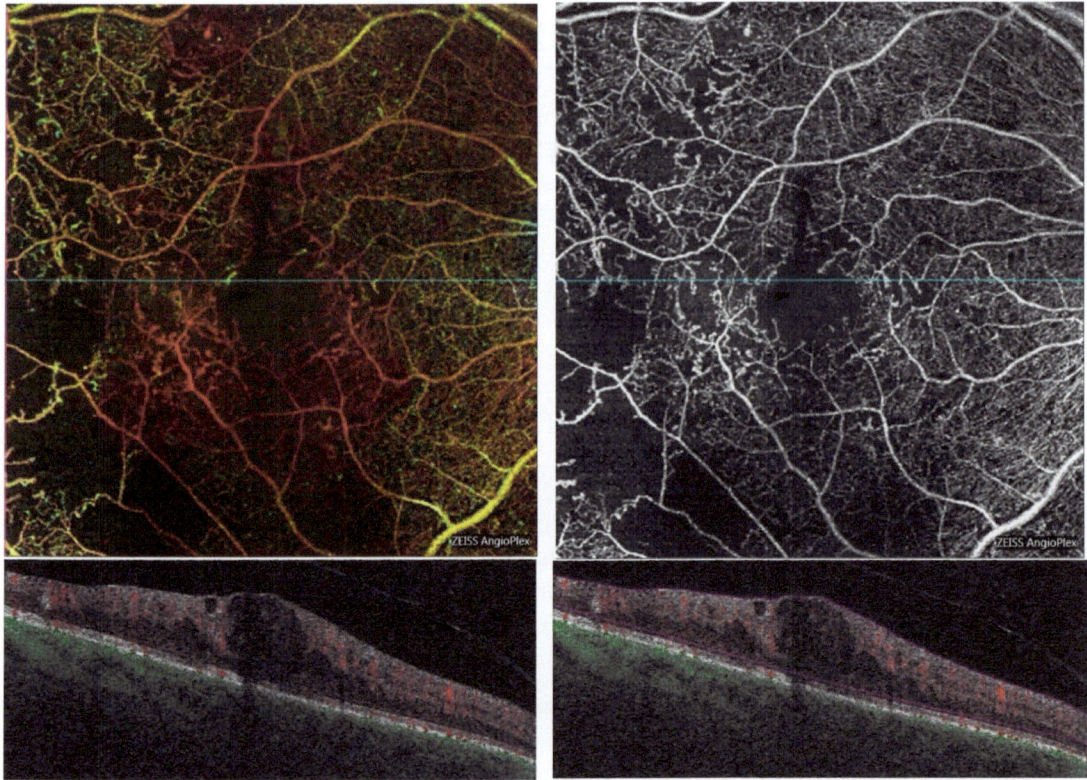

C1   C2

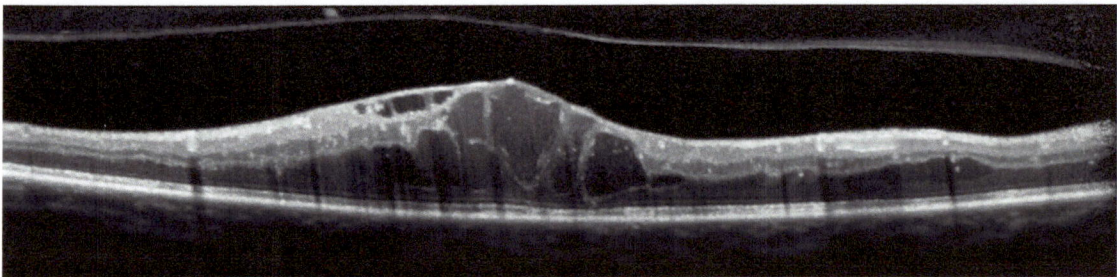

D1

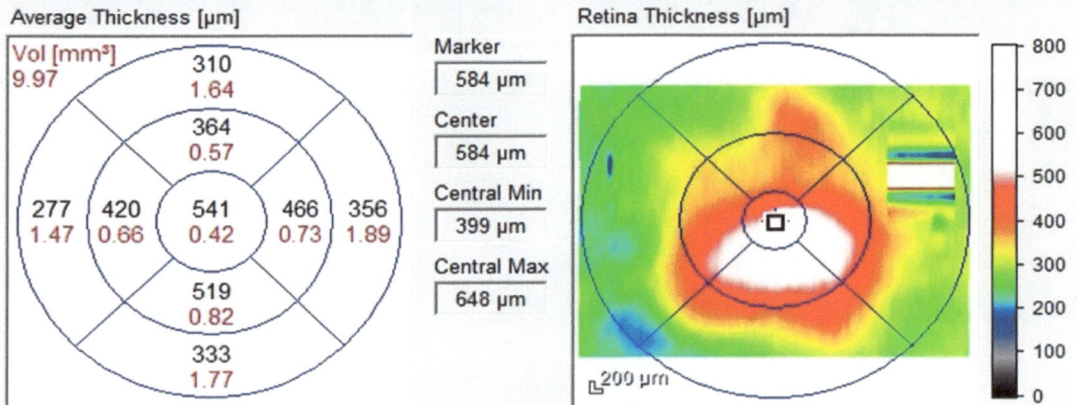

D2

Case 13: *Proliferative Diabetic Retinopathy*

Clinical Summary

(Same as the previous case)

Image Summary

A. Color Fundus: Shows several intraretinal hemorrhages. There is a sclerotic vessel in the inferotemporal macula and the temporal macula appears ischemic.

B. Fluorescein Angiography: B1: Early to mid phase fluorescein angiogram shows a very large area of impaired perfusion involving almost the entire temporal half of the macula. There are numerous pinpoint areas of hyperfluorescence consistent with microaneurysms. **B2**: Late phase fluorescein angiogram shows similar findings to the earlier image the addition of late hyperfluorescence and leakage that is consistent with multiple areas of neovascularization.

C. OCT Angiography: C1: Depth encoded OCTA with corresponding B-scan shows that the temporal half of the macula has essentially no perfusion. The corresponding B-scans show loss of the inner retina. There is a small tuft of neovascularization in the bottom right of the image. **C2**: Superficial retinal layer OCTA with corresponding B-scan confirms previous findings. **C3**: Depth encoded OCTA of NVE. **C4**: Magnified depth encoded OCTA of NVE. **C5**: Superficial retina OCTA of NVE. **C6**: Vitreo-retinal interface (VRI) layer OCTA of NVE

D. OCT: D1: B-scan of NVE from OCTA shows perfusion in the tissue that is overlying the retina consistent with active NVE. The large area of red signal corresponds to a large vessel passing through that region of the B-scan. **D2**: Volumetric OCT shows thinning of the retina temporal to the fovea and extending into the periphery, consistent with the findings of non-perfusion seen in the other imaging modalities.

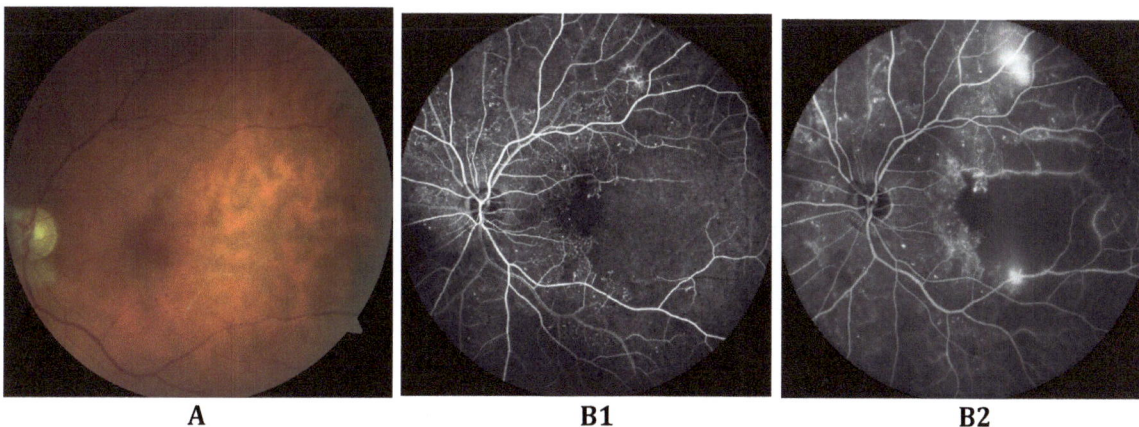

A   B1   B2

206

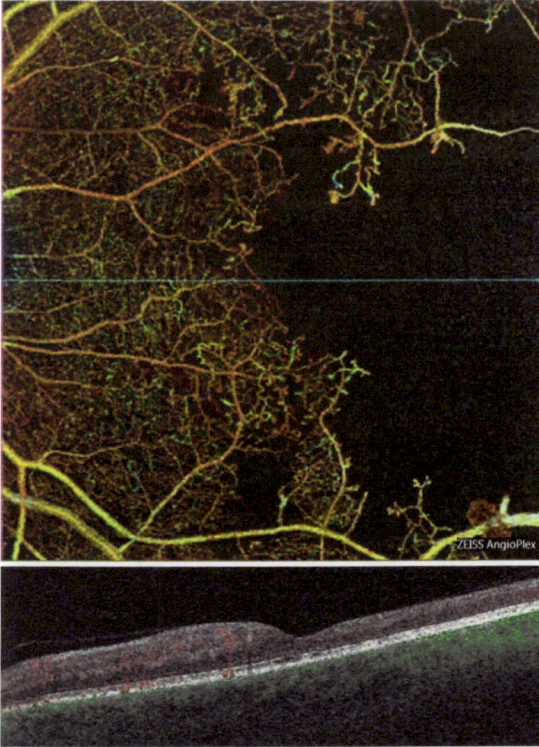

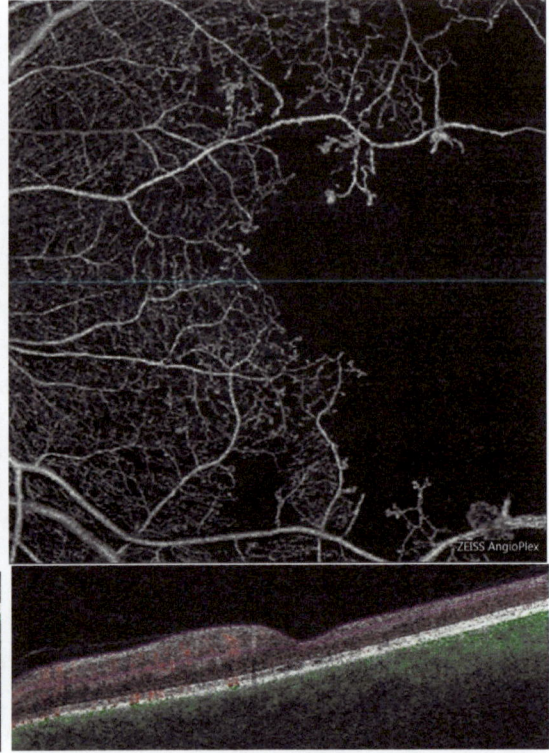

C1

C2

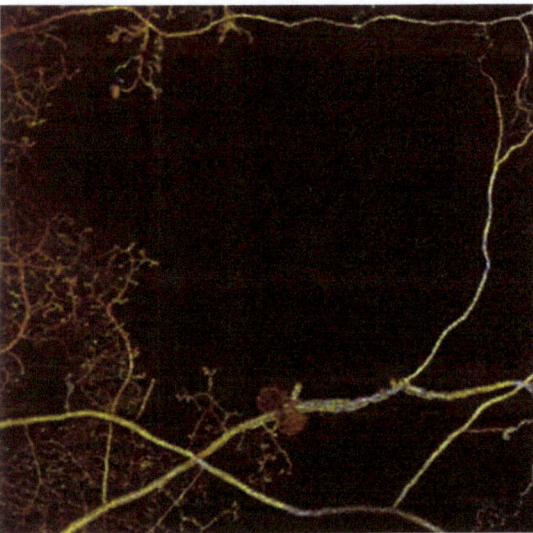

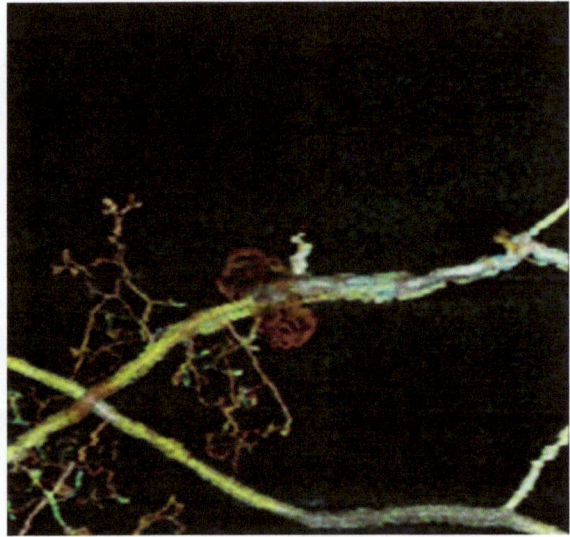

C3

C4

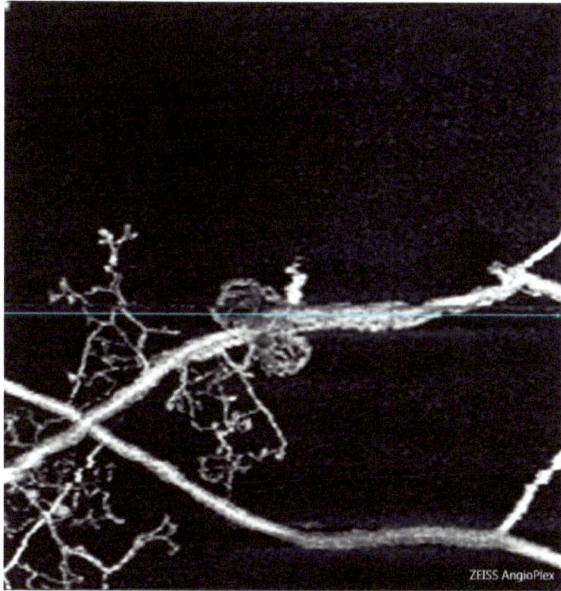

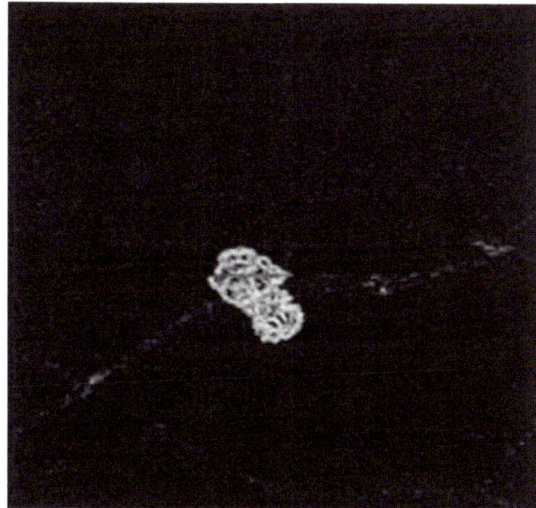

C5

C6

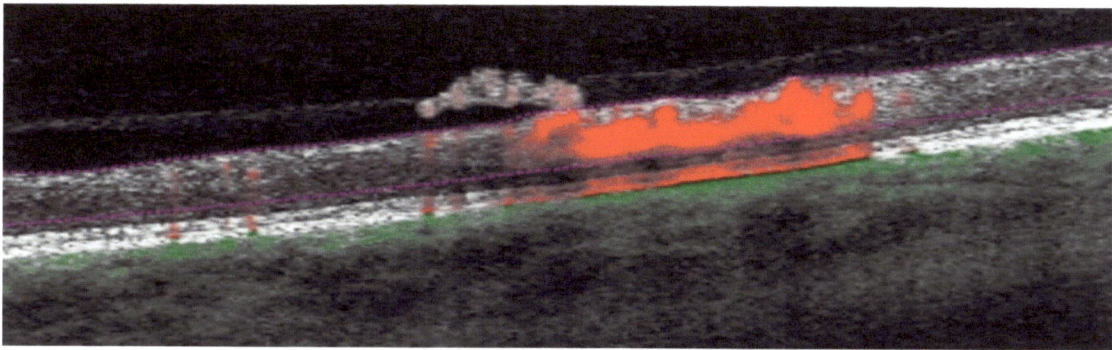

D1

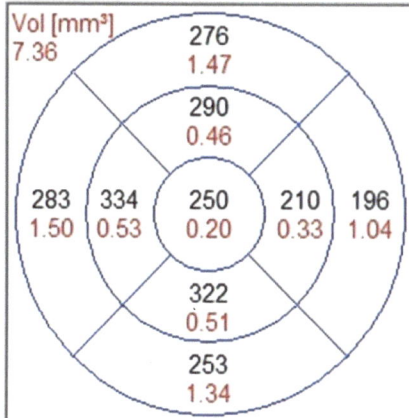

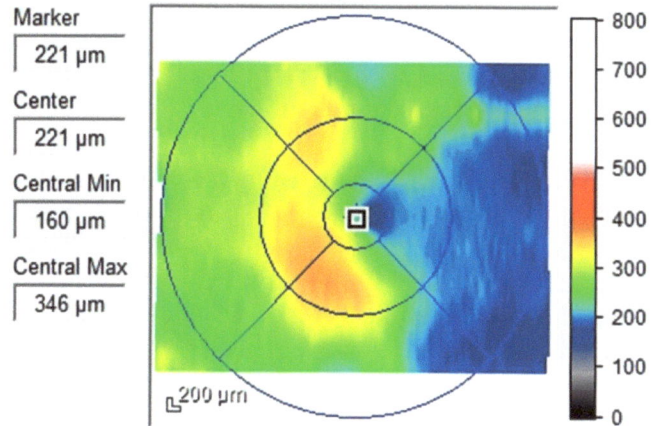

D2

Case 14: *Proliferative Diabetic Retinopathy*

Clinical Summary

28-year-old white male with Type1 IDDM presents with complaints of decrease vision OU for "years". Visual acuity is 20/30 OU.

Image Summary

A. Color Fundus: A1: Color montage fundus image OD shows attenuated arteries, dilated veins, and sclerotic vessel superotemporally. There are numerous white and pigmented lesions in the periphery that are consistent with old laser scars, and there are numerous intraretinal hemorrhages throughout. **A2**: Color montage fundus image OS shows similar findings to OD with the addition of a boat shaped hemorrhage overlying the inferior arcade.

B. Fluorescein Angiography: B1: Mid-phase fluorescein angiogram OD shows mild staining of old laser scars and a large area of impaired capillary perfusion temporal to the disc. There is hyperfluorescence around the disc indicating NVD. **B2**: Late phase angiogram OD shows similar findings with much more late phase leakage. **B3**: Mid-phase fluorescein angiogram OS shows similar findings to OD. There is a shadow in the lower left of the image consistent with a vitreous hemorrhage. **B4**: Late phase fluorescein angiogram shows continued hyperfluorescence in the areas of neovascularization, and staining of the retinal vessels.

C. OCT Angiography: C1: Depth encoded OCTA with corresponding B-scan OD shows large area of impaired perfusion involving almost the whole temporal macula. The nasal macula has very abnormal and reduced capillary density in both the superficial and deep capillary layers. There is a patch of superficial perfusion (red) in the upper right of the image that is consistent with NVD. Note the paucity of perfusion signal on the B-scan as well. **C2**: Full thickness retina composite with corresponding B-scan OD shows similar findings. **C3**: Depth encoded OCTA of disc with corresponding B-scan shows peripheral regions of impaired perfusion. There is a significant amount of NVD involving almost the whole image and appearing red. **C4**: Vitreo-retinal interface OCTA with corresponding B-scan shows the NVD more clearly. The pattern of capillaries in this image is consistent with NVD rather than the normal peripapillary vasculature. The corresponding B-scans clearly show the perfusion in the membrane overlying the retina consistent with NVD.
C5: Depth encoded OCTA with corresponding B-scan OS shows similar findings to OD. **C6**: Deep retinal layer OCTA with corresponding B-scan OS shows similar findings to OD.

D. OCT: D1: B-scan OCT OD shows numerous intraretinal cystoid spaces and a few hyperreflective foci consistent with hard exudates. **D2**: B-scan OCT OS shows similar findings to OD with numerous pinpoint hyperreflective spots in the vitreous consistent with vitreous hemorrhage in the color photo. **D3**: Volumetric OCT OD shows fairly thin-normal retinal thickness, with the exception of the presence of NVD. **D4**: Volumetric OCT OS shows thickening temporal to the fovea, consistent with the cystic fluid seen on OCT.

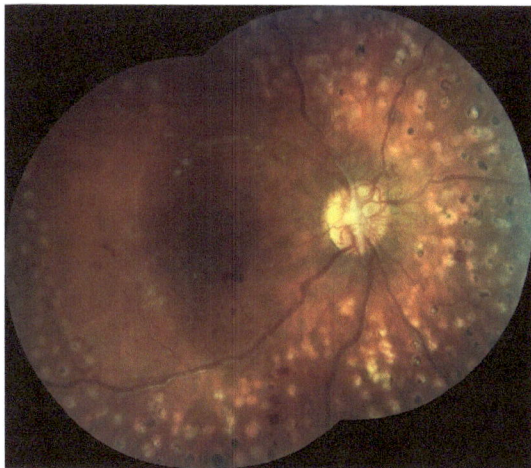

A1

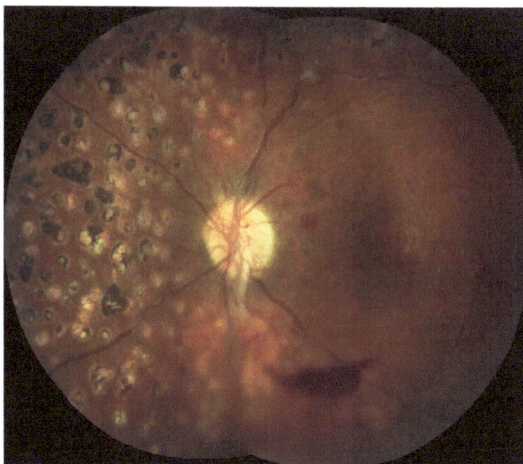

A2

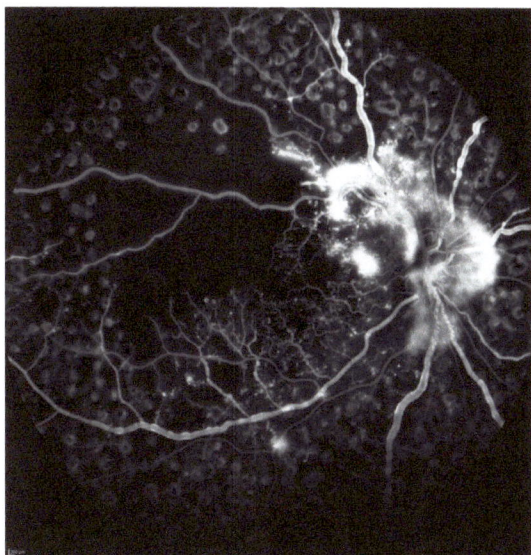

B1

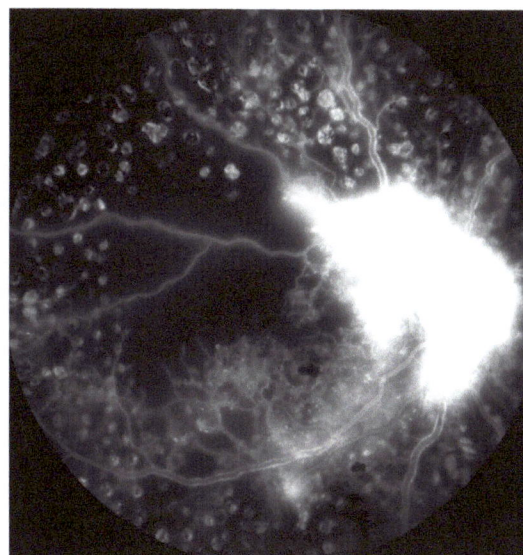

B2

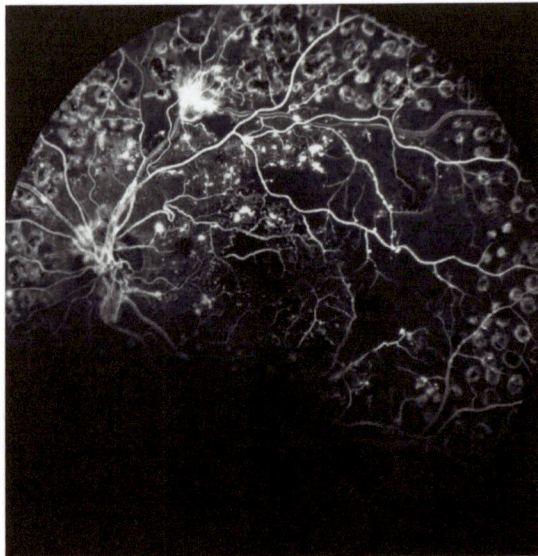

B3

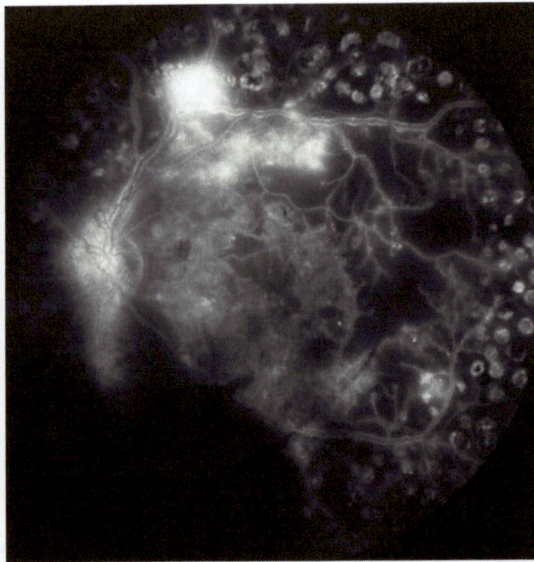

B4

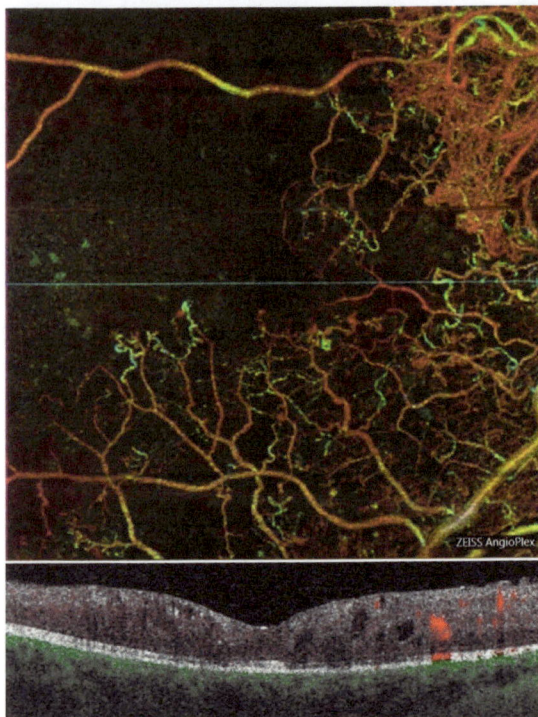

C1

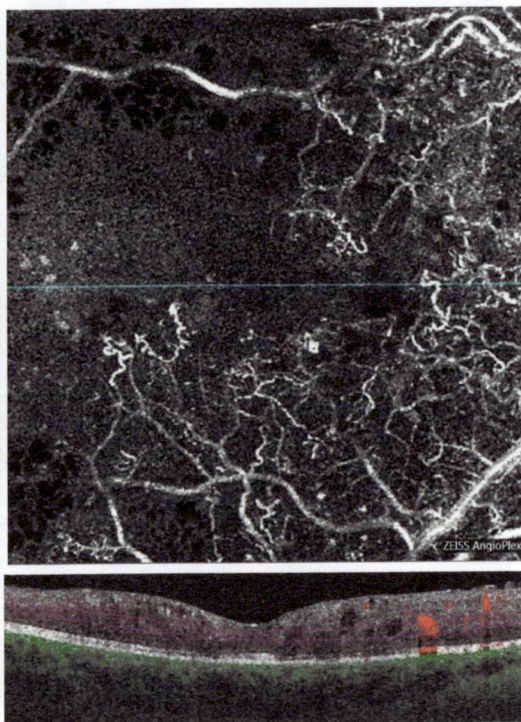

C2

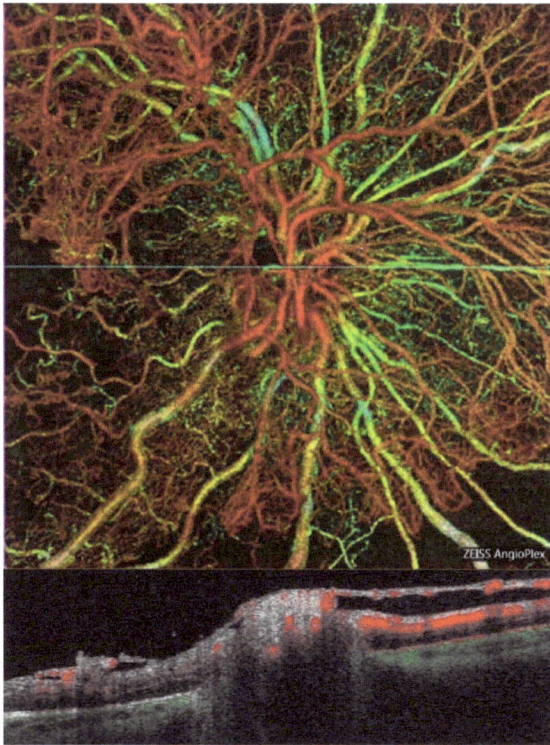

C3

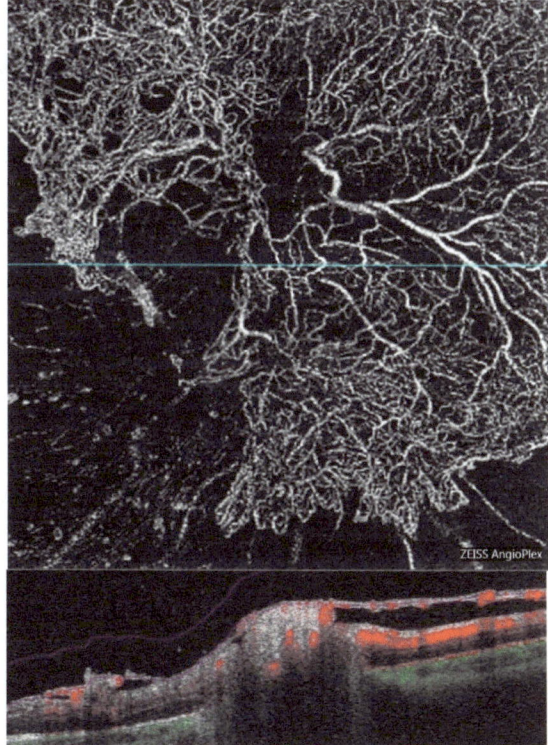

C4

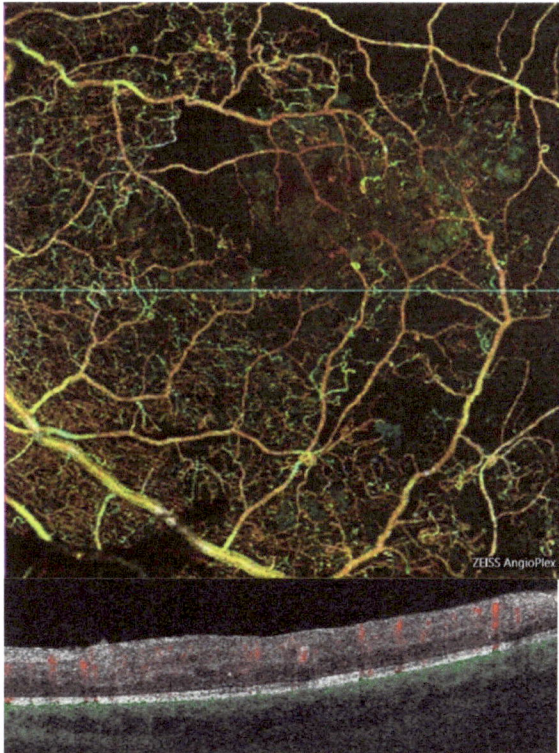

C5

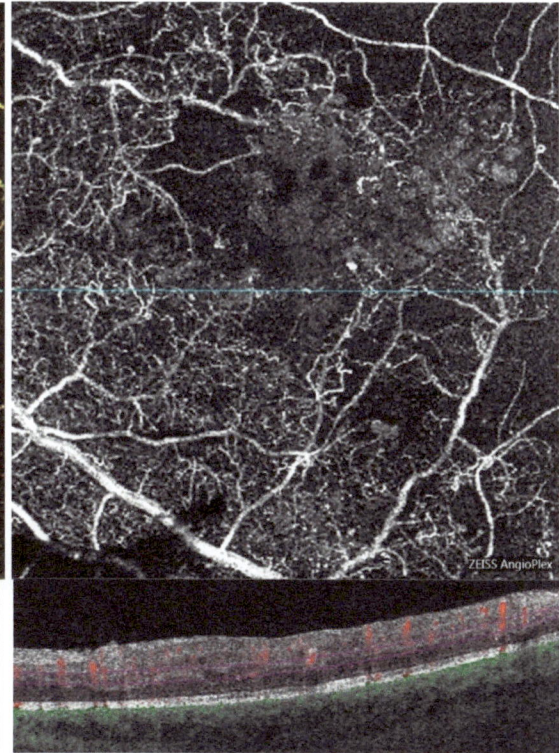

C6

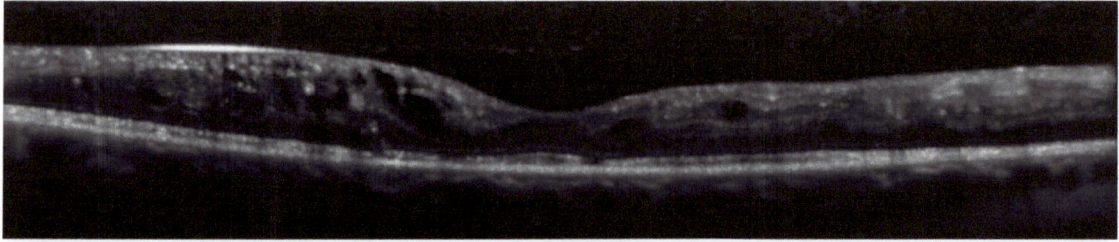
D1

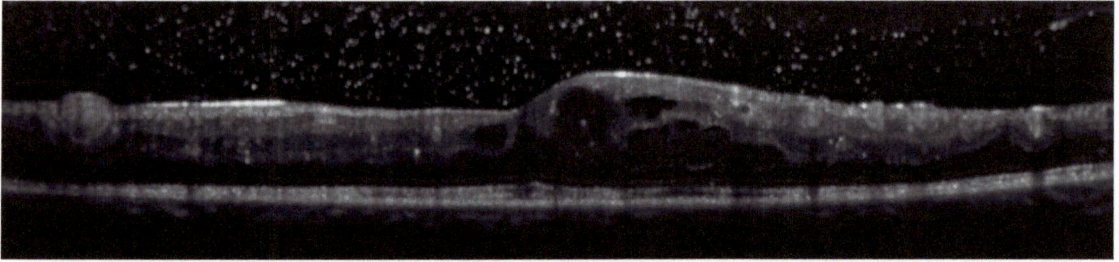
D2

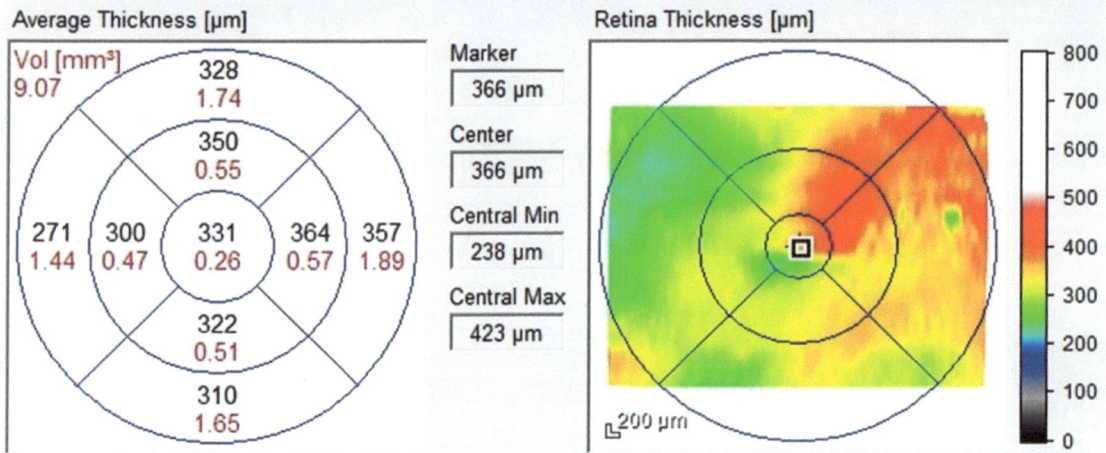
D3

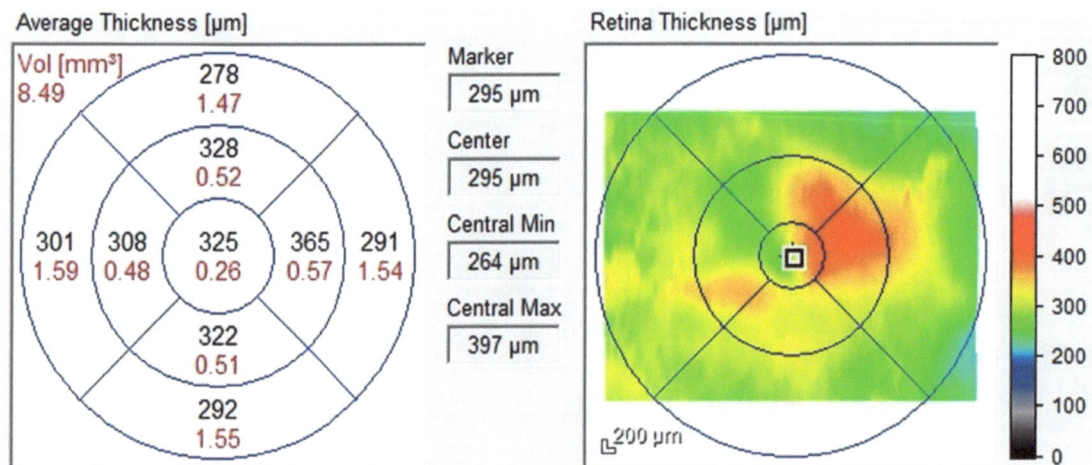
D4

Case 15: *Proliferative Diabetic Retinopathy*

Clinical Summary

41-year-old Type-2 DM presents with complaints of decrease vision OU for a period of 5 years. Visual acuity is 20/200 OD and count fingers at 3 feet OS. The patient has a history of hypertension and kidney failure.

Image Summary

A. Color Fundus: A1: Color fundus image OD shows old vitreous hemorrhage layered along the inferior arcade. There is a pale white sheen overlying the disc and arcades consistent with old NV that is regressed, and there are numerous intraretinal hemorrhages. The retina has fine striae throughout which suggest an ERM, and there are focal scars seen around the fovea. **A2**: Color fundus image OS shows similar findings to OD. In this eye, the vitreous hemorrhage has been very chronic and de-hemoglobinized, which makes it appear white.

B. Fluorescein Angiography: B1: Late phase fluorescein OD shows large areas with late leakage consistent with old NV. The hemorrhage along the inferior arcade blocks any underlying fluorescence. **B2**: Late phase fluorescein OS shows similar findings. The retina in both eyes appears very ischemic with minimal perfusion of the capillary beds.

C. OCT Angiography: C1: Depth encoded OCTA of NVE with corresponding B-scan OS shows perfusion in the superficial retinal layer (red) consistent with NVE. The perfusion in the B-scan reveals that the NVE is actually above the retina. **C2**: Depth encoded OCTA with corresponding B-scan OD shows very low capillary perfusion signal. There is a large tuft of NVE at the top of the image, and the B-scan shows an atrophic retina with overlying vitreous separation. Note the presence of red dots in the sub-hyaloid space, indicating movement and likely hemorrhage.

D.OCT: D1: B-scan OCT OD shows blunted foveal contour and an irregular retinal surface, likely due to an ERM. There is no macular edema but there are numerous hyperreflective spots suggestive of hard exudates. **D2**: B-scan OCT OS shows similar findings. The overlying vitreous is separated and appears more hyperreflective than normal, which likely reflects the vitreous hemorrhage.
D3: Volumetric OCT OD shows irregular thickness throughout, due to areas of edema, impaired perfusion and neovascularization. **D4**: Volumetric OCT OS shows similar findings as OD.

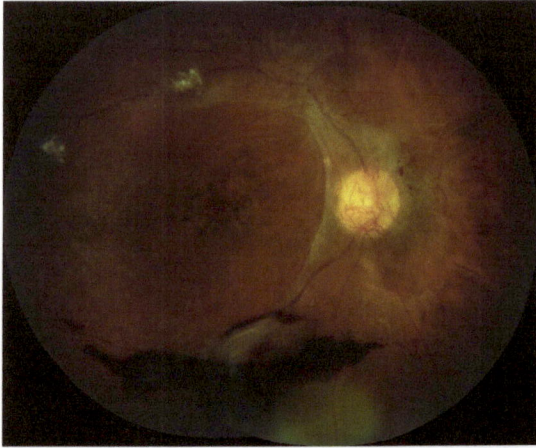
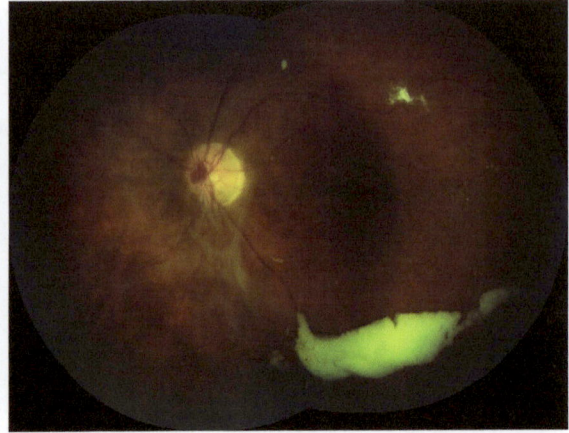

A1

A2

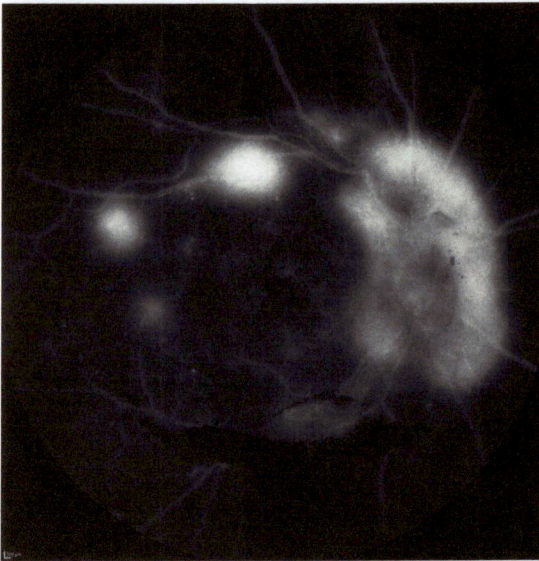
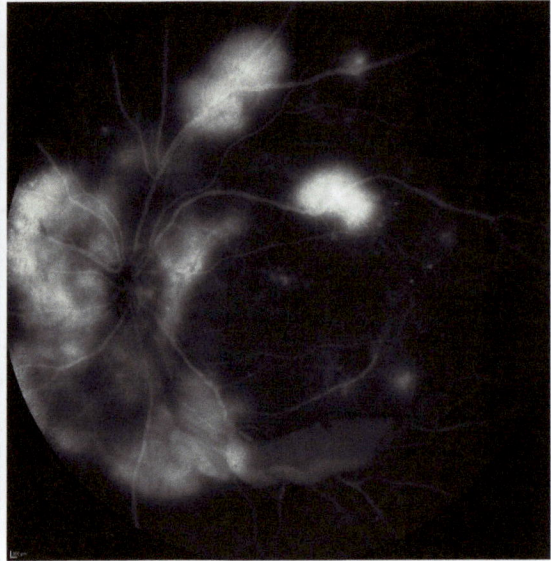

B1

B2

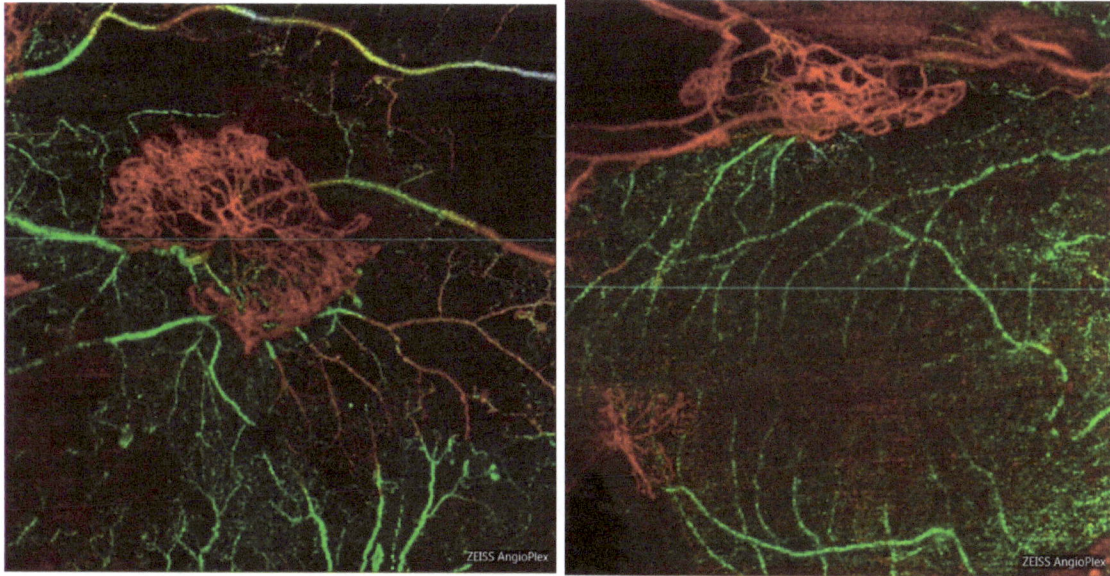

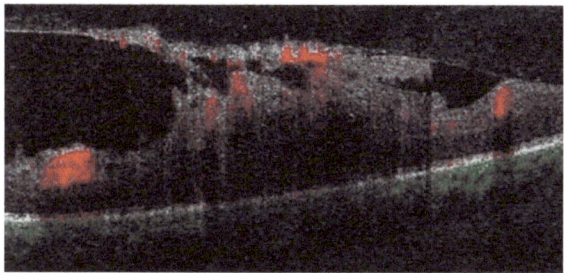
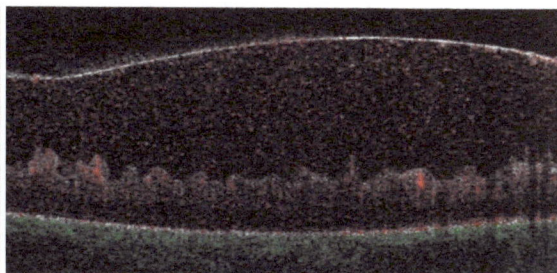

C1   C2

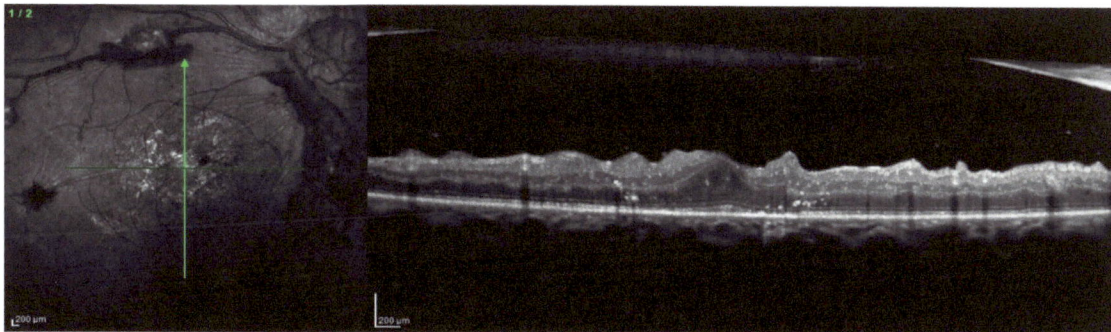

D1

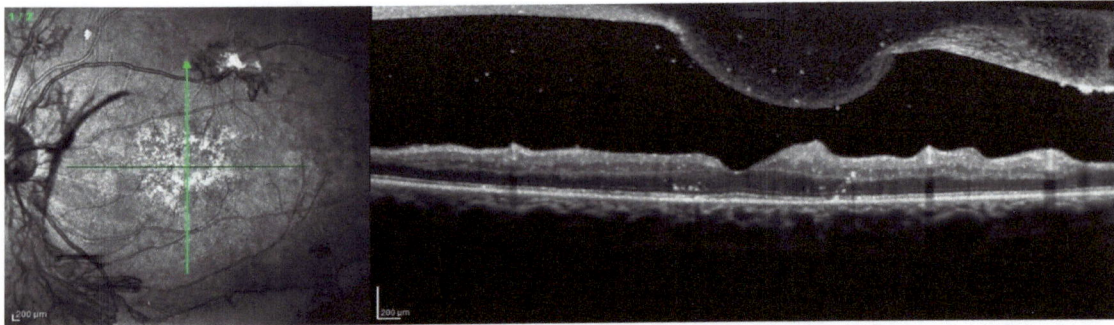

D2

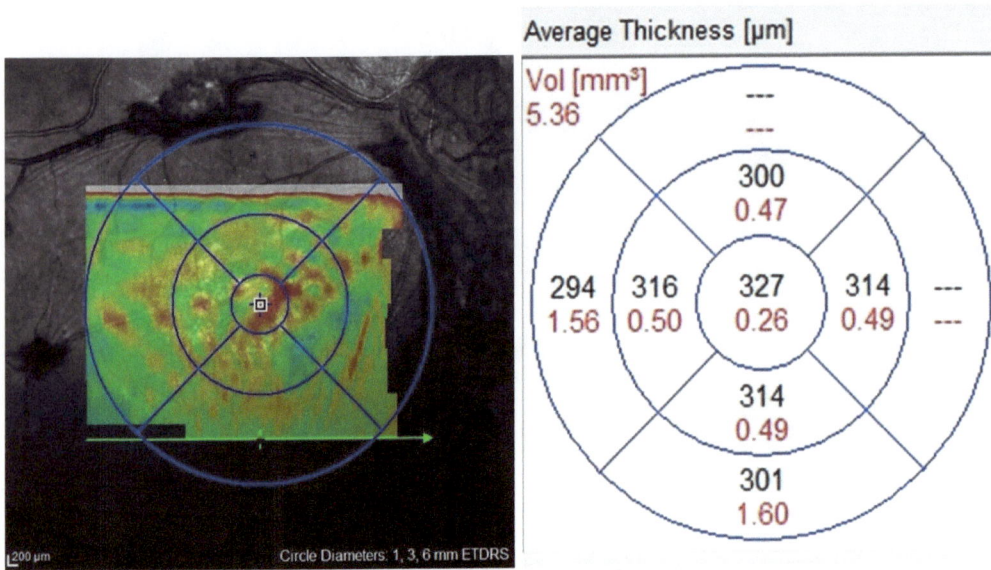

D3

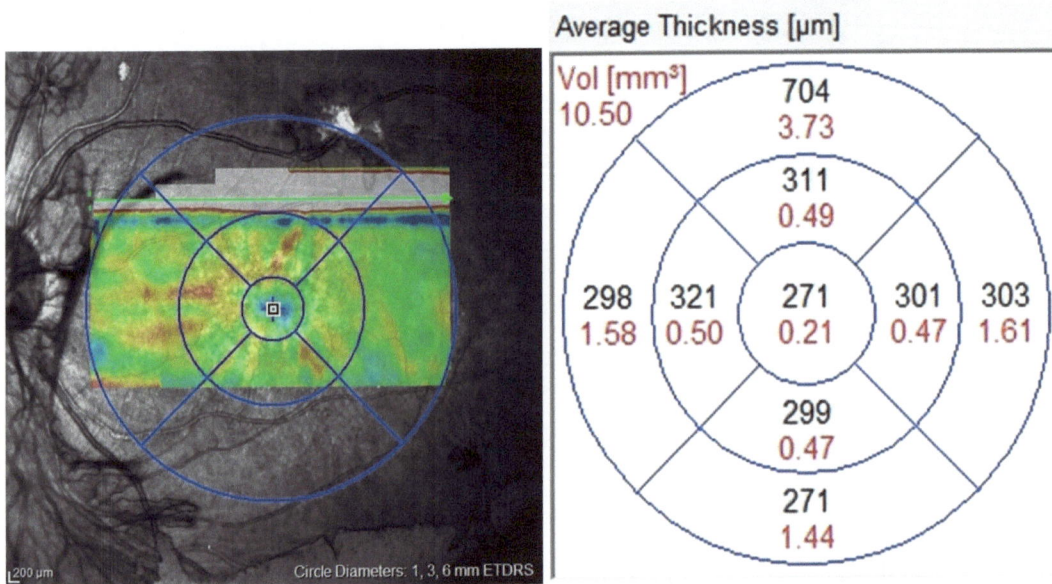

D4

Case 16: *Proliferative Diabetic Retinopathy*

Clinical Summary

47-year-old white male with history of Type-1 IDDM, lost to follow up from previous retinal exam x 4 years. Patient referred by optometrist after presenting with complaints of floaters. No other vision complaints and vision is 20/25 OU. We present the left eye findings here.

Image Summary

A. Color Fundus: Color fundus image shows several intraretinal hemorrhages and yellow deposits consistent with hard exudates in the temporal periphery.

B. Fluorescein Angiography: B1: Early to mid phase fluorescein angiogram OS shows numerous areas of impaired perfusion and microaneurysms in the periphery. The foveal avascular zone appears irregular and slightly enlarged. **B2**: Late phase fluorescein angiogram shows diffuse leakage throughout the entire image and intense hyperfluorescence in the inferotemporal aspect of the image, suggestive of NVE.

C. OCT Angiography: C1: Depth encoded OCTA of macula with corresponding B-scan shows a small tuft of NVE in the upper right side of the image. The superficial layer appears to have some perfusion defects in the lower right edge of the image. **C2**: Vitreo-retinal interface (VRI) level OCTA of the disc shows NVD with corresponding B-scan illustrating vitreous traction on the disc.

D. OCT: D1: B-scan OCT of macula is relatively unremarkable. **D2**: B-scan OCT of disc shows the vitreous traction on the disc.

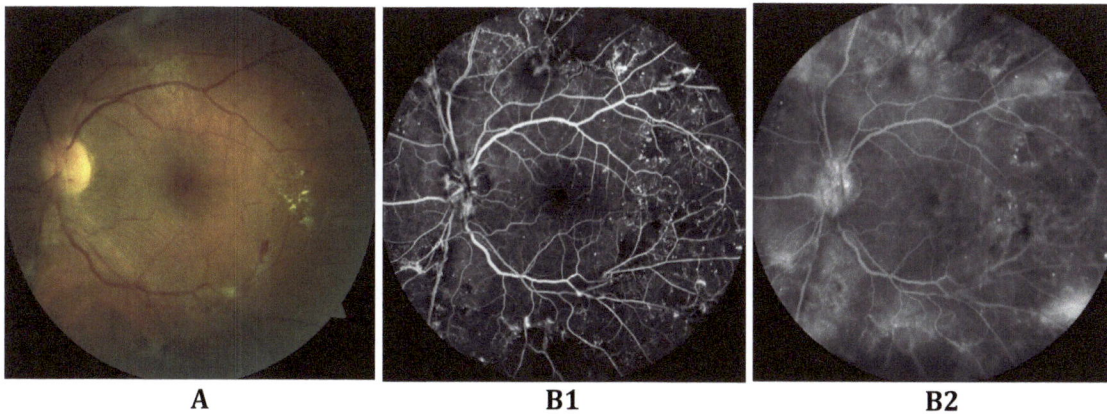

A   B1   B2

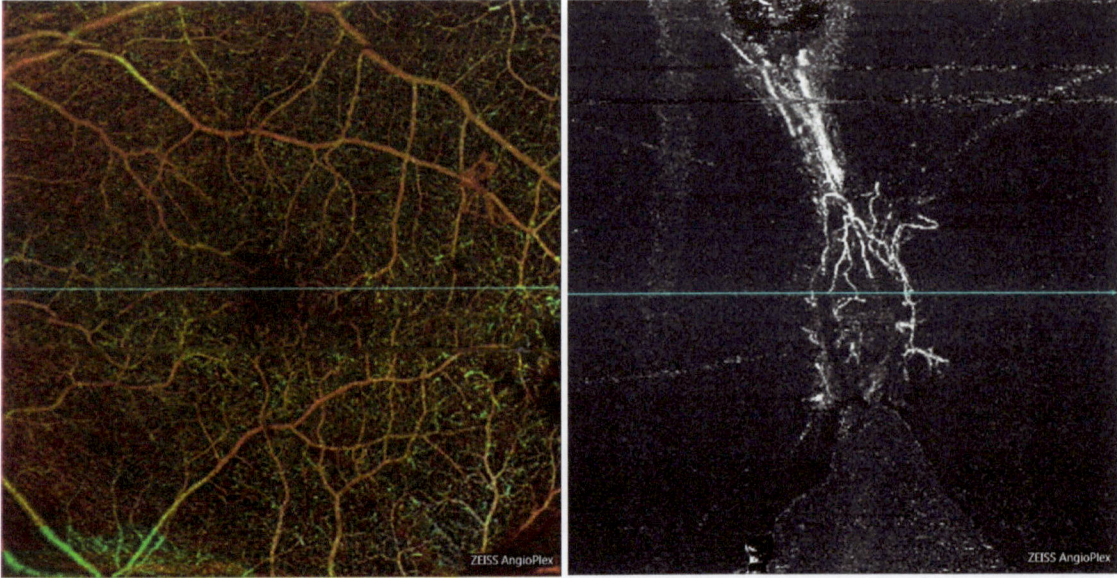

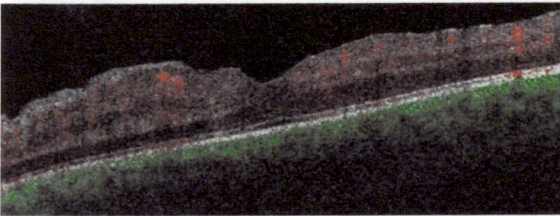

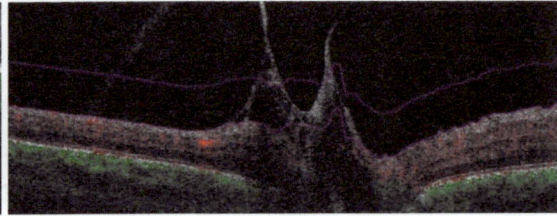

C1

C2

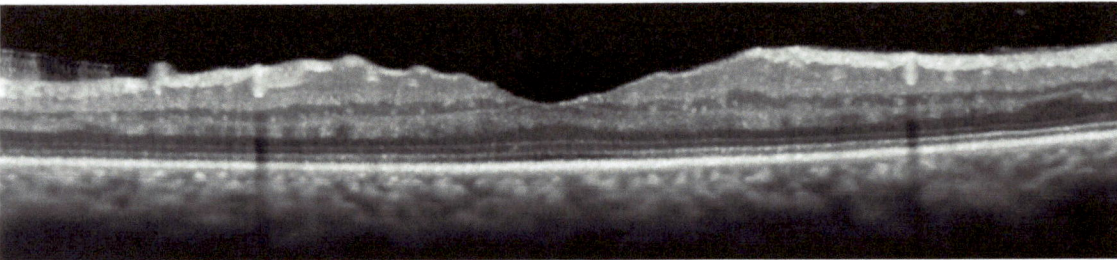

D1

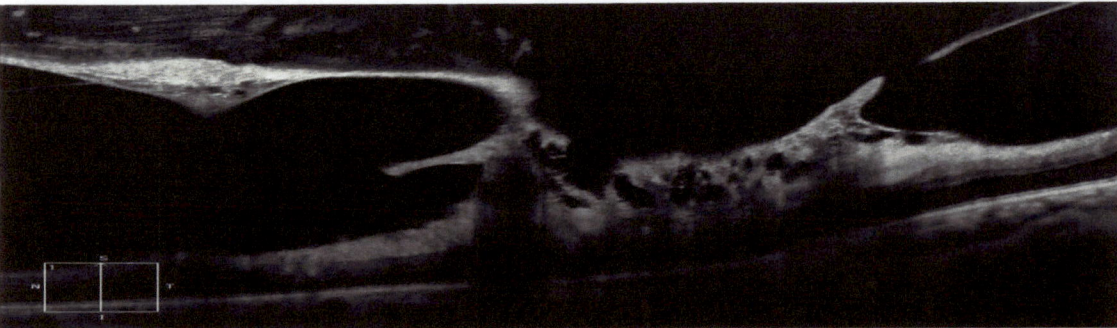

D2

Case 17: *Branch Retinal Vein Occlusion*

Clinical Summary

87-year-old white male with history of NIDDM x 17 years, hypertension and atrial fibrillation. Past treatments include pan-retinal photocoagulation. Presents with sudden onset of blurred vision centrally and superiorly OD. Vision OD is 20/80-.

Image Summary

A. Color Fundus: Shows several intraretinal hemorrhages inferonasal to the fovea. Some of these hemorrhages appear to be flame shaped and located in the nerve fiber layer, and there are numerous white and pigmented round lesions in the periphery consistent with old laser scars.

B. Fluorescein Angiography: B1: Mid-phase fluorescein angiogram shows similar findings to color image. The foveal avascular zone appears enlarged and irregular, and the vessels appear tortuous. The intraretinal hemorrhages block the underlying fluorescence. **B2**: Late-phase fluorescein angiogram shows staining of the laser scars, and there is mild leakage in the macula consistent with macular edema. Portions of the macula appear to have impaired perfusion.

C. OCT Angiography: C1: Depth encoded OCTA with corresponding B-scan shows large sections of impaired perfusion, most evident superior to the fovea and involving the fovea. **C2**: Full thickness retina composite OCTA with corresponding B-scan confirms the same findings. **C3**: Deep retinal plexus OCTA with corresponding B-scan shows diffuse areas of impaired perfusion inferior and superior to the fovea.

D. OCT: D1: B-scan OCT shows a large hyporeflective space immediately to the left of the fovea consistent with macular edema. **D2**: Volumetric OCT illustrates thickening in the area of edema.

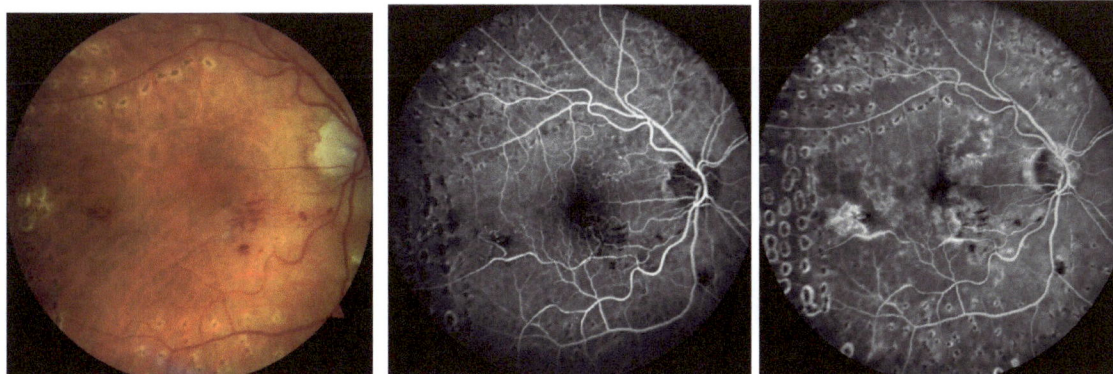

A   B1   B2

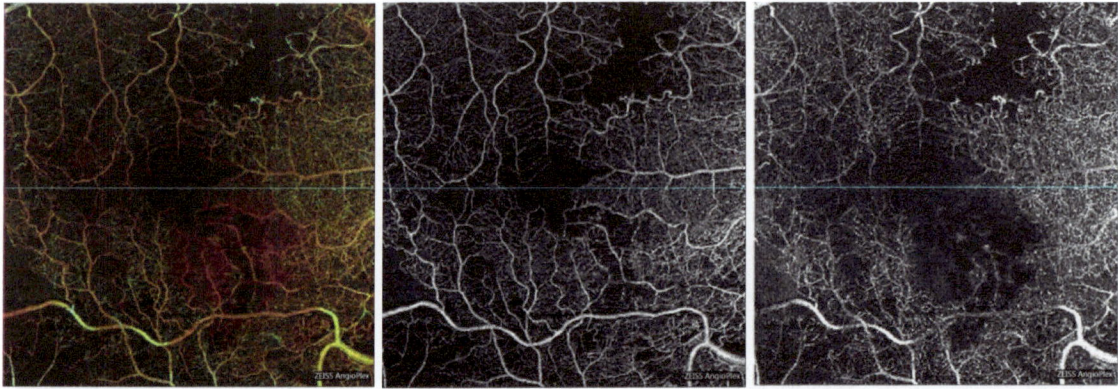

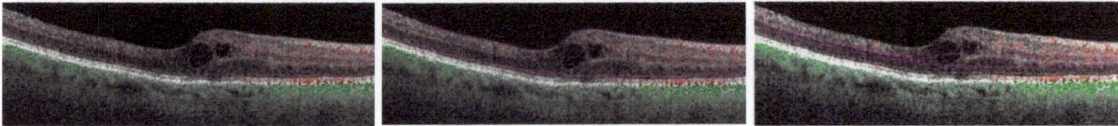

C1   C2   C3

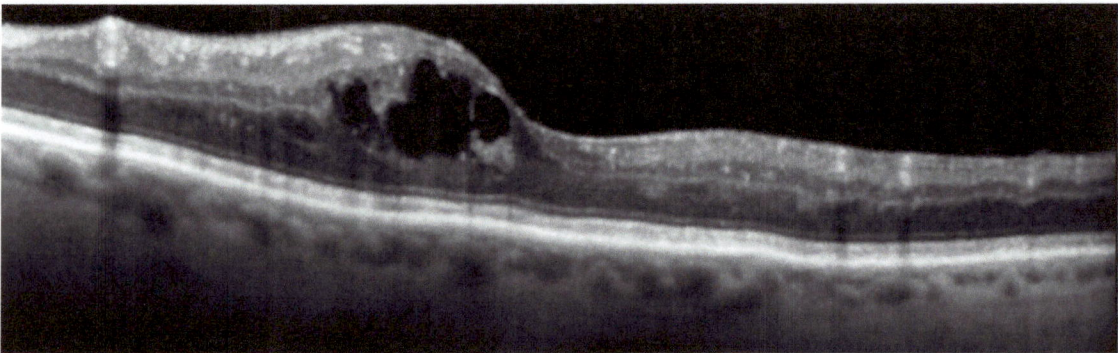

D1

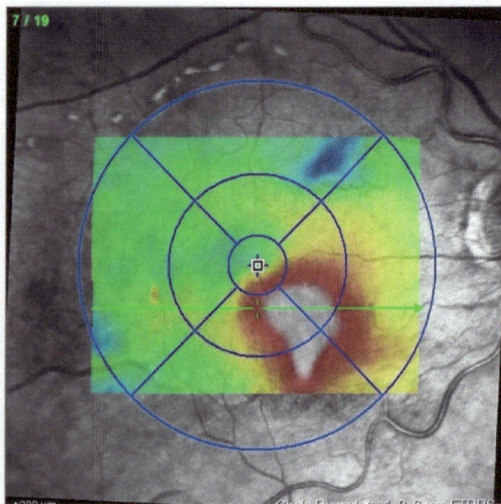

D2

Case 18: *Branch Retinal Vein Occlusion*

Clinical Summary

73-year-old white male with history of hypertension, hypercholesterolemia, presents with sudden onset blurred vision OD. Vision OD is 20/30-.

Image Summary

A. Color Fundus: Color montage shows intraretinal hemorrhage in the nerve fiber layer in the superior nasal macula. There are a few cotton wool spots as well.

B. Fluorescein Angiography: B1: Early to mid phase fluorescein angiogram shows that the intraretinal hemorrhage blocks the underlying fluorescence. **B2**: Late phase fluorescein angiogram shows staining of the retina and vessels involved in the hemorrhage, and the staining extends to the fovea and likely indicates cystoid edema.

C. OCT Angiography: C1: Depth encoded OCTA of macula with corresponding B-scan shows impaired perfusion in the superonasal quadrant of the macula. The superficial retina layer shows the peripapillary capillaries that travel with the nerve fiber layer well, however there is no perfusion signal from the deep retinal layer (lack of green). This may be due to either true impairment in the perfusion or blockage of the deep retinal layer signal by the hemorrhage. **C2**: Deep retinal plexus OCTA with corresponding B-scan showing the full extent of the lesion. The B-scan shows that the retina is edematous and the details of the deep retina are shadowed by the overlying hemorrhage in the nerve fiber layer.

D. OCT: D1: B-scan OCT shows large intraretinal cystoid spaces and retinal thickening on the right side of the image. The overlying vitreous is still adherent to the retina at the fovea and nasally. **D2**: Volumetric OCT illustrates the edema superiorly that extends into the fovea.

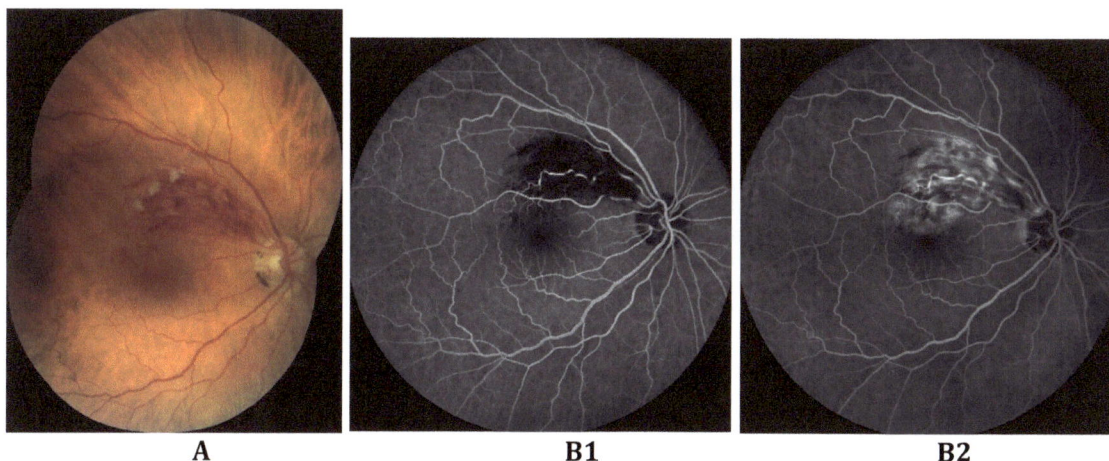

A   B1   B2

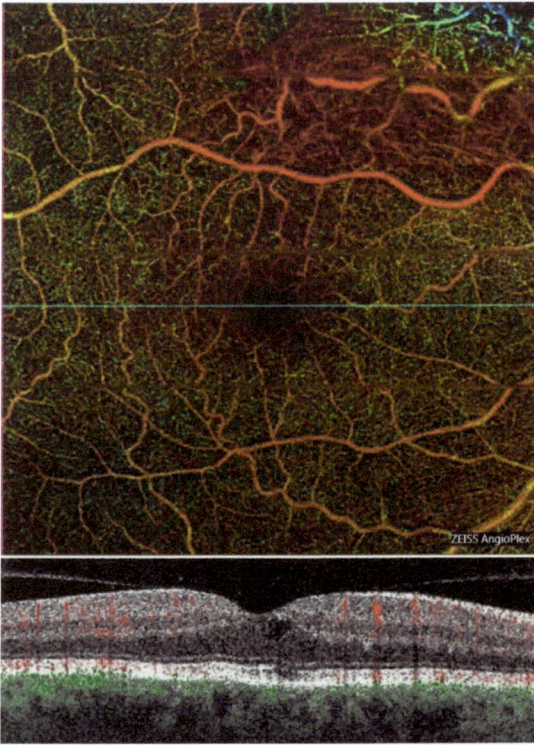

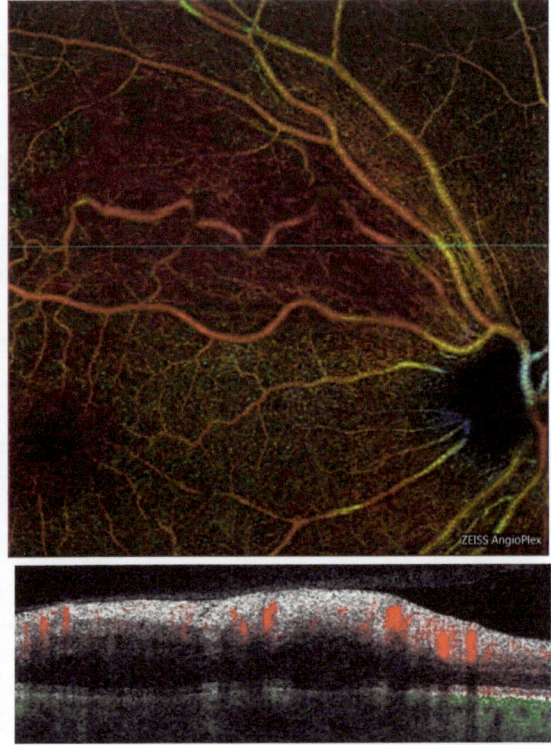

C1

C2

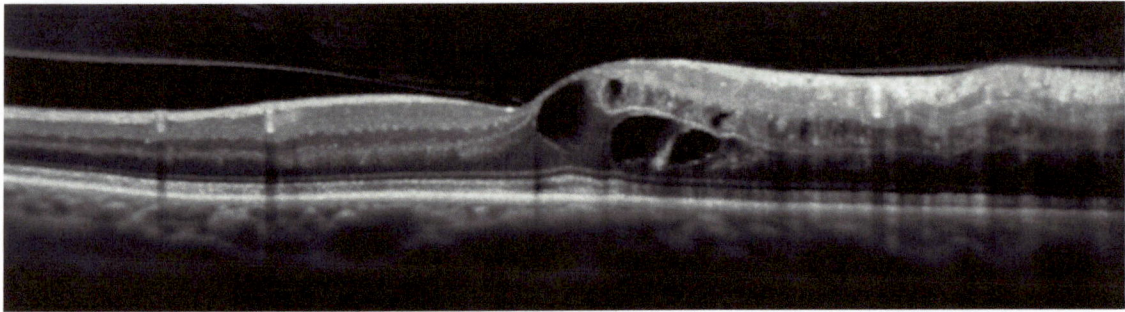

D1

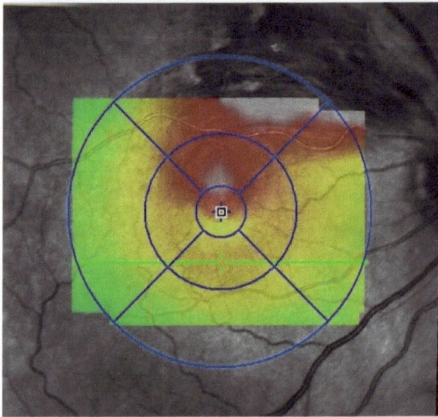

D2

Case 19: *Branch Retinal Vein Occlusion*

Clinical Summary

78-year-old white female with history of hypertension and NIDDM x 20 years, who presents with complaints of sudden onset of blurred vision OS. Vision is 20/40- OS.

Image Summary

A. Color Fundus: Shows diffuse intraretinal hemorrhages and retinal edema in the superotemporal quadrant extending to the fovea. The vessels appear tortuous throughout the image and the superior temporal vein is engorged.

B. Fluorescein Angiography: Late phase fluorescein angiogram shows dilated and tortuous veins in the superotemporal quadrant, with the majority of the superior temporal retina showing impaired perfusion. The overlying hemorrhage blocks some of the underlying fluorescence, and there is late staining of the some of the retinal veins.

C. OCT Angiography: C1: Depth encoded OCTA of the macula with corresponding B-scan shows a large area of impaired perfusion in the superior temporal macula. The remaining vessels are dilated and arteriovenous anastomoses are evident, with the foveal avascular zone involved. The B-scan shows thinning of the inner retina temporally, which is suggestive of a chronic process and retinal atrophy. **C2:** Deep retinal layer OCTA of the macula with corresponding B-scan illustrates the extent of non-perfusion. **C3:** Depth encoded OCTA superotemporal with corresponding B-scan show almost no intact capillaries. **C4:** Deep retinal layer OCTA superotemporal with corresponding B-scan.

D. OCT: D1: B scan OCT of macula shows severe intraretinal hyporeflective spaces consistent with macular edema and large amount of subretinal fluid. **D2:** Volumetric OCT of macula.

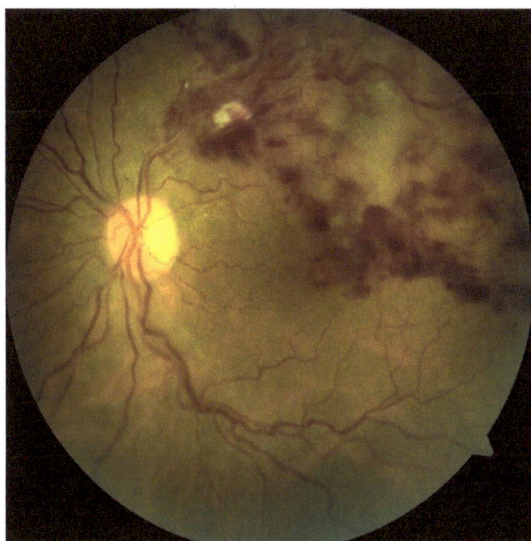

A

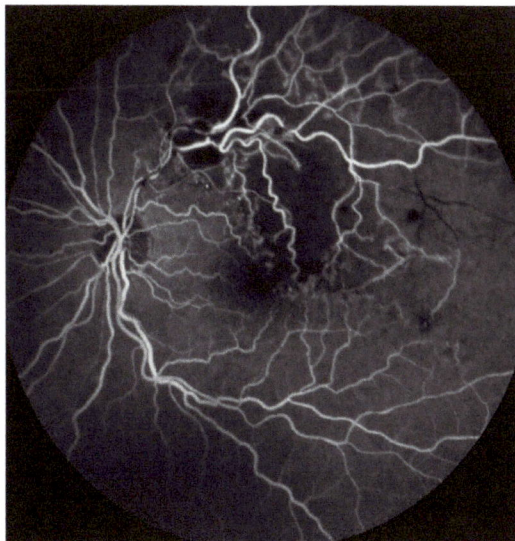

B

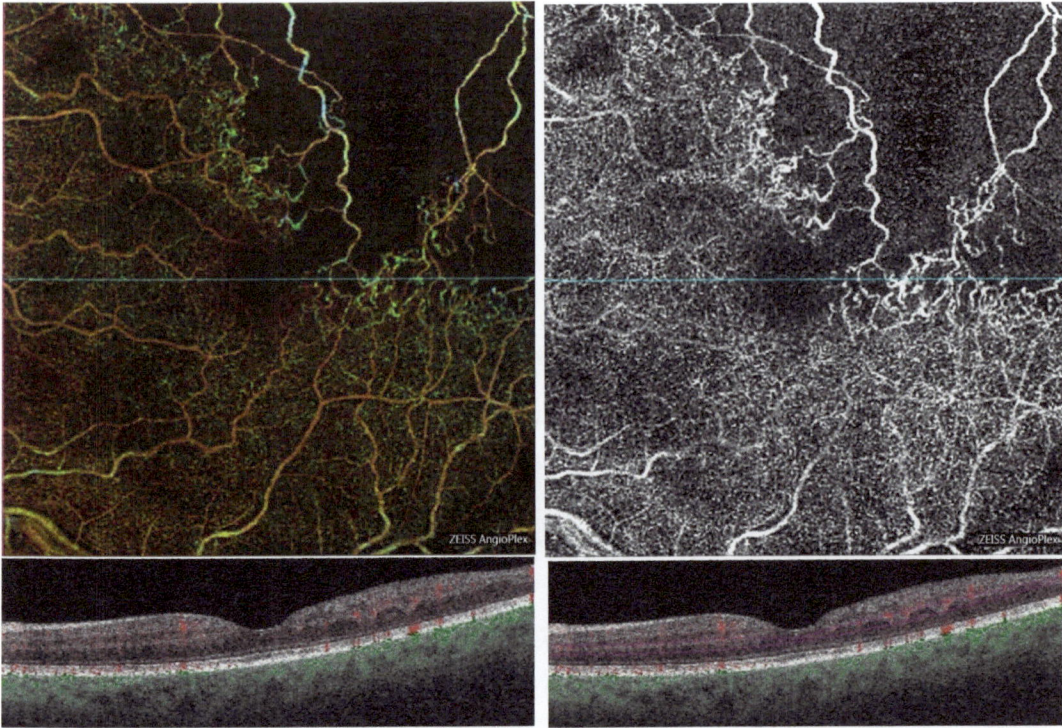

C1

C2

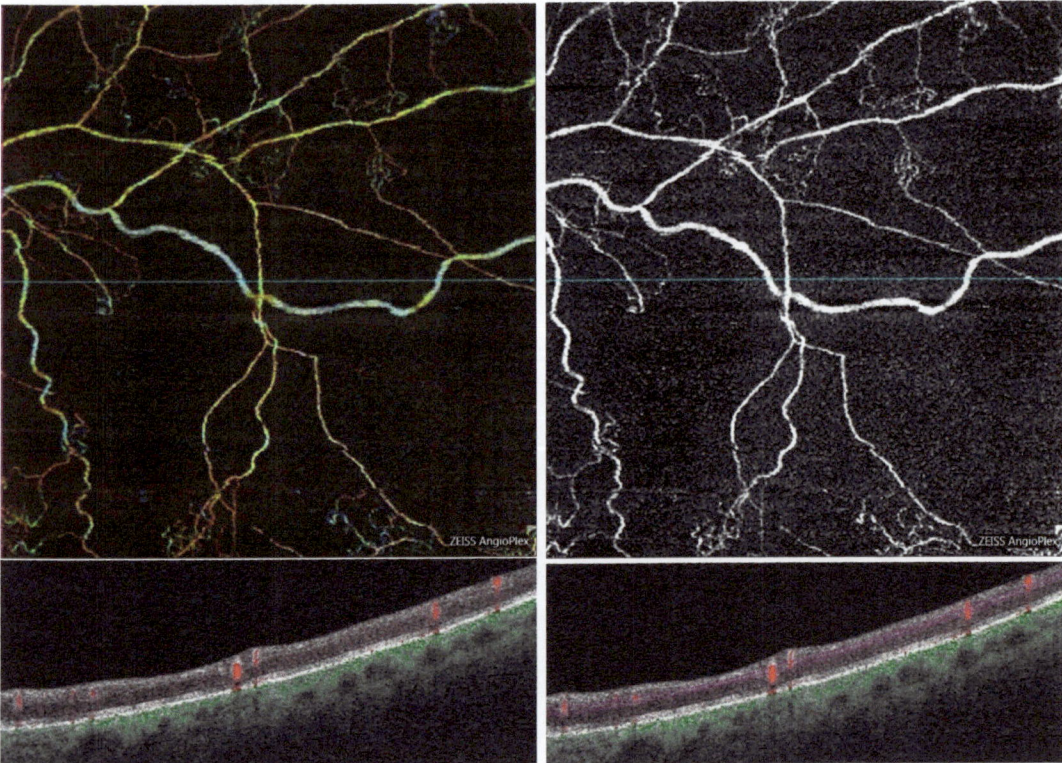

C3

C4

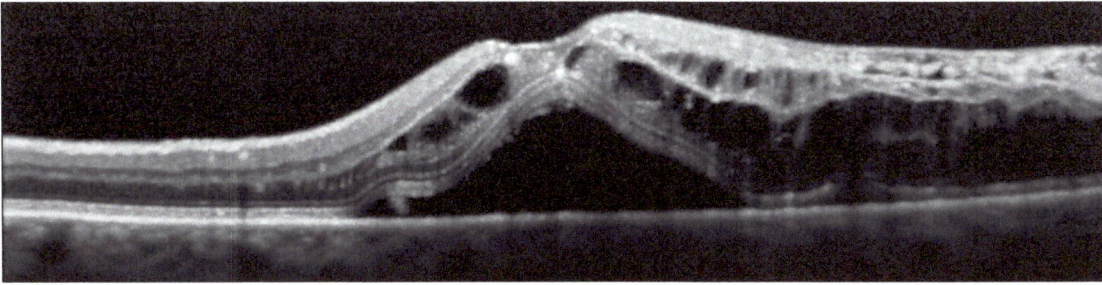

D1

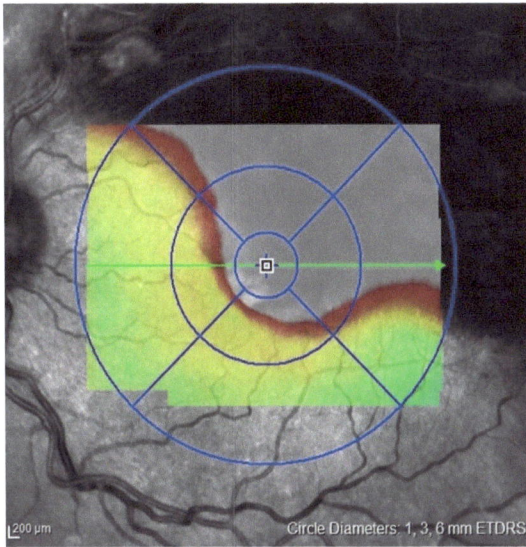

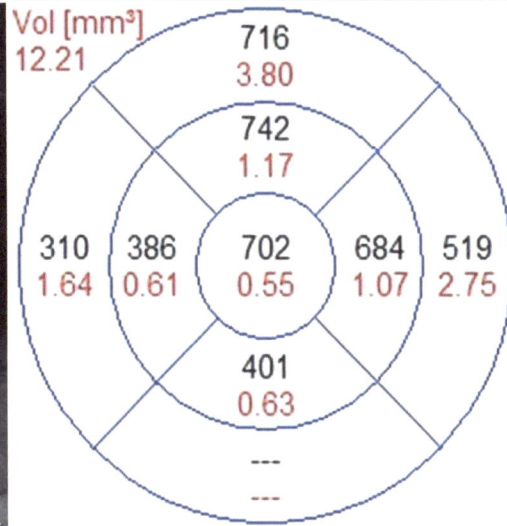

D2

Case 20: *Branch Retinal Vein Occlusion*

Clinical Summary

62-year-old white female with history of hypertension and s/p CVA presents with complaints of sudden onset of decreased, blurry vision OD x 3 days. Vision is 20/60- OD.

Image Summary

A. Color Fundus: Shows yellow deposits in the temporal macula consistent with hard exudates. The inferotemporal vessels are sclerotic (white appearing) suggesting a chronic vascular process, and the inferior retina appears ischemic.

B. Fluorescein Angiography: B1: Mid-phase fluorescein angiogram OD shows tortuous vessels and numerous pinpoint hyperfluorescent lesions consistent with microaneurysms. The inferior retina shows impaired perfusion extending to the fovea. **B2**: Late phase fluorescein angiogram shows similar findings with more prominent staining of the vessels.

C. OCT Angiography: C1: Depth encoded OCTA with corresponding B-scan shows impaired perfusion extending to the fovea. The remaining vessels are dilated and there is arteriovenous shunting across the horizontal meridian typical of a chronic vascular process. **C2**: Deep retinal plexus OCTA with corresponding B-scan shows similar findings.

D. OCT: D1: B scan OCT shows abnormal retinal layering in the left half of the image and intraretinal cystoid spaces. The outer retinal layers are broken immediately to the left of the fovea. **D2**: Volumetric OCT illustrates thinning inferiorly, corresponding to the area of impaired perfusion.

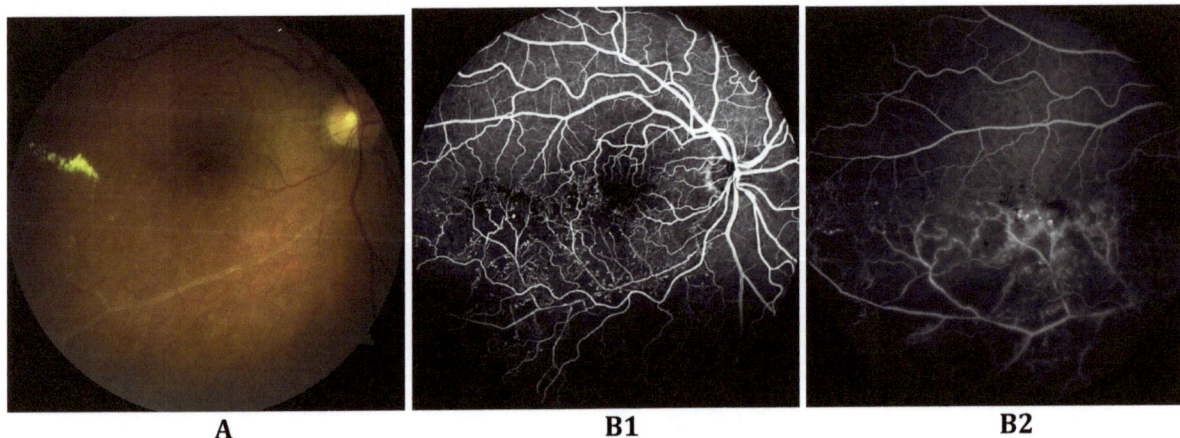

A   B1   B2

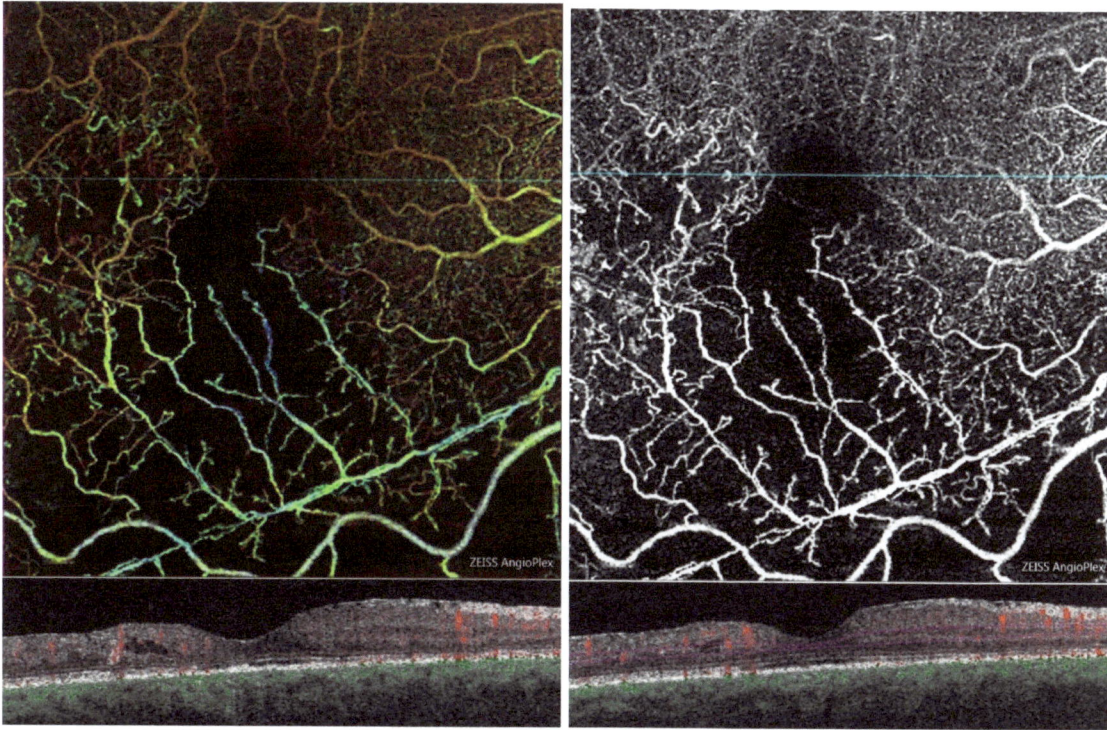

C1   C2

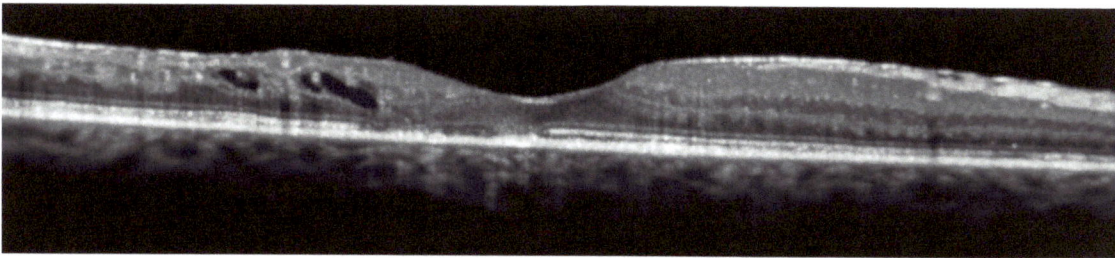

D1

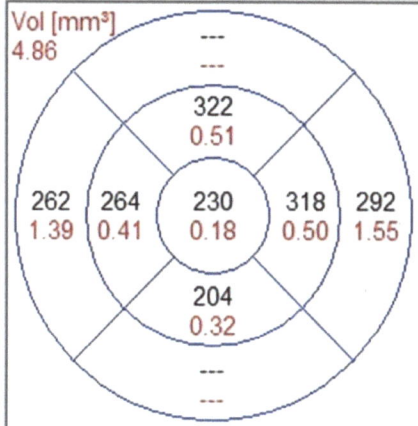
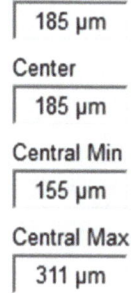
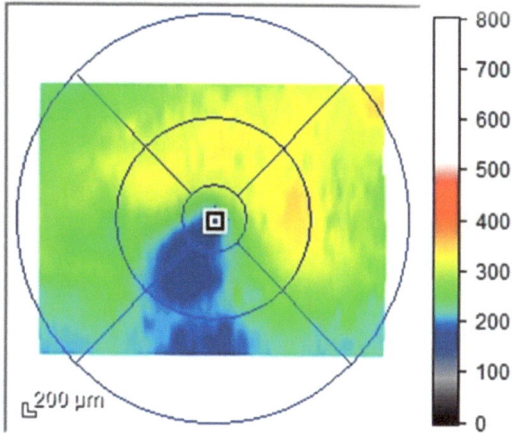

D2

Case 21: *Branch Retinal Vein Occlusion*

Clinical Summary

57-year-old white female with a history of IDDM x 6 years, hypertension and atrial fibrillation, presents with complaints of blurred vision OD x 1 week. Vision OD is 20/50.

Image Summary

A. Color Fundus: "Blood and thunder" appearance of the superotemporal retina. There are numerous hemorrhages in the nerve fiber layer (flame shaped hemorrhages) and in the deeper retinal layers (dot-blot hemorrhages).

B. Fluorescein Angiography: B1: Early phase fluorescein angiogram shows impaired perfusion in the superior temporal retina up to and including the fovea. The fluorescein is not from the same time point as the color image, as the patient refused angiography initially. On return visit, fluorescein was performed and the intraretinal hemorrhages have resolved. **B2**: Late phase fluorescein angiogram shows similar findings.

C. OCT Angiography: C1: Depth encoded OCTA of the macula with corresponding B-scan shows large areas of impaired perfusion in the superior macula involving the fovea. **C2**: Superficial retina layer OCTA of the macula with corresponding B-scan shows impaired flow in the left half of the image. **C3**: Deep retinal layer OCTA of the macula with corresponding B-scan shows similar findings. **C4**: Depth encoded OCTA of the superior arcade with corresponding B-scan shows impaired perfusion. **C5**: Superficial retina layer OCTA of the superior arcade with corresponding B-scan. **C6**: Deep retinal plexus OCTA of the superior arcade with corresponding B-scan.

D. OCT: D1: Vertical B-scan OCT shows retinal thickening of the superior macula. **D2**: Volumetric OCT confirms the extent of thickening in the fovea and superiorly.

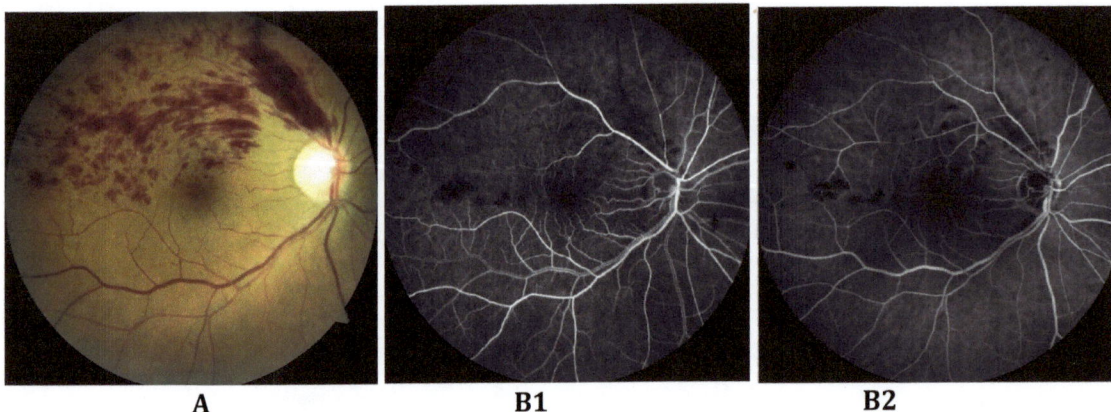

A   B1   B2

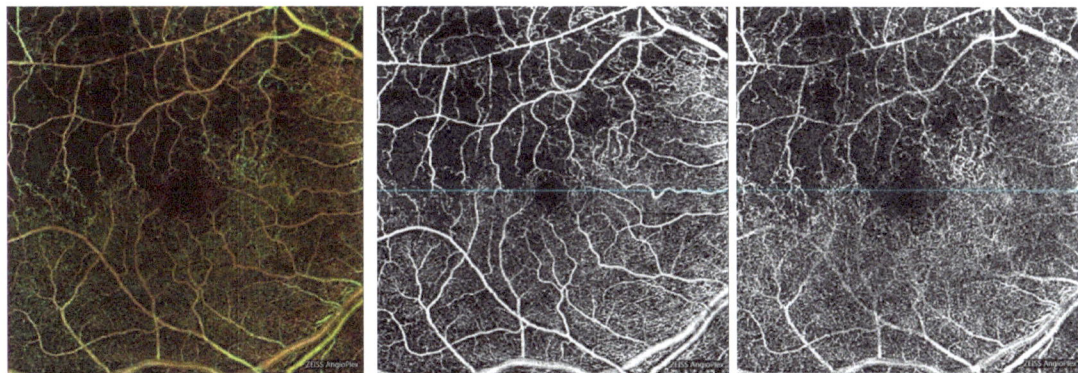

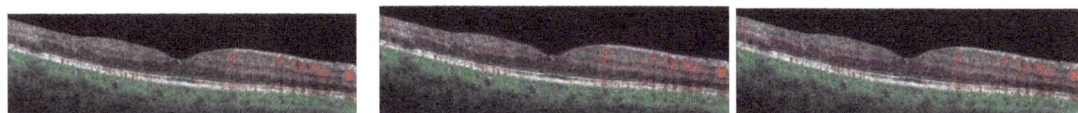

C1   C2   C3

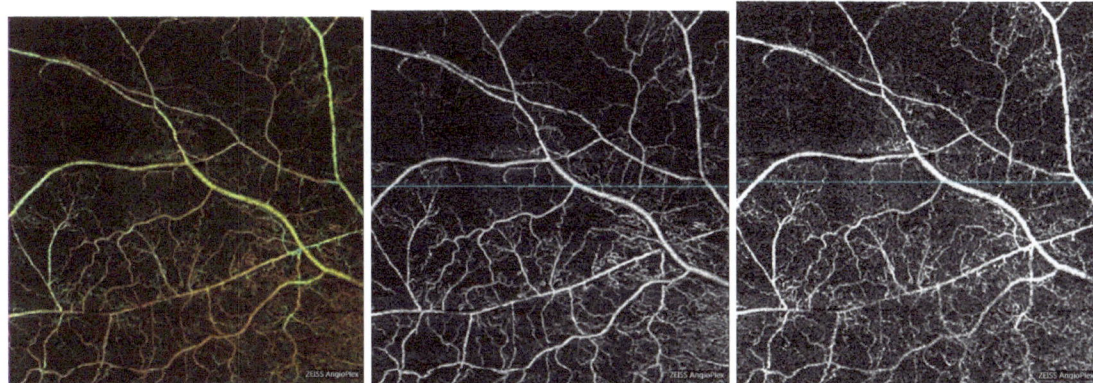

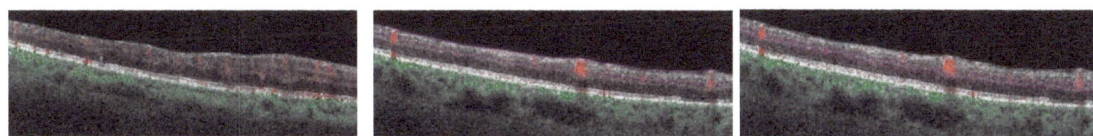

C4   C5   C6

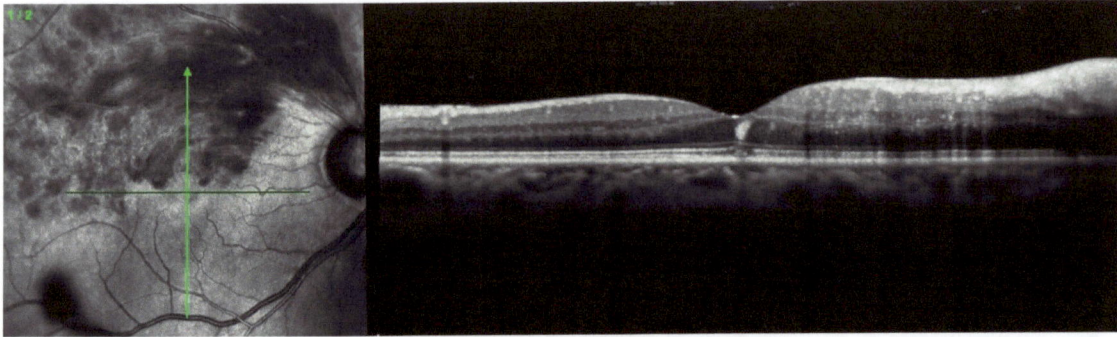

D1

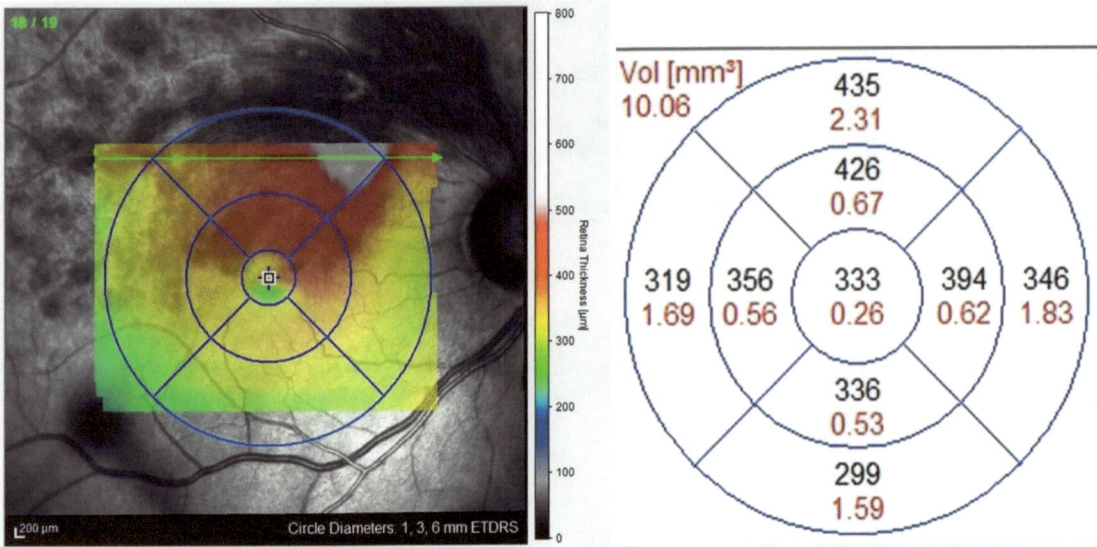

D2

Case 22: *Central Retinal Vein Occlusion*

Clinical Summary

66-year-old white male with history of hypertension who presents with a complaint of sudden on-set blurred vision OS x 2 days. Vision OD is 20/200.

Image Summary

A. Color Fundus: Shows dilated veins and multiple intraretinal hemorrhages throughout the macula and temporal retina.

B. Fluorescein Angiography: B1: Early phase fluorescein angiogram confirms tortuous vessels and dilated veins. **B2**: Late phase fluorescein angiogram shows staining throughout the macula consistent with macular edema. Parts of the macula and peripheral retina appear ischemic.

C. OCT Angiography: C1: Depth encoded OCTA with corresponding B-scan shows very asymmetric perfusion in the superficial retinal layer (red), and there are numerous pockets of impaired perfusion as well. **C2**: Full thickness retina composite OCTA with corresponding B-scan shows similar findings. **C3**: Deep retina layer OCTA with corresponding B-scan confirms lack of perfusion in the deep retinal layer, however the B-scan shows that the retinal anatomy is severely distorted due to intraretinal edema, and the deep retinal layer segmentation maybe inaccurate. Overall the perfusion throughout the retina is decreased compared to a normal case.

D. OCT: D1: B-scan OCT shows diffuse intraretinal edema and subretinal fluid, and the foveal depression is completely blunted. **D2**: Volumetric OCT shows diffuse thickening.

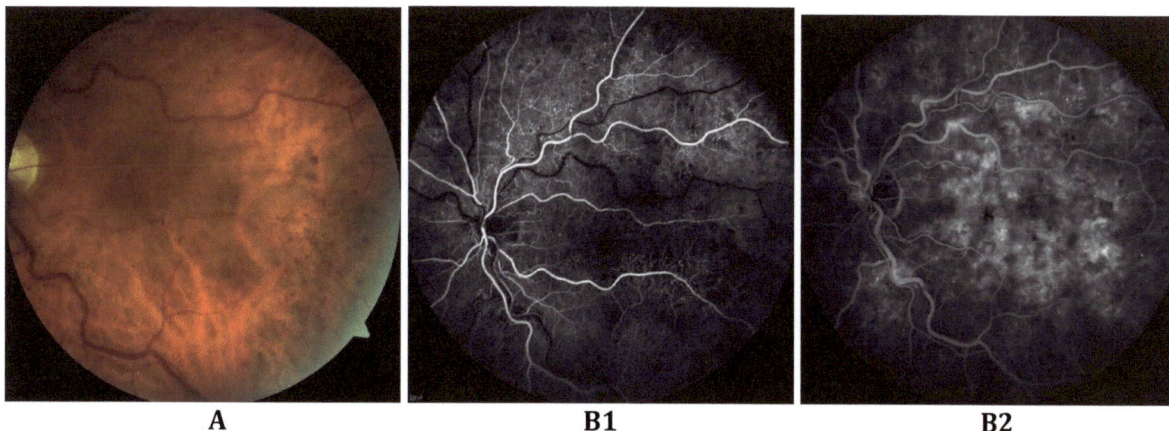

A   B1   B2

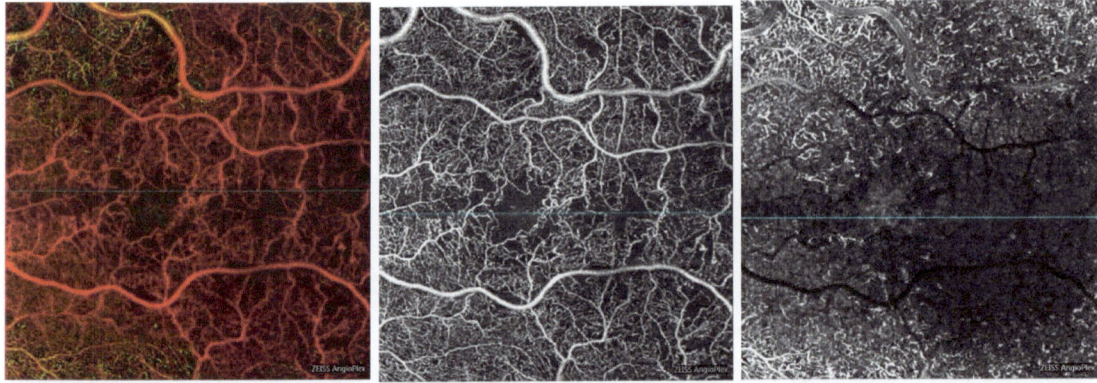

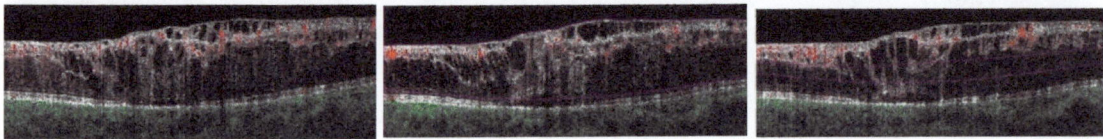

C1　　　　　**C2**　　　　　**C3**

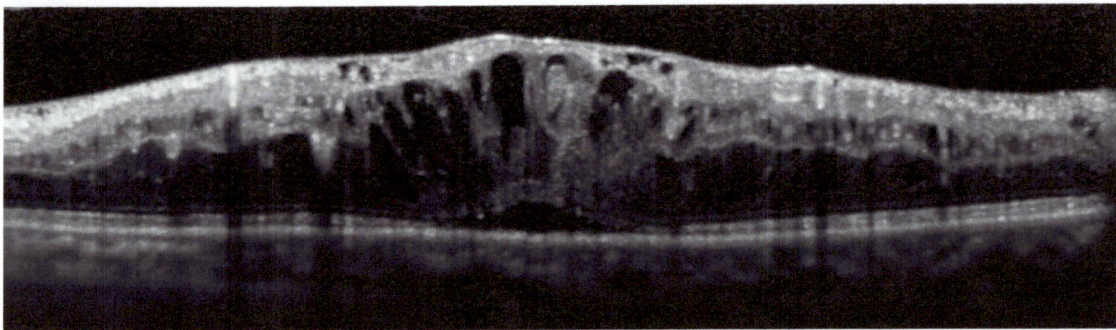

D1

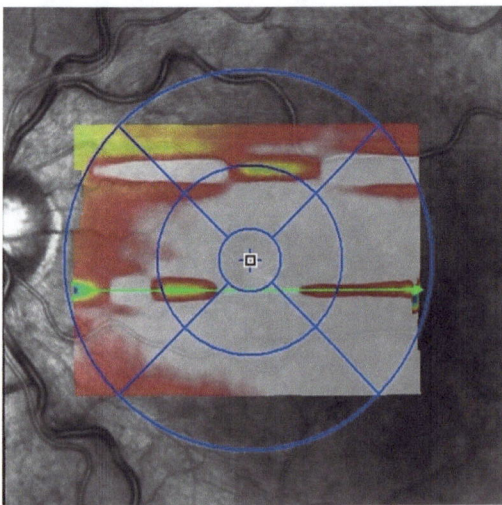

Average Thickness [µm]

Vol [mm³]
13.69

	404 2.14	
	492 0.77	
440 2.33	579 0.91	738 0.58	712 1.12	469 2.49
	456 0.72	
	496 2.63	

D2

Case 23: *Central Retinal Vein Occlusion*

Clinical Summary

70-year-old white male with a history of hypertension, hypercholesterolemia, and NIDDM x 10 years presents with complaint of vision "diminished" suddenly x 2 days. Vision OD is 20/25.

Image Summary

A. Color Fundus: Color montage image shows dilated and tortuous veins. There are numerous dot-blot hemorrhages throughout the image, and a few cotton wool spots are present.

B. Fluorescein Angiography: B1: Early phase fluorescein angiogram shows tortuous vessels and a shadow over the macula suggestive of a media opacity. The numerous hemorrhages throughout the macula block the underlying fluorescence. **B2**: Late phase fluorescein angiogram confirms earlier findings. There are a few foci of late staining in the macula consistent with macular edema.

C. OCT Angiography: C1: Depth encoded OCTA with corresponding B-scan shows severe impairment in the capillary perfusion throughout the macula. Arteriovenous shunts can be seen at multiple points, and the fovea avascular zone is completely destroyed. The B-scan shows limited perfusion throughout. **C2**: Full thickness retinal composite OCTA with corresponding B-scan shows similar findings. **C3**: Superficial retina layer OCTA with corresponding B-scan confirms earlier findings. **C4**: Deep retinal plexus OCTA with corresponding B-scan shows more severe involvement of the deeper layers. The B-scan demonstrates severe distortion of macular anatomy which makes the segmentation unreliable, nevertheless the perfusion throughout the retina is clearly abnormal.

D: En Face: Deep retina layer en face intensity image shows many hyporeflective lesions consistent with cystoid spaces on the B-scans.

E. OCT: E1: Retinal nerve fiber analysis shows possible diminished nerve fiber thickness.
E2: B-scan OCT illustrates diffuse edema throughout the scan. **E3**: volumetric OCT analysis shows thickening in the central portion of the volume analysis.

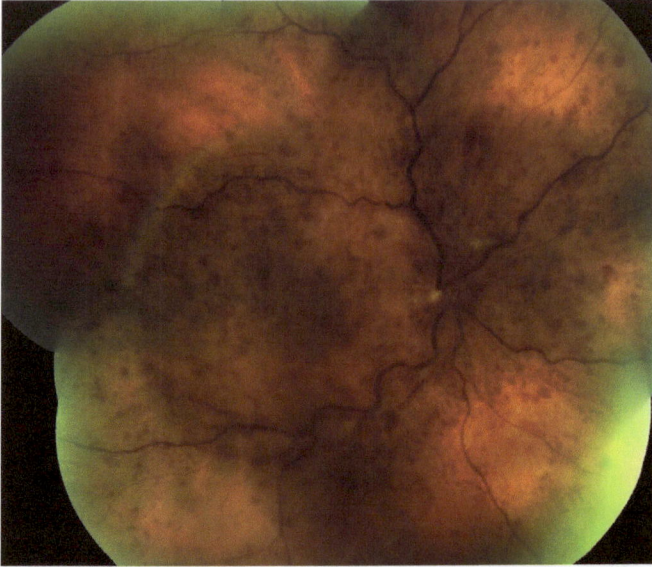

A

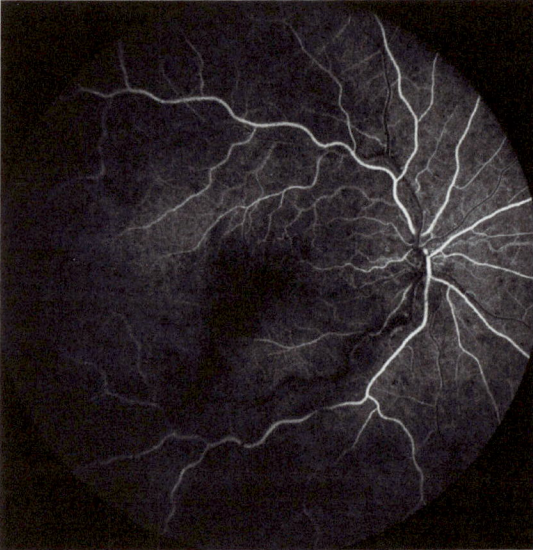

B1

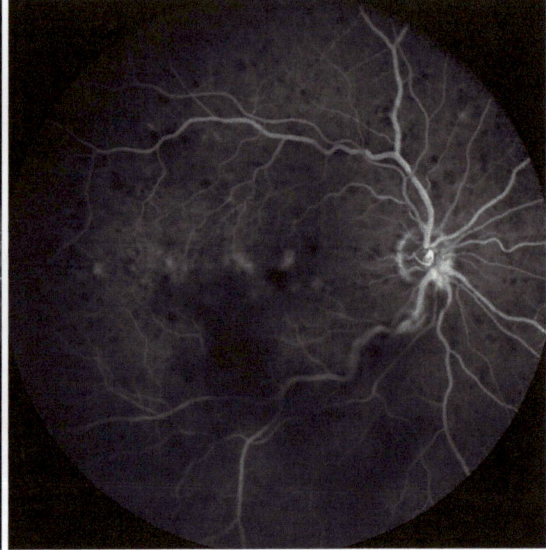

B2

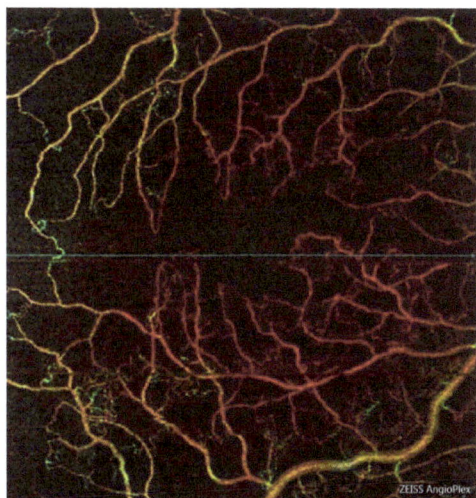
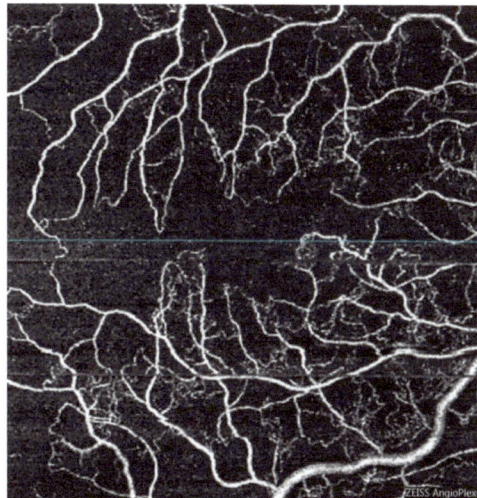
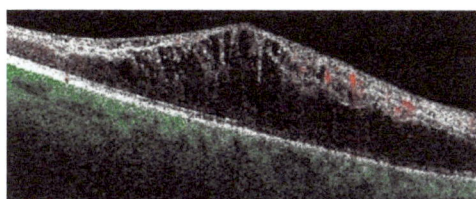
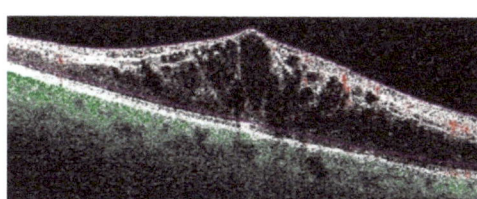

C1

C2

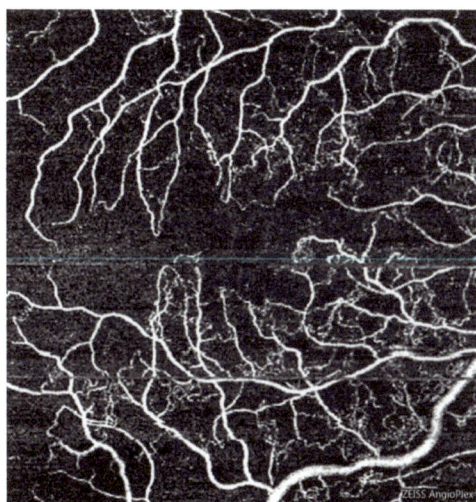
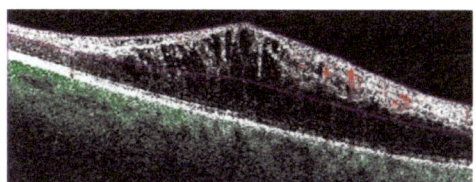
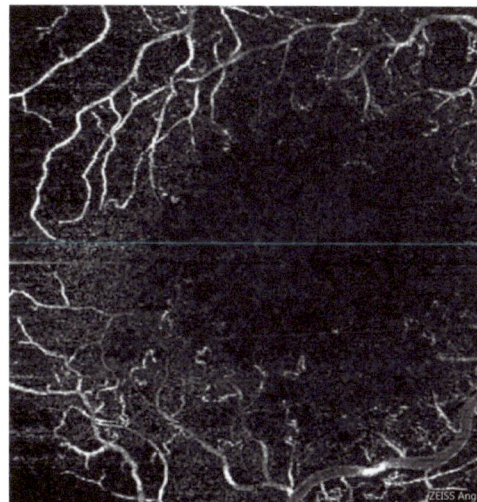
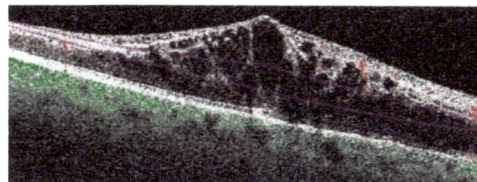

C3

C4

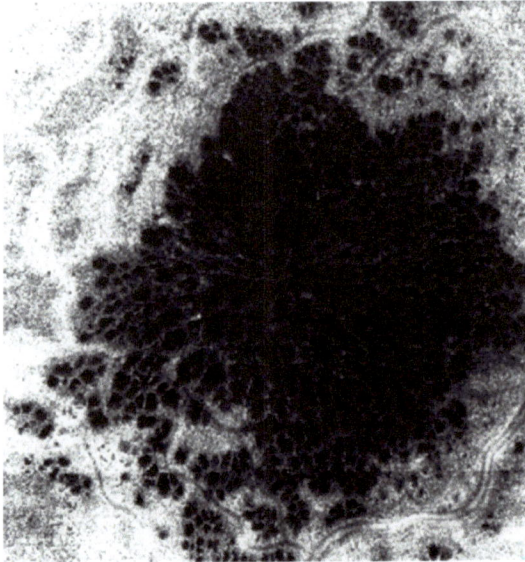

D

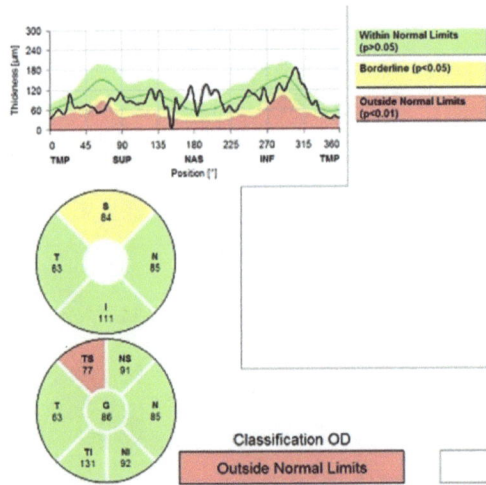

E1

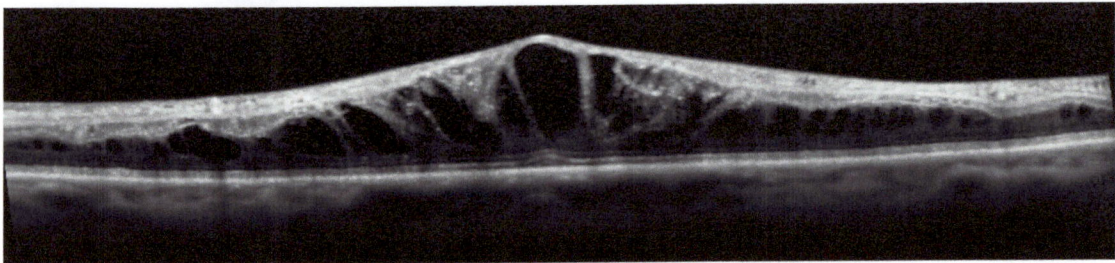

E2

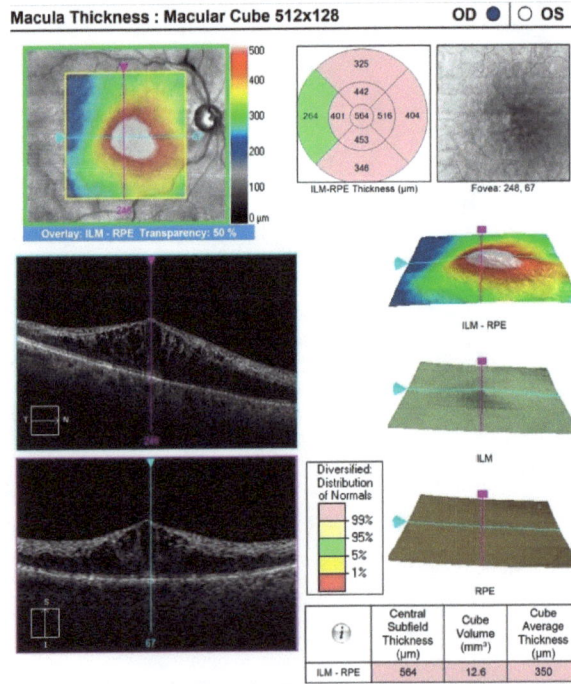

E3

Case 24: *Central Retinal Vein Occlusion and Cilioretinal Artery Occlusion*

Clinical Summary

62-year-old white female with history of NIDDM x 12 years, presents with complaints of blurred vision OS x 6 months. Vision OS is 20/200.

Image Summary

A. Color Fundus: Shows several large into retinal hemorrhages along the arcades that are consistent with nerve fiber layer infarcts. The veins appeared to be dilated and the arteries are relatively attenuated. The retina between the optic disc and fovea appears slightly opaque and is consistent with a cilioretinal artery occlusion in the setting of a CRVO.

B. Fluorescein Angiography: Shows several areas of blocked florescence consistent with the hemorrhages in the color image. There are numerous focal areas of late hyper-florescent staining in the superior macula that are consistent with old focal scars, and the foveal avascular zone appears irregular and enlarged.

C. OCT Angiography: C1: Depth encoded OCTA with corresponding B-scan confirms cilioretinal artery occlusion involving the nasal half of the macula. There is also a prominent loss of the deep retinal layer perfusion. The retina is thickened overall with evidence of numerous intraretinal cystoid spaces on the accompanying B-scan. **C2**: Full thickness retina composite OCTA with corresponding B-scan essentially illustrates the same findings as in the depth encoded OCTA.
C3: Deep retinal layer OCTA with corresponding B-scan shows that the edema has displaced the deep retinal layers superiorly and that some of the decreased signal in the en face image is likely an artifact of this displacement. Nevertheless, overall there is severe reduction in the perfusion signal throughout the retina in this image.

D. OCT: Volumetric OCT analysis illustrating both B-scan OCT images with diffuse cystic pockets, along with a fine epiretinal membrane. The volumetric OCT shows central thickening of the retina.

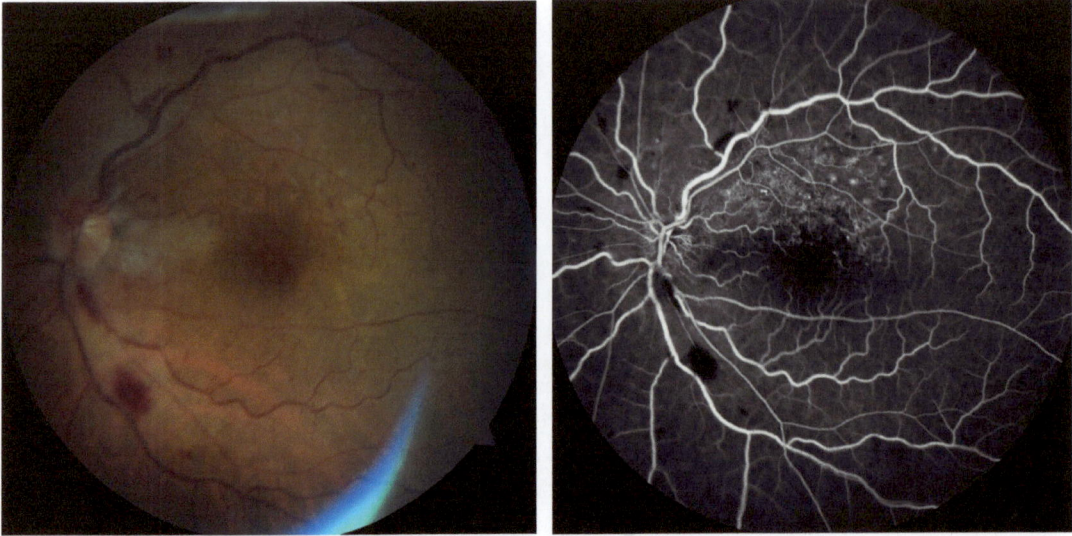

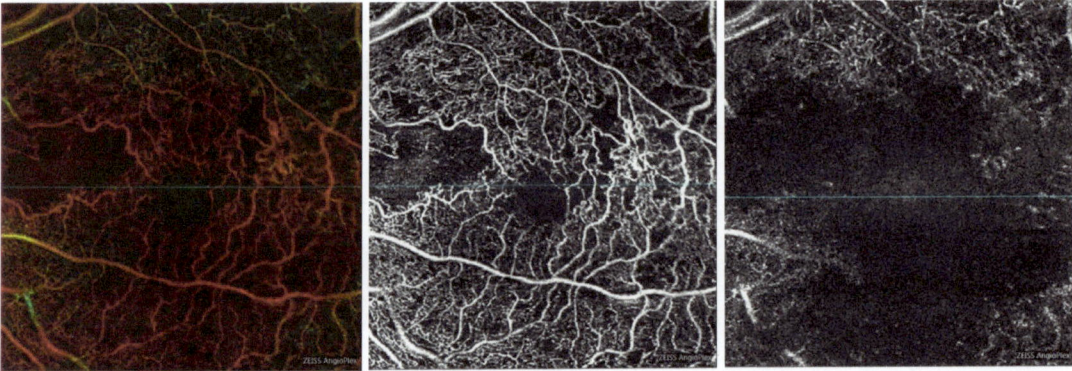

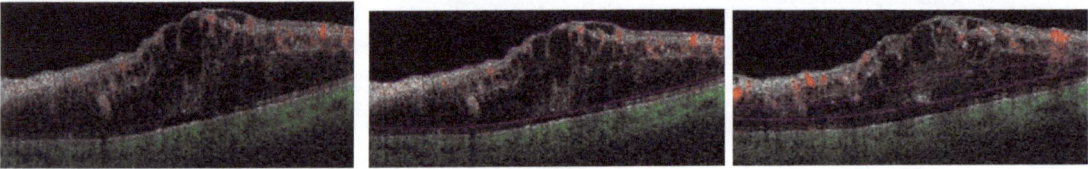

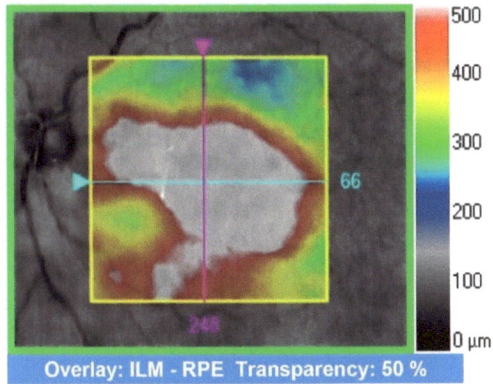

Overlay: ILM - RPE Transparency: 50 %

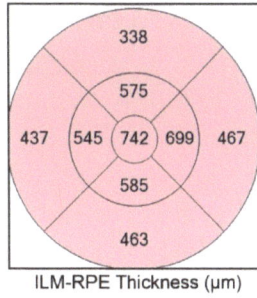

ILM-RPE Thickness (µm)

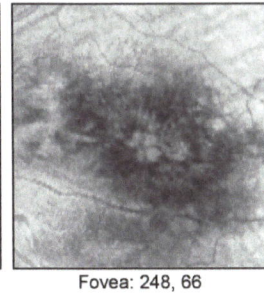

Fovea: 248, 66

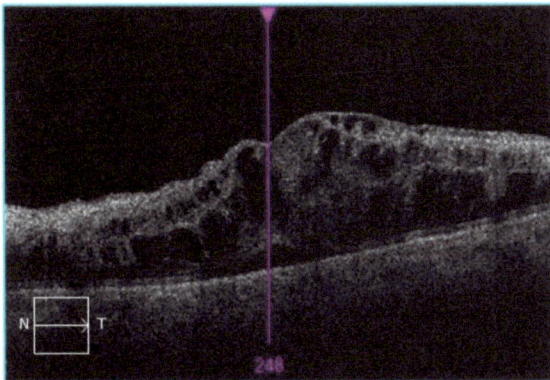

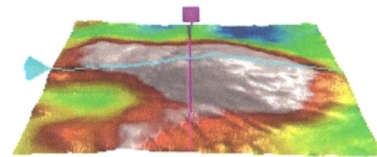

ILM - RPE

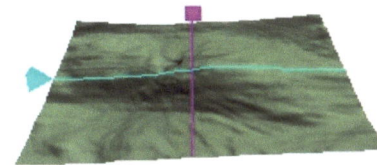

ILM

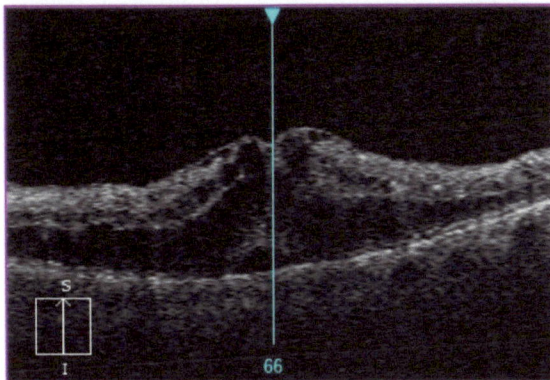

Diversified:
Distribution
of Normals

99%	
95%	
5%	
1%	

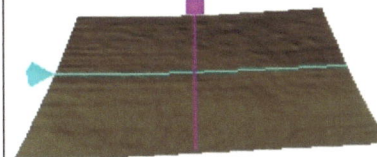

RPE

(i)	Central Subfield Thickness (µm)	Cube Volume (mm³)	Cube Average Thickness (µm)
ILM - RPE	742	16.0	445

D

Case 25: *Central Retinal Vein Occlusion and Central Retinal Artery Occlusion*

Clinical Summary

74-year-old white male with a history of hypertension and hypercholesterolemia presented initially with sudden decrease vision OD x 2 days. Vision is 20/200 OD.

Image Summary

A. Color Fundus: Shows dilated and tortuous veins. There are numerous intraretinal hemorrhages, and severe arteriovenous nicking at multiple crossing points.

B. Fluorescein Angiography: B1: Early phase fluorescein angiogram shows the numerous retinal hemorrhages which block the underlying fluorescence. **B2**: Late phase fluorescein angiogram confirms the dilation of the retinal veins and the late staining of the nasal macula suggests severe macular edema.

C. OCT Angiography: C1: Depth encoded OCTA with corresponding B-scan shows severe impairment of perfusion involving the majority of the macula. **C2**: Full thickness retina composite with corresponding B-scan shows similar findings. **C3**: Deep retina plexus OCTA with corresponding B-scan shows the extent of perfusion impairment. **C4**: Deep retina layer en face intensity image shows hyporeflective spots consistent with intraretinal fluid pockets (edema). There are some horizontal lines along the bottom of the image consistent with movement artifacts.

D. OCT: D1: Volumetric OCT shows diffuse intraretinal edema in the fovea and inferiorly. **D2**: B-scan OCT shows many hyporeflective intraretinal spaces consistent with severe intraretinal edema, and the fovea depression is completely blunted.

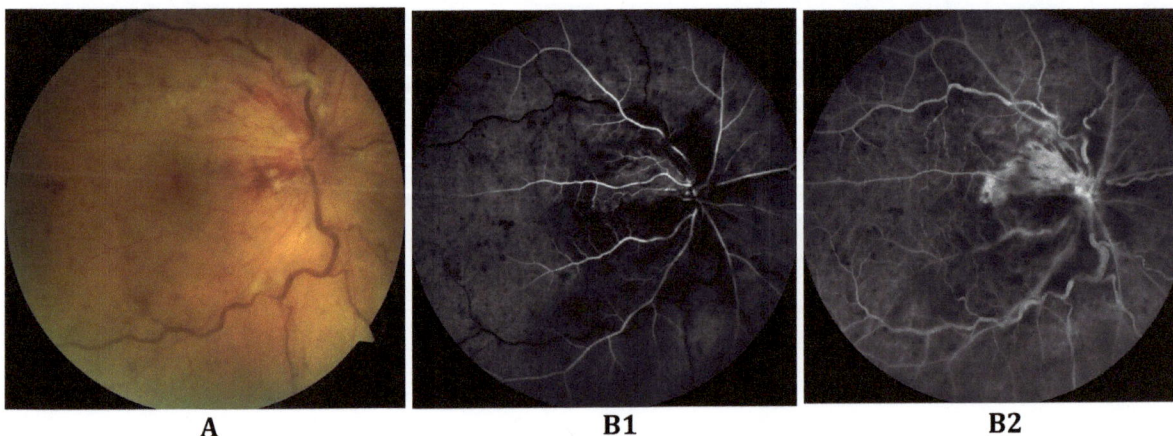

A　　　　　　　　　B1　　　　　　　　　B2

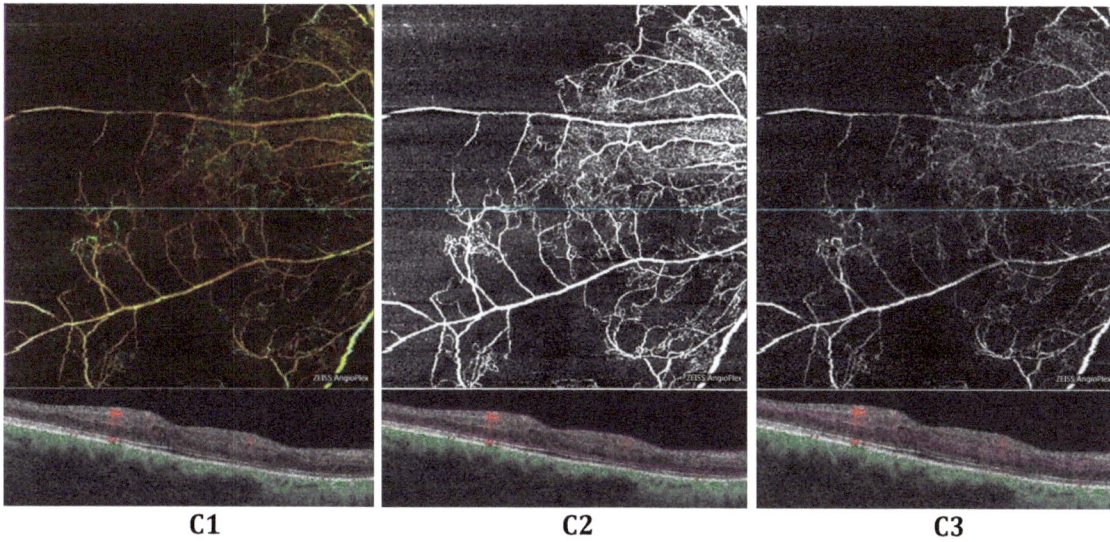

C1   **C2**   **C3**

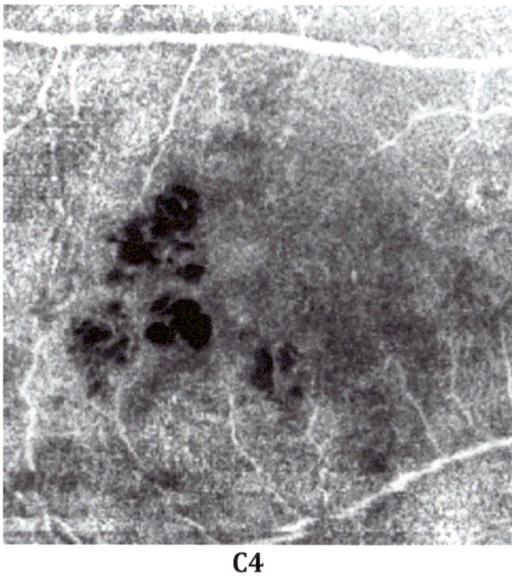

C4   **D1**

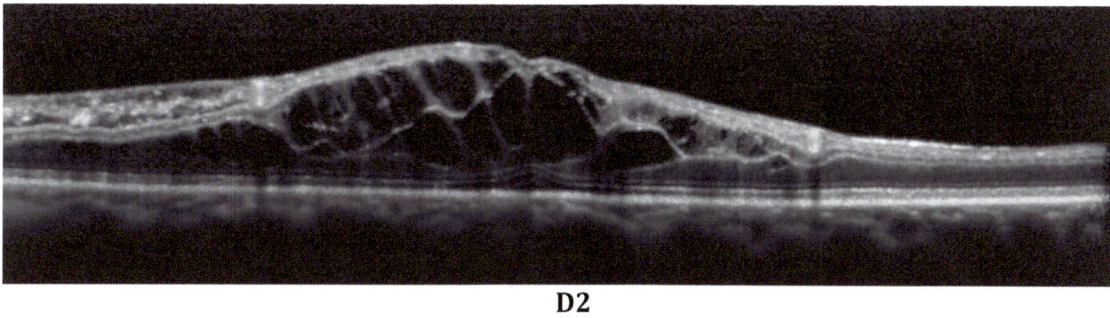

D2

Case 26: *Branch Retinal Artery Occlusion*

Clinical Summary

69-year-old white male with history of hypertension, hypercholesterolemia, heart disease and kidney failure presents with complaints of sudden onset of "curtain" in vision inferiorly OS with diminished vision and blurred spot in vision OD x 1 week. Vision is 20/30- OD and 20/100 OS.

Image Summary

A. Color Fundus: A1: Color fundus image OD is hazy due to cataract. There is intraretinal hemorrhage along the inferior arcade. **A2**: Color fundus image OS shows sclerotic vessels along the superotemporal arcade, and there are numerous hemorrhages along that region as well. The superior retina appears ischemic.

B. Fluorescein Angiography: B1: Mid-phase fluorescein angiogram OD shows several pinpoint hyperfluorescent spots in the area corresponding to the hemorrhage on color image. **B2**: Late phase fluorescein angiogram OD shows late staining corresponding to the retinal hemorrhage area seen on the color image. **B3**: Mid-phase fluorescein angiogram OS shows severe impairment in perfusion involving the whole superior retina. **B4**: Late phase fluorescein angiogram OS shows staining of the retinal vessels in the affected region.

C. OCT Angiography: C1: Depth encoded OCTA with corresponding B-scan OD shows asymmetric perfusion of the superficial retinal layer in the inferior nasal macula. The peripapillary capillaries appear perfused, but the deep retinal layer perfusion is severely impaired. **C2**: Deep retina layer OCTA with corresponding B-scan OD confirms the severe impairment in perfusion. The B-scan shows diffuse intraretinal edema that has artifactually displaced the retinal layers anteriorly and likely explains some of decreased perfusion signal in the deep retinal layer.
C3: Depth encoded OCTA with corresponding B-scan OS shows impaired perfusion involving most of the superior macula. **C4**: Full thickness retina composite OCTA with corresponding B-scan OS. There are several horizontal motion artifacts. **C5**: Deep retina layer OCTA with corresponding B-scan OS shows impaired perfusion superiorly and several pockets of intraretinal edema near the fovea.

D. OCT: D1: B-scan OCT OD shows diffuse retinal edema in the nasal macula. **D2**: B-scan OCT OS shows diffuse macular edema in the nasal macula and subretinal fluid. **D3**: Volumetric OCT OD illustrates thickened retina associated with intraretinal edema nasal to the fovea. **D4**: Volumetric OCT OS shows thickening superiorly with extension into the fovea.

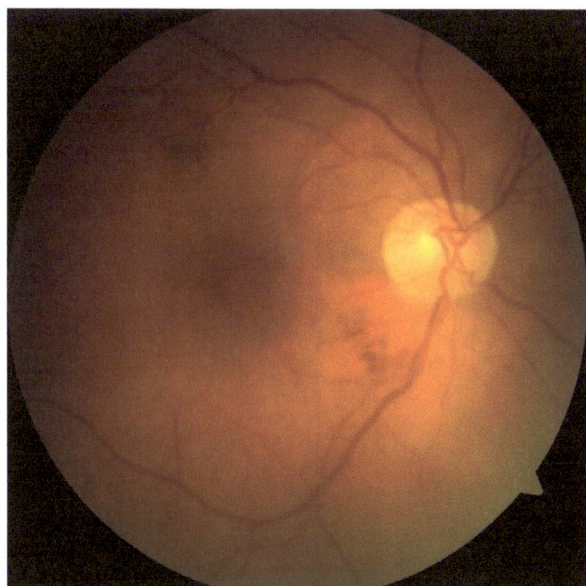

A1

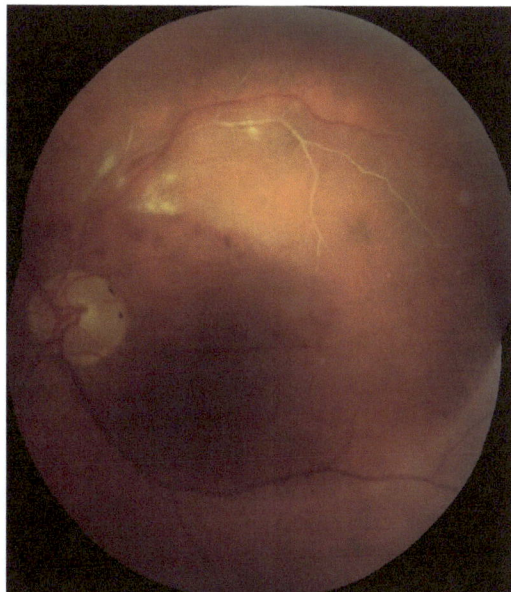

A2

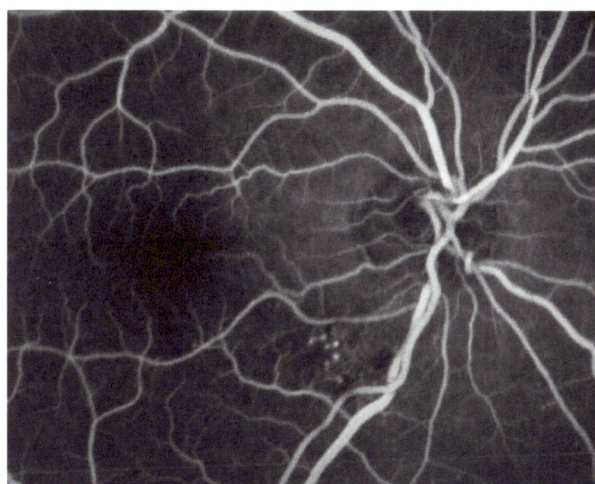

B1

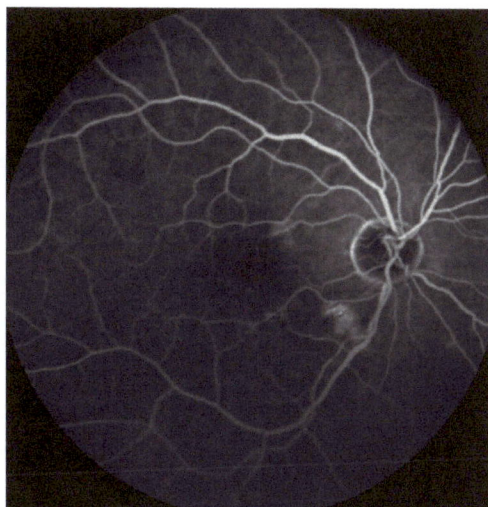

B2

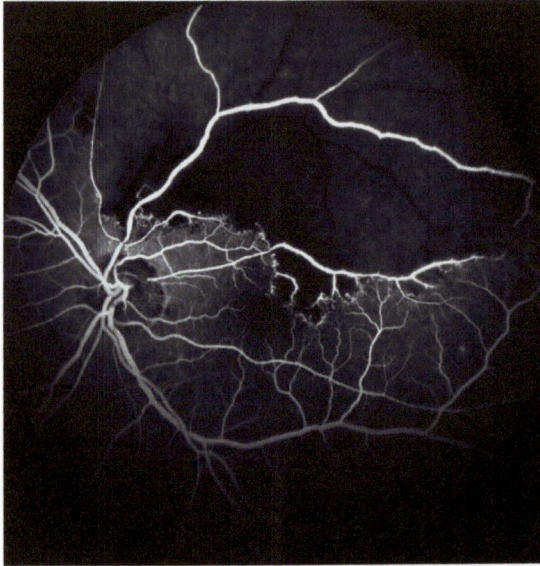

B3

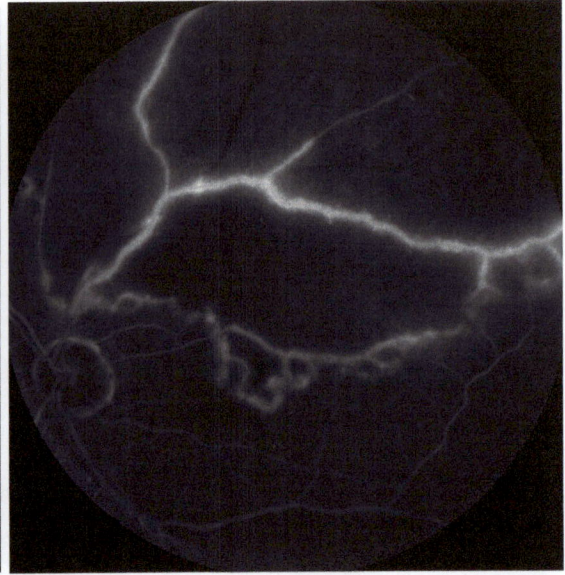

B4

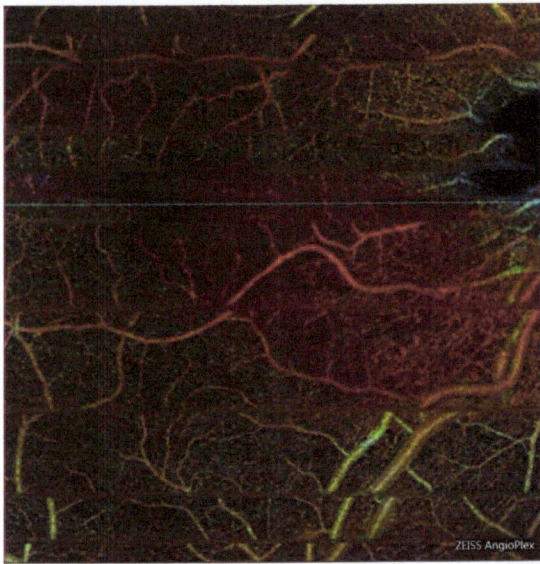

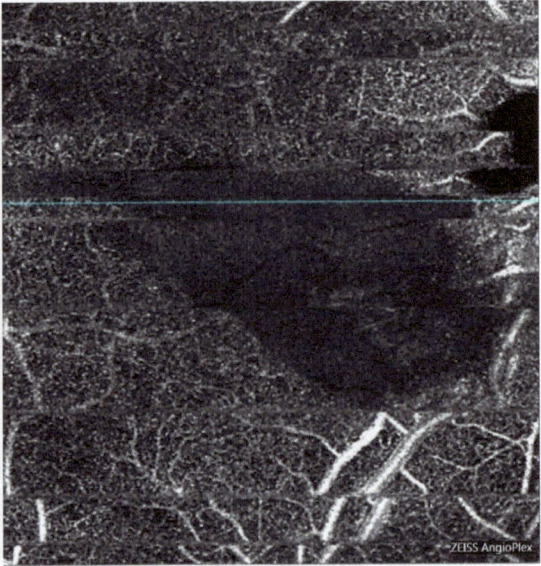

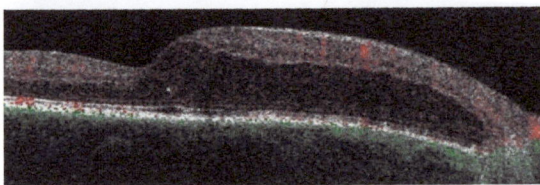

C1

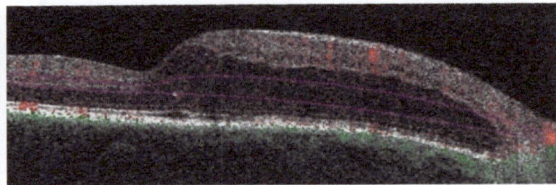

C2

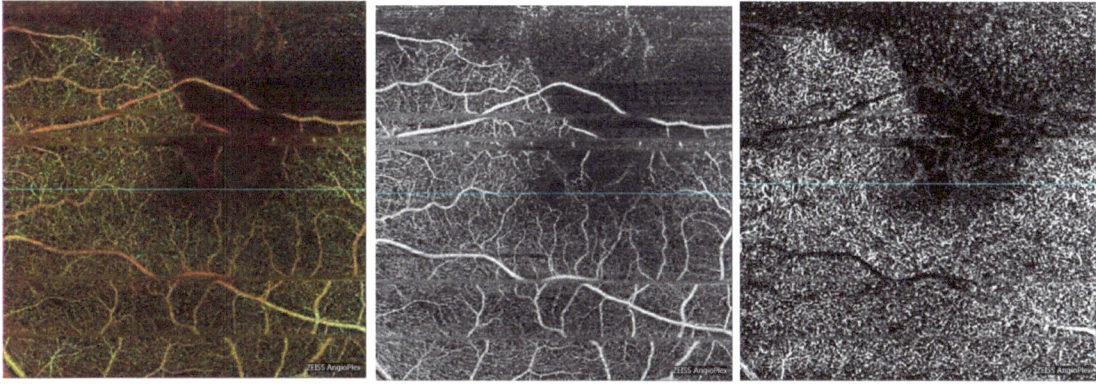

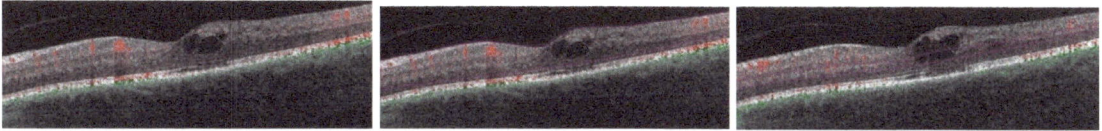

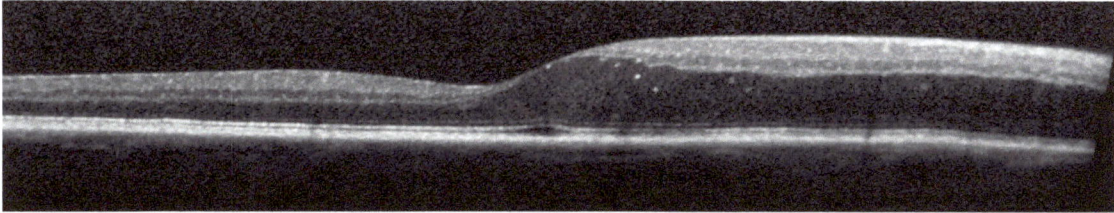

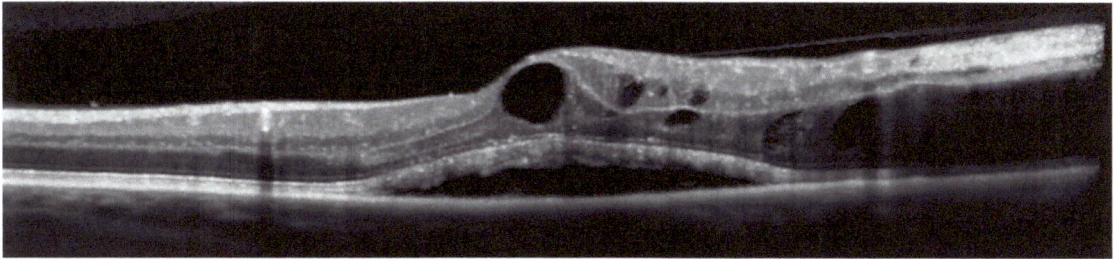

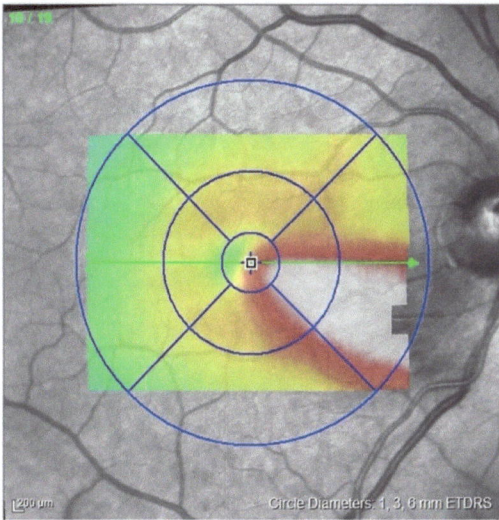

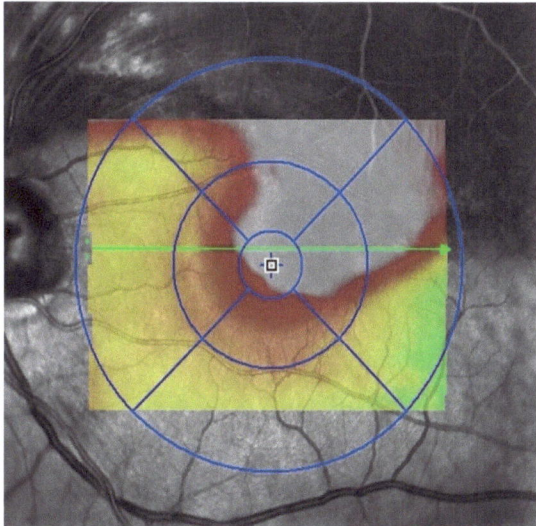

C3　　　　　　　C4　　　　　　　C5

D1

D2

D3　　　　　　　　　　　D4

Case 27: *Central Retinal Artery Occlusion*

Clinical Summary

80-year-old white female with history of hypertension, congestive heart failure and atrial fibrillation presents with complaint of sudden loss of vision x 2 days. Vision OD is hand motion.

Image Summary

A. Color Fundus: Shows diffuse retinal whitening that spares the nasal macula. There are intra-arterial plaques in the superonasal vessels suggestive of arterial occlusion. The nasal macula is spared in the distribution of the cilioretinal artery.

B. Fluorescein Angiography: B1: Early phase fluorescein angiogram shows sparing of the cilioretinal artery distribution and delayed filling of the majority of the retina. **B2**: Late phase fluorescein angiogram shows incomplete filling of the retinal vessels throughout the retina consistent with an arterial occlusion. The lack of choroidal filling and the poor vision may also suggest ophthalmic artery occlusion.

C. OCT Angiography: C1: Depth encoded OCTA with corresponding B-scan shows almost no perfusion in the macula, and the retina appears thin and atrophic temporally. **C2**: Full thickness retina composite OCTA with corresponding B-scan shows similar findings. **C3**: Deep retina plexus OCTA with corresponding B-scan illustrates more extensive non-perfusion.

D. OCT: B-scan OCT shows hyperreflectivity of the inner retina throughout the whole image and thickening more temporally than nasally.

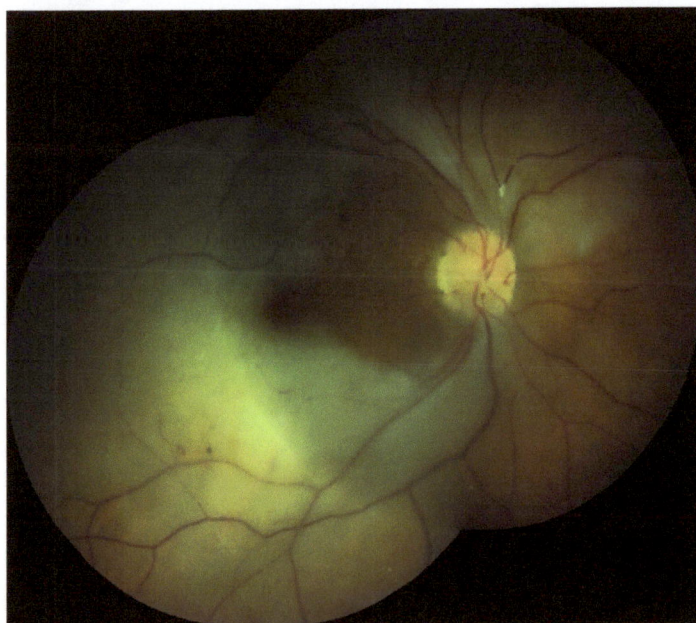

A

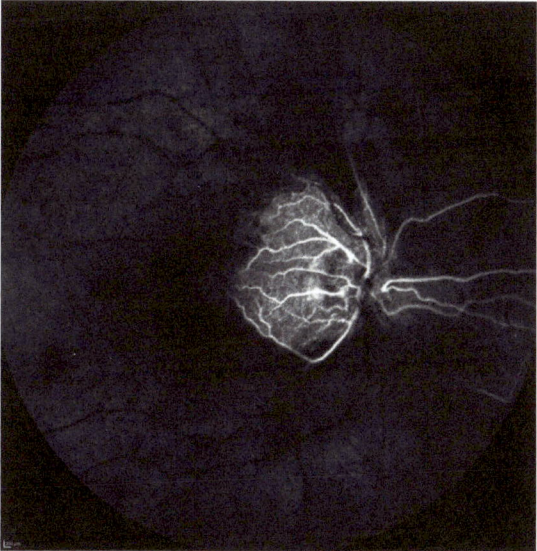
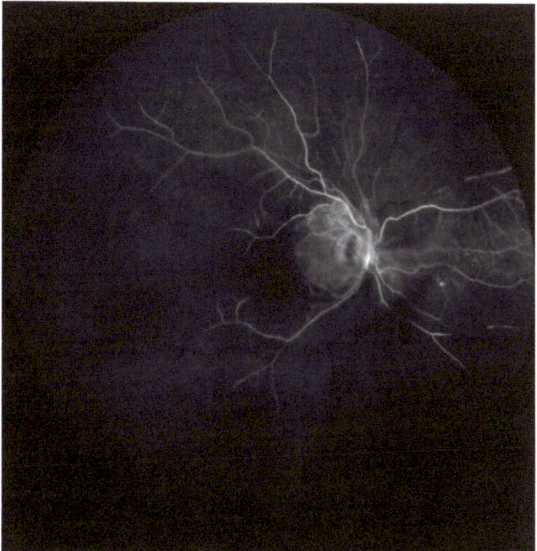

B1

B2

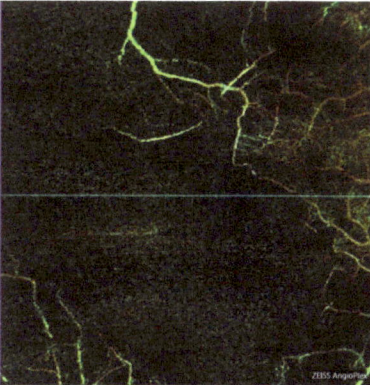
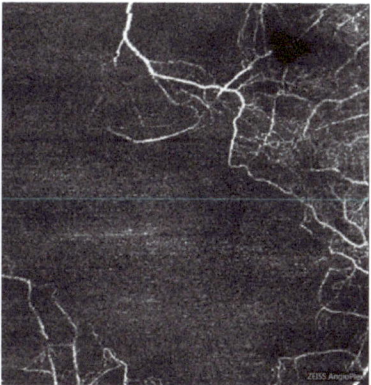
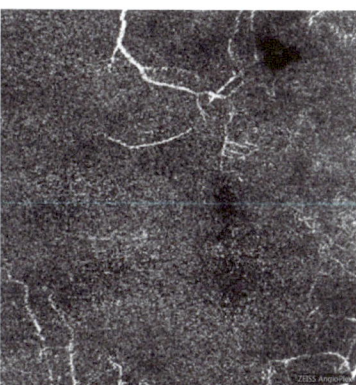

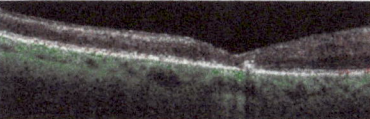
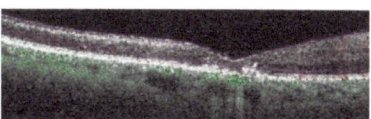
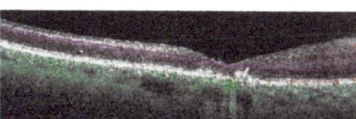

C1

C2

C3

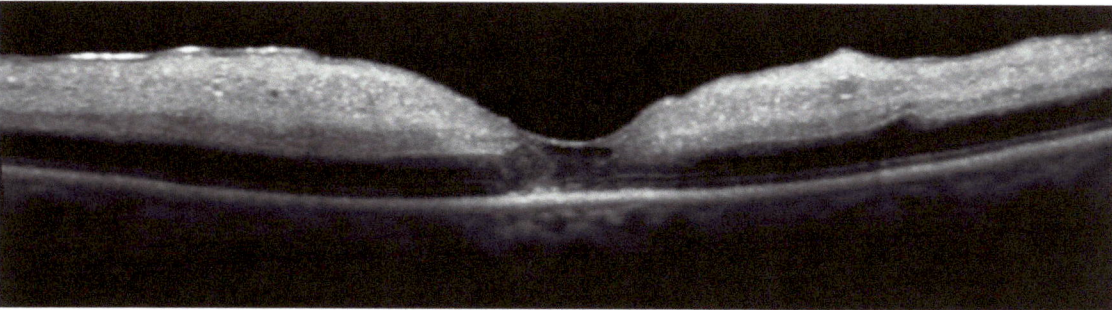

D

Subretinal- Choroidal Diseases

- **Drusen**

- **Exudative Macular Degeneration**

- **Polypoidal Choroidal Vasculopathy**

- **Retinal Angiomatous Proliferation**

- **Central Serous Chorioretinopathy**

Case 28: *High Risk Drusen vs Early CNV*

Clinical Summary

69-year-old healthy white male with pseudophakia presents with no vision complaints for annual retinal exam. Vision is 20/25 OU.

Image Summary

A. Color Fundus: **A1**: Color image OD shows numerous soft drusen throughout the macula. There is a focal area of RPE change temporal to the fovea, and no hemorrhage is noted. **A2**: Color image OS shows similar changes to OD.

B. Fundus Autofluorescence: B1: FAF OD shows hypoautofluorescence throughout the macula corresponding to the drusen lesions. **B2**: FAF OS shows similar findings to OD.

C. OCT Angiography: **C1**: Depth encoded OCTA with corresponding B-scan OD shows a normal fovea avascular zone. There are apparent focal regions of perfusion in the avascular retinal layer (blue) that corresponds to shallow PEDs on the B-scan. **C2**: Choriocapillaris level OCTA with corresponding B-scan OD shows a non-homogenous layer with numerous areas of apparent hypoperfusion. **C3**: Avascular level OCTA OD shows focal areas of apparent perfusion in the outer retina. These areas correspond to perfusion signal from below the level of the RPE on the corresponding B-scan consistent with early choroidal neovascularization. **C4**: Avascular level en face OD intensity image with B-scan shows no image artifacts. Note the green perfusion signal on the B-scan in the region of the PEDs. These suggest that there is flow signal and neovascularization within the PEDs. **C5**: Depth encoded OCTA with corresponding B-scan OS shows similar findings to OD. **C6**: Choriocapillaris level OCTA OS with corresponding B-scan shows similar findings to OD. **C7**: Avascular level OCTA OS shows similar findings OD. **C8**: Avascular level en face OS with avascular level B-scan shows similar findings to OD.

D. OCT: D1: B-scan OCT OD shows numerous PEDs with hypo and hyperreflective internal contents. The appearance of some of the PEDs is consistent with underlying CNV. **D2**: B-scan OCT OS shows similar findings to OD.

Note: The OCTA findings and OCT findings in this case strongly suggest that there is early CNV. However, there is no evidence of active CNV (i.e. intraretinal fluid). This type of case should prompt the provider to consider an FA/ICG and retinal consultation to confirm or further evaluate the possible CNV. Although in the past, this case would have been considered non-neovascular or dry AMD, the use of OCTA will start to identify sub-clinical CNV, such as this case, and this warrants earlier referral and evaluation by retinal specialists.

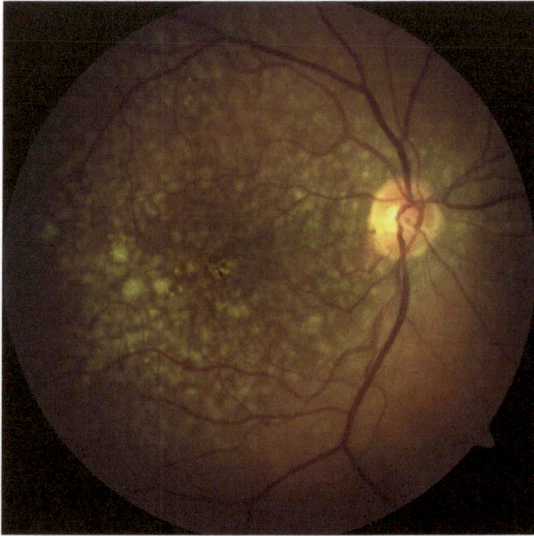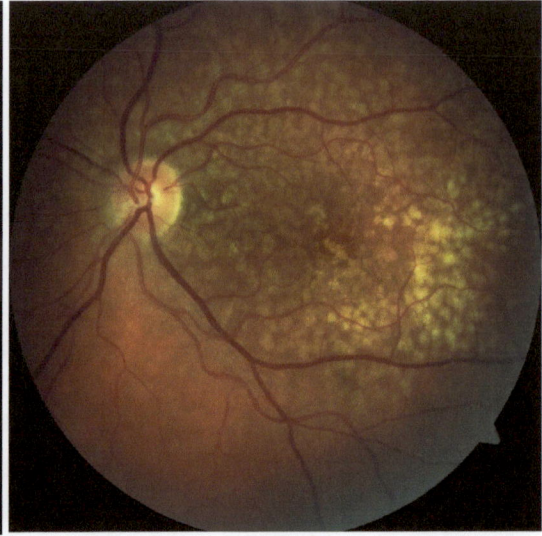

A1 **A2**

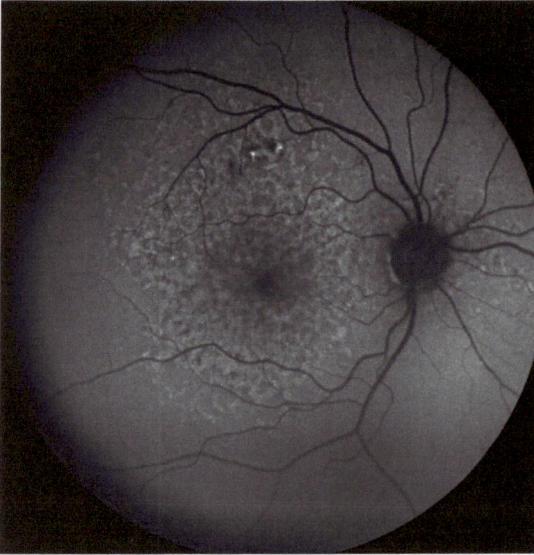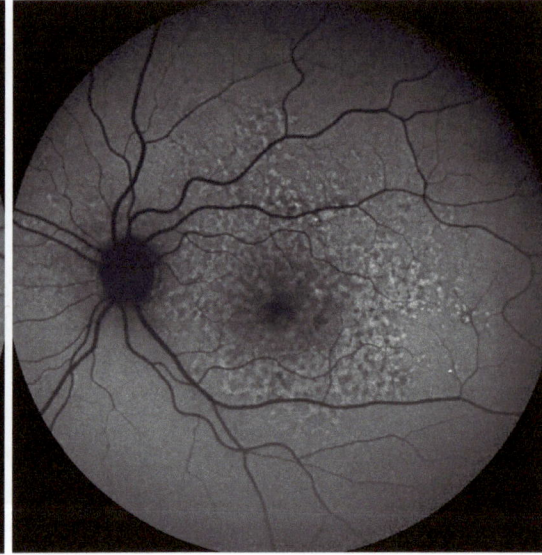

B1 **B2**

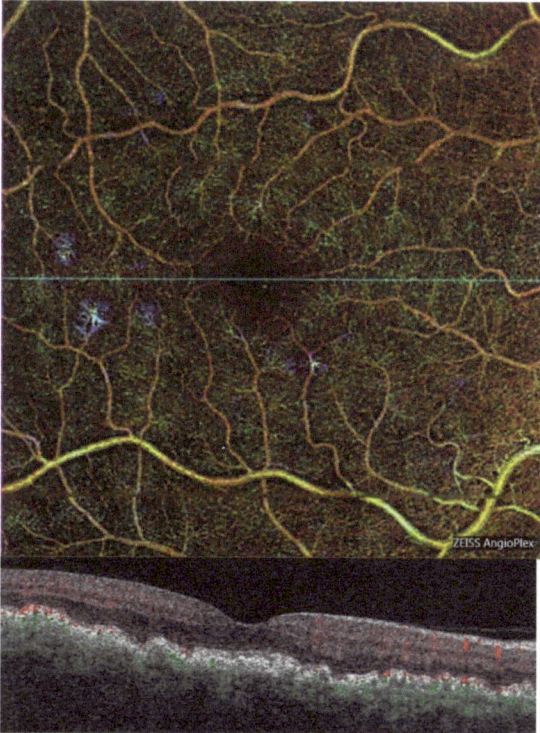

C1

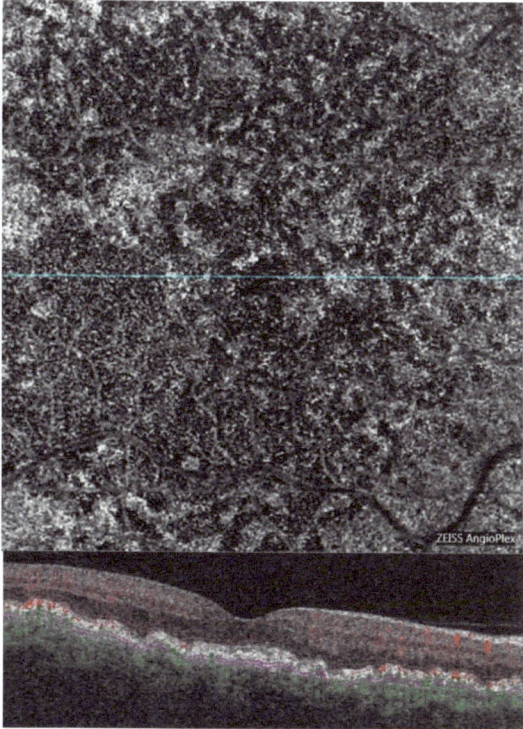

C2

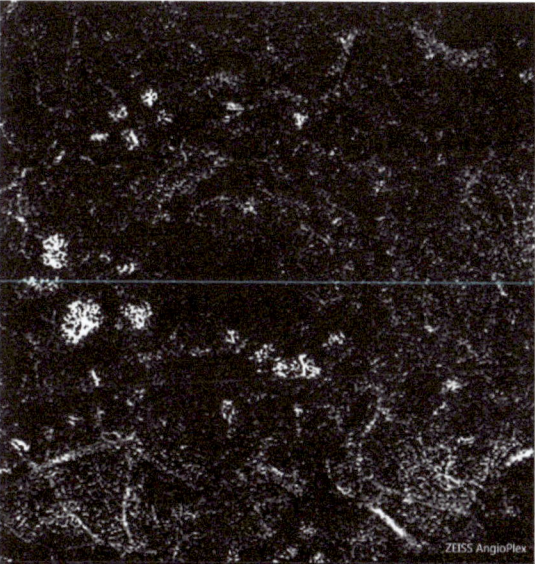

C3

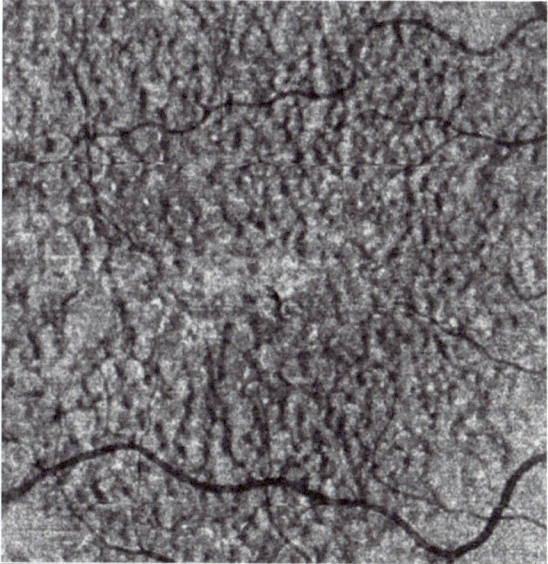

C4

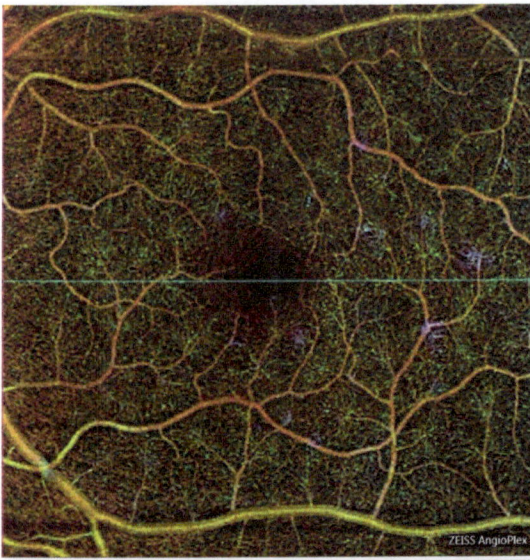

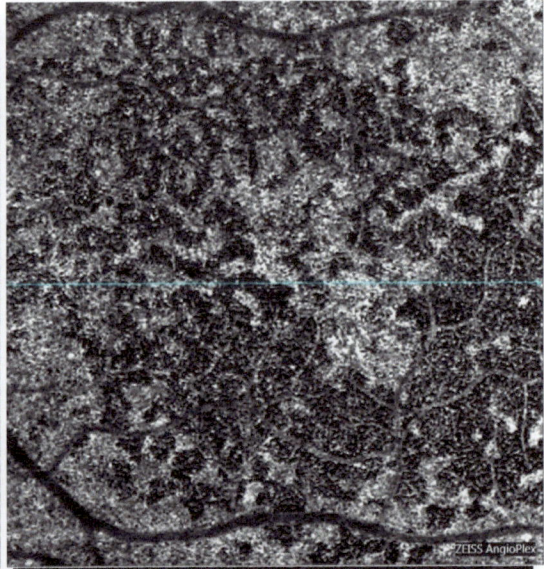

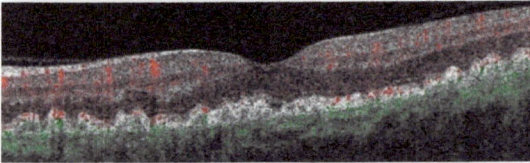

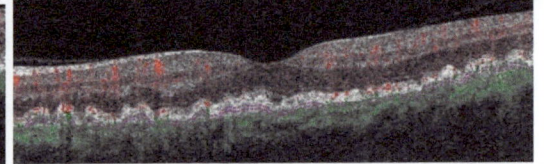

C5

C6

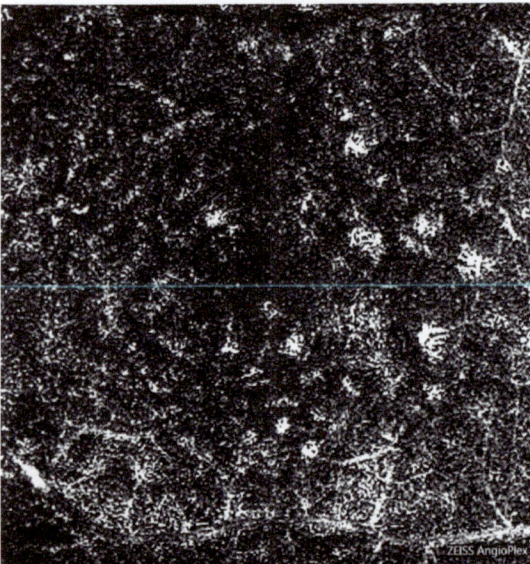

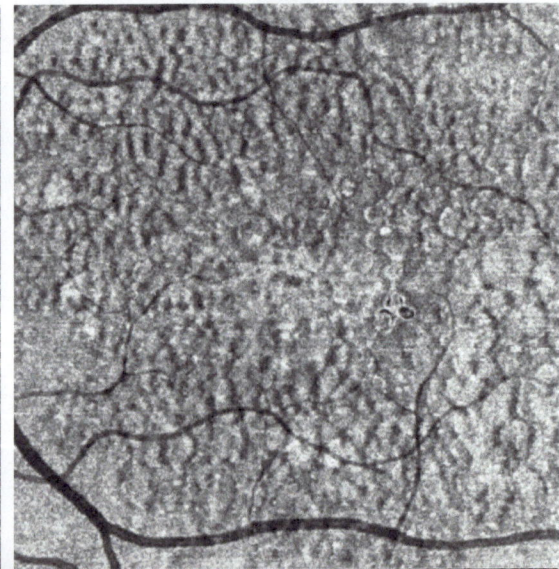

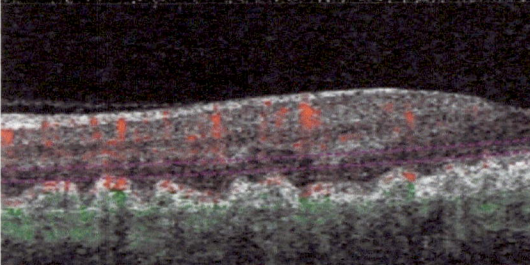

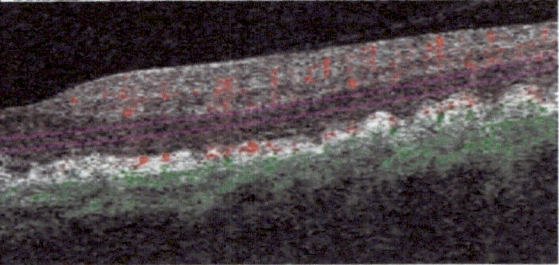

C7

C8

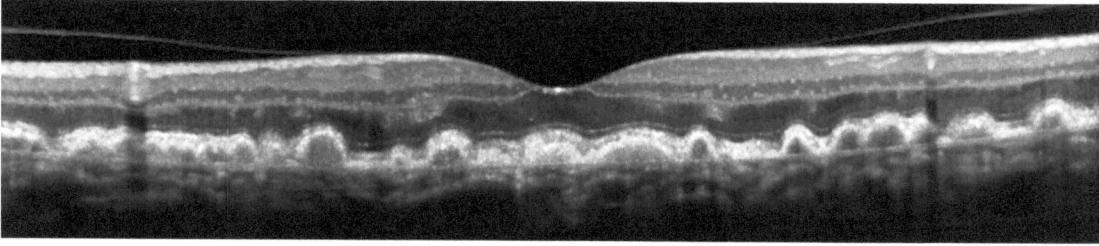

D1

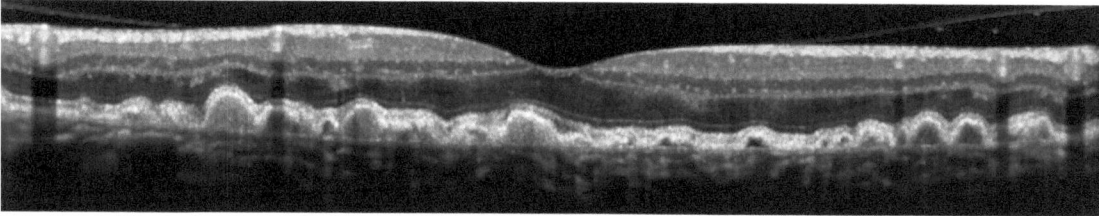

D2

Case 29: *Drusen*

Clinical Summary

67-year-old referred for sudden decrease vision OS (case in RAP section). Vision is 20/40- OD and 20/200 OS. OD is asymptomatic.

Image Summary

A. Color Fundus: Color image OD shows multiple, large, confluent drusen and mild RPE changes in the central macula.

B. Fundus Autofluorescence: Shows areas of hyper- and hypo-autofluorescence corresponding to some of the drusen on the color image. FAF does not always correlate with drusen on color images.

C. Fluorescein Angiography: C1: Early-mid phase fluorescein angiogram shows numerous fine hyperfluorescent spots consistent with small drusen. **C2**: Late phase fluorescein angiogram shows additional staining of some of the larger drusen.

D. ICG Angiography: D1: Early phase ICG angiogram shows blockage of fluorescence in the region of the large drusen. **D2**: Late phase angiogram shows similar findings. There is no evidence of choroidal neovascularization.

E. OCT Angiography: E1: Depth encoded OCTA with corresponding B-scan shows some perifoveal areas that appear to have perfusion in the avascular layer. The corresponding B-scan does not confirm perfusion within the PEDs in these regions and therefore these are likely artifacts. Close examination of the B-scan shows that the perfusion signal is coming from the RPE and not the internal contents of the PEDs. Perfusion signal that originates from the RPE layer on the B-scan is in most cases projection artifacts of the OCTA. **E2**: Chorioretinal level OCTA with corresponding B-scan shows the choriocapillaris is largely homogenous in appearance and unremarkable.

F. OCT: B-scan OCT shows multiple large drusen with medium reflectivity of internal contents. There is no evidence of intraretinal edema; however, there appears to be SRF overlying the central drusen. The lack of CNV on the ICG/FA and OCTA suggests that this is not CNV (or SRF) and may represent an atypical looking drusen with a defect in the overlying RPE. Referral to a retinal specialist in atypical cases is warranted.

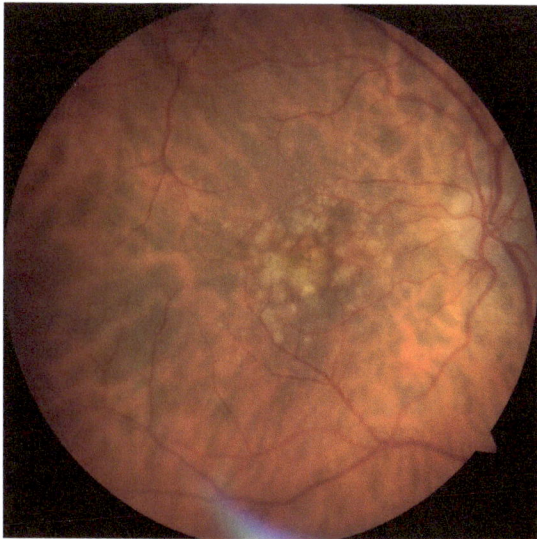

A

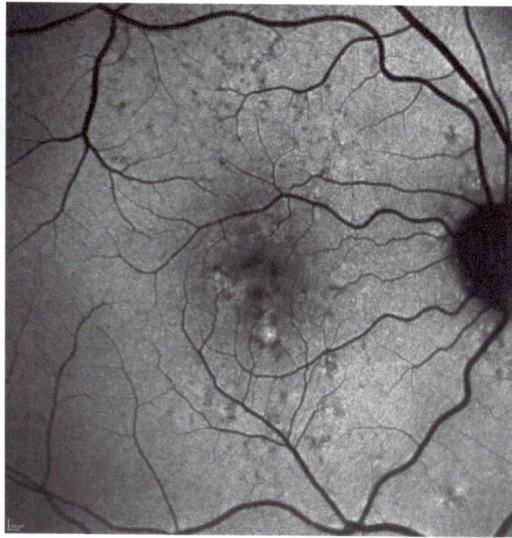

B

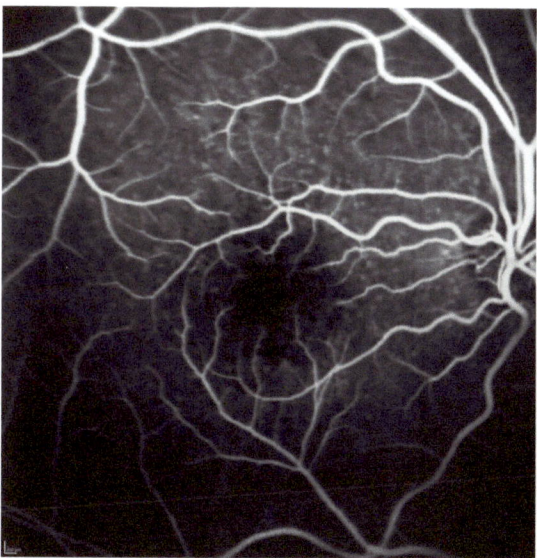

C1

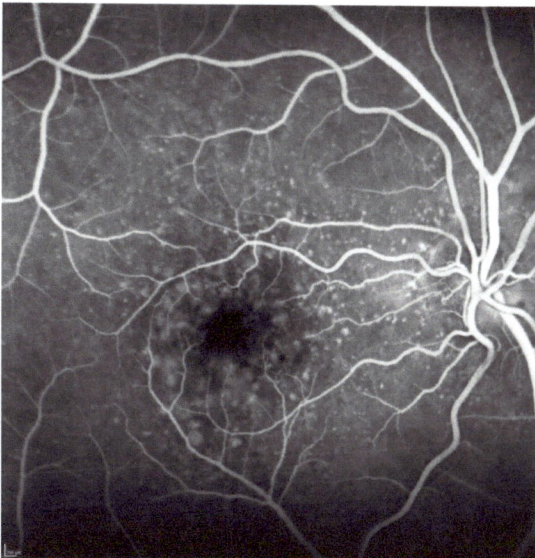

C2

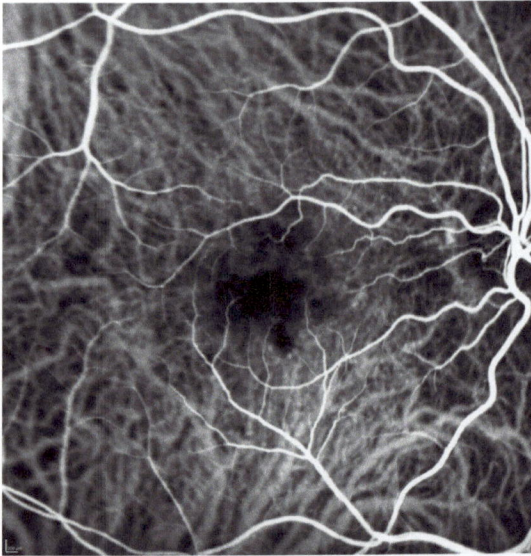
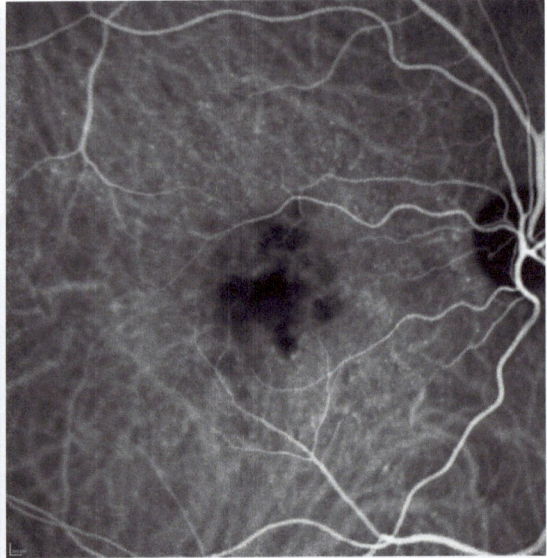

D1 **D2**

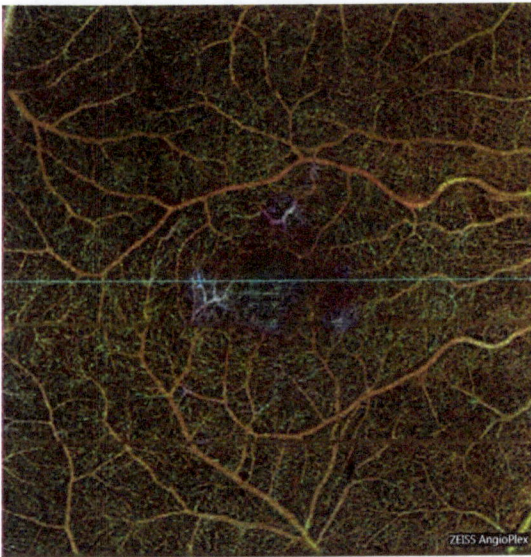
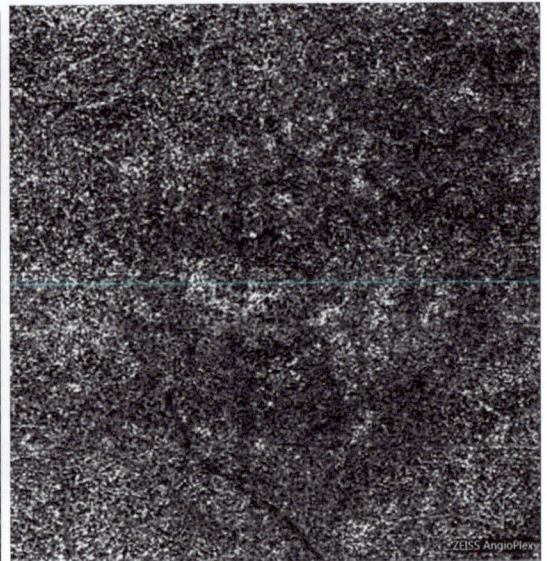

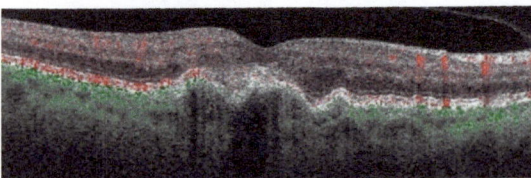
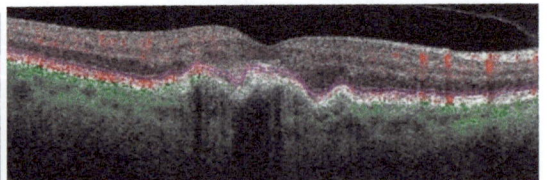

E1 **E2**

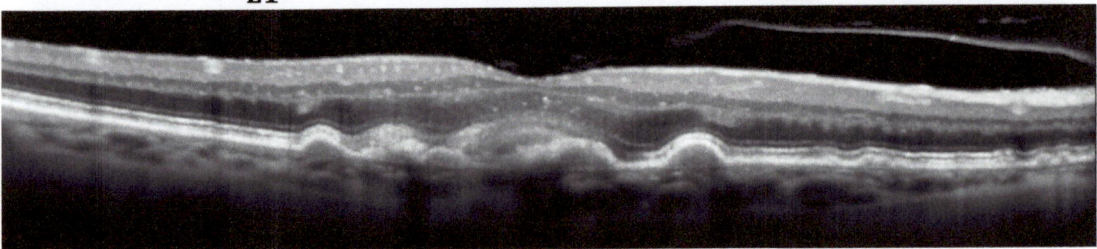

F

Case 30: *Exudative Macular Degeneration*

Clinical Summary

82-year-old white female presents with sudden blurred central vision OD with metamorphopsia x 1 week, progressively worsening since onset. Vision is 20/100-.

Image Summary

A. Color Fundus: not available

B. Fluorescein Angiography: B1: Mid phase fluorescein angiogram shows intense staining of subretinal lesions inferior to the fovea. There is also mild hyperfluorescence surrounding the fovea suggesting macular edema, and there are numerous pinpoint hyperfluorescent spots surrounding the fovea. **B2**: Late phase fluorescein angiogram confirms the same findings.

C. OCT Angiography: C1: Depth encoded OCTA with corresponding B-scan shows abnormal perfusion throughout the central macula. The corresponding B-scan reveals a large PED that is distorting the retina and likely causing significant segmentation artifacts. Interpretation of this image may be difficult due to the distorted retinal contour. **C2**: Deep retinal plexus OCTA with corresponding B-scan shows similar findings and highlights the choroidal neovascular complex within the PED. **C3**: Avascular level OCTA with corresponding B-scan shows the outline of the PED at a deeper level, which reveals a ring of CNV. In this case, the color-coding scheme on the image is not reliable and a very careful evaluation of the individual B-scans are necessary for an accurate understanding of the image.

D. OCT: B-scan OCT shows a large lobulated PED with hyporeflective and hyperreflective internal contents.

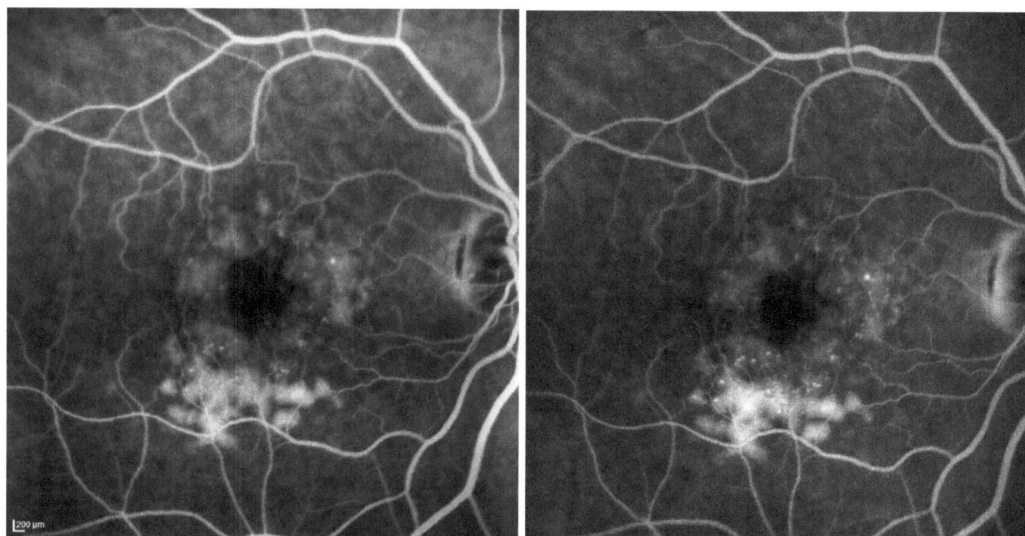

B1

B2

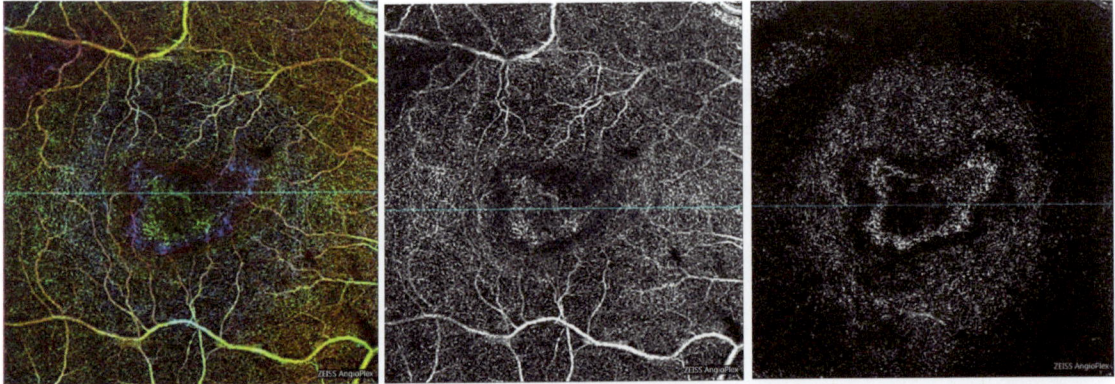

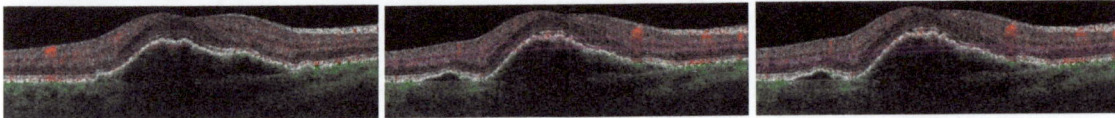

C1   C2   C3

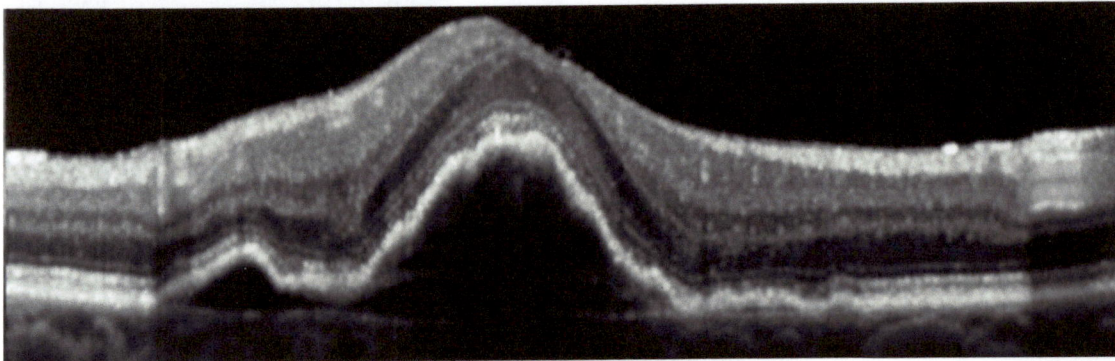

D

Case 31: *Exudative Macular Degeneration*

Clinical Summary

52-year-old healthy white male presents with sudden onset of decreased vision OD. Vision is count fingers.

Image Summary

A. Color Fundus: Shows a large subretinal hemorrhage with an associated yellow-green appearing lesion consistent with a CNV.

B. Fluorescein Angiography: **B1**: Early phase fluorescein angiogram shows blockage in the region of the hemorrhage and staining of a lesion that is similar in size and shape to the area of likely of CNV in the color image. **B2**: Late phase fluorescein angiogram shows similar findings to early phase image.

C. OCT Angiography: C1: Depth encoded OCTA with corresponding B-scan shows a large subretinal neovascular complex (blue) that is consistent with the lesion in the FA above. **C2**: Full thickness retina composite OCTA with corresponding B-scan shows similar findings. **C3**: Deep retina plexus OCTA with corresponding B-scan shows similar findings. **C4**: Avascular level OCTA with corresponding B-scan shows similar findings. **C5**: Choriocapillaris level OCTA with corresponding B-scan shows further extent of the CNV and surrounding area of impaired perfusion. The corresponding B-scans show that the subretinal lesion has perfusion associated with it, consistent with the CNV. Notice that the segmentation around the lesion is not accurate however interpretation of the images is still useful if the segmentation artifacts are accounted for.

D. OCT: D1: B-scan OCT shows a subretinal lesion and associated subretinal fluid.

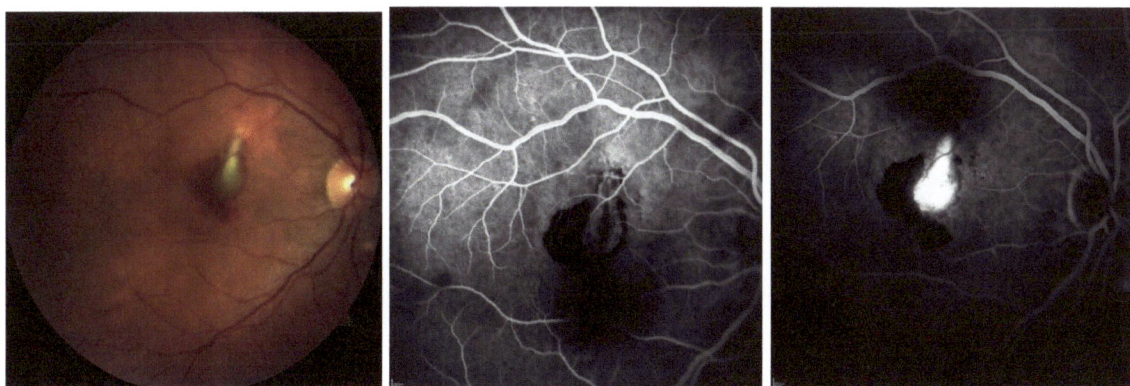

A   B1   B2

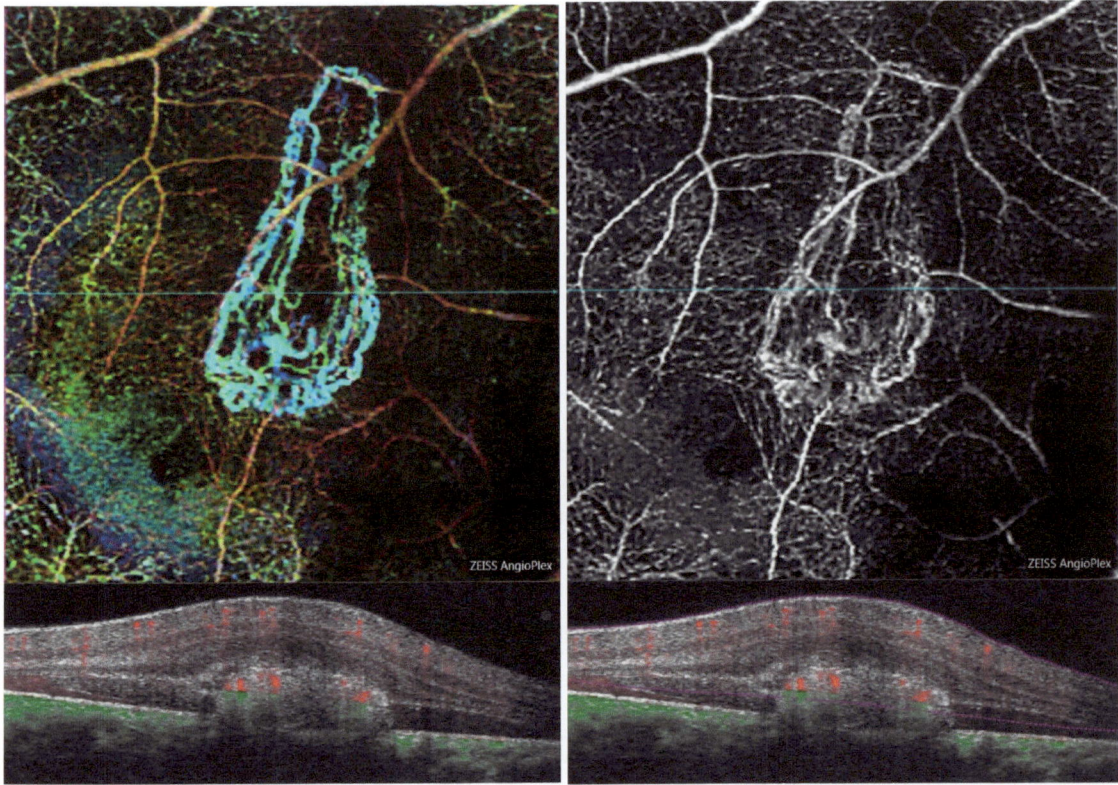

C1　　　　　　　　　　　　　C2

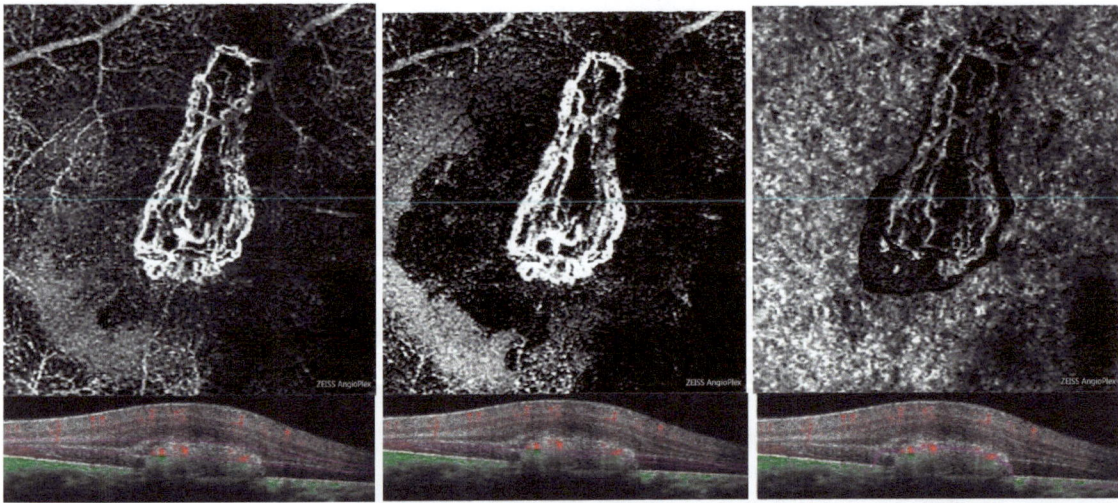

C3　　　　　　C4　　　　　　C5

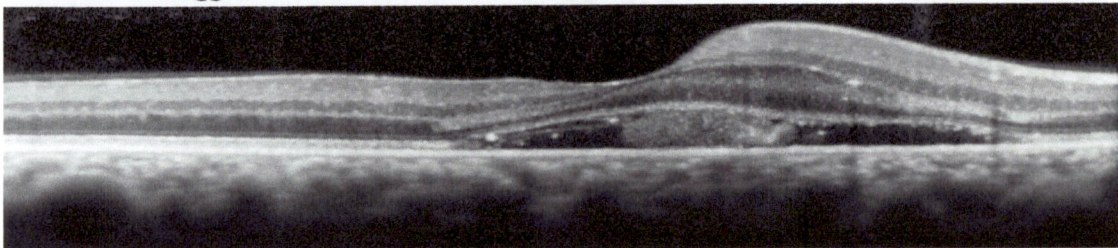

D

Case 32: *Exudative Macular Degeneration*

Clinical Summary

65-year-old white male with history of hypertension and heart disease presents with complaints of gradual decline in central vision OS with metamorphopsia x 1 month. Vision OS is 20/60.

Image Summary

A. Color Fundus: Shows fine yellow deposits consistent with drusen and RPE changes. There is a small area of intraretinal hemorrhage superotemporal to the disc with surrounding RPE changes.

B. Fluorescein Angiography: B1: Mid to late phase fluorescein angiogram shows staining of drusen and some leakage associated with the region of RPE changes on the color image. **B2**: Late phase fluorescein angiogram confirms the same findings as the early with the addition of late hyperfluorescence around the superotemporal aspect of the disc that may be consistent with CNV.

C. OCT Angiography: **C1**: Depth encoded OCTA with corresponding B-scan shows a neovascular complex inferior to the macula. **C2**: Deep retinal plexus OCTA with corresponding B-scan confirms the earlier finding of a neovascular complex. **C3**: Avascular level OCTA with corresponding B-scan shows that the lesion is clearly present in the avascular layer of the retina. **C4**: Choriocapillaris level OCTA with corresponding B-scan shows irregular choriocapillaris perfusion in the region surrounding the lesion. The corresponding B-scans of all the images do not show perfusion inside the PED, however the presence of subretinal fluid in the scans below strongly suggests that the PED has a neovascular component.

D. OCT: D1: B scan OCT shows PED with associated subretinal fluid. There is one drusen in the far left of the image. **D2**: Volumetric OCT illustrates the extent of retinal elevation associated with the lesion.

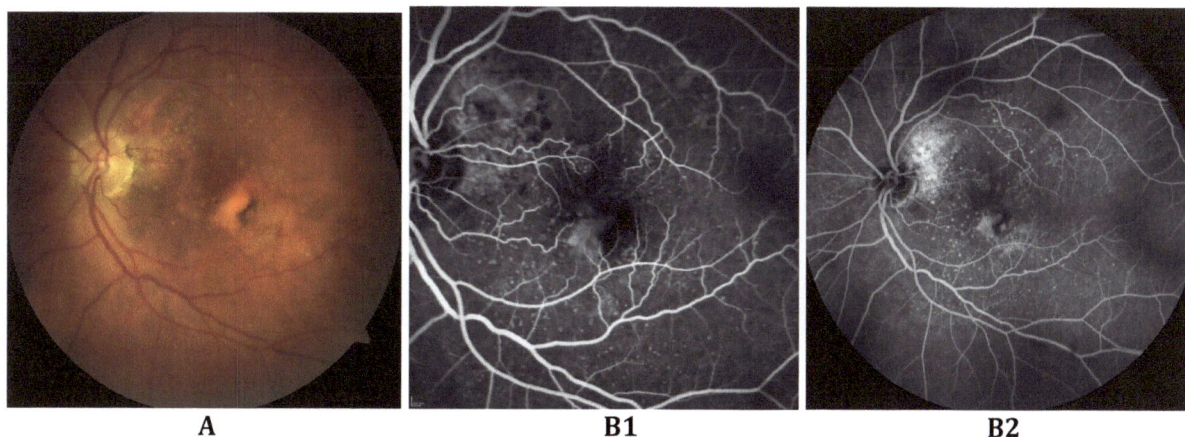

A   B1   B2

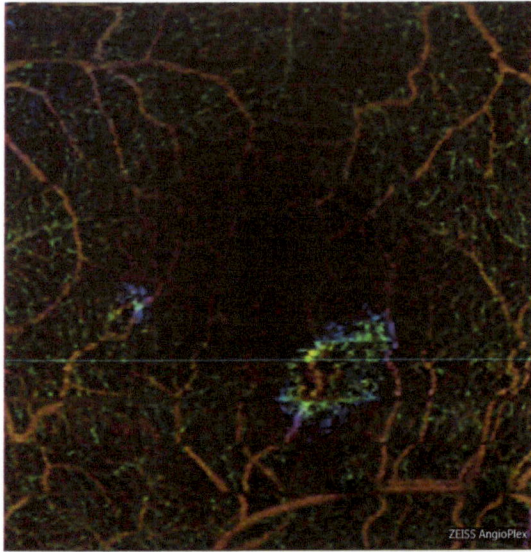
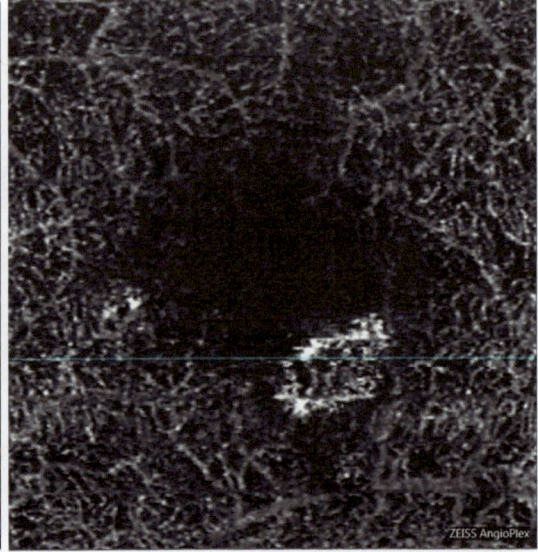
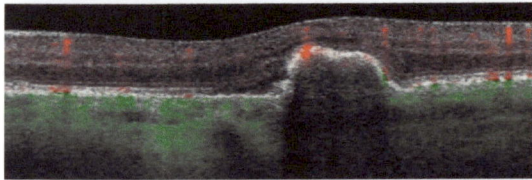
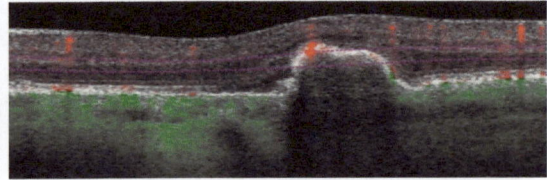

C1

C2

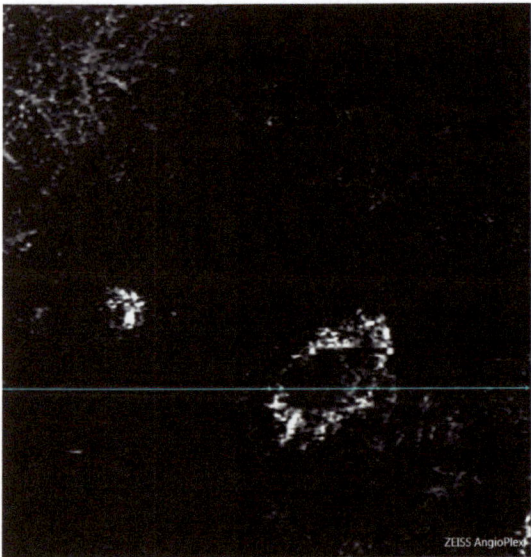
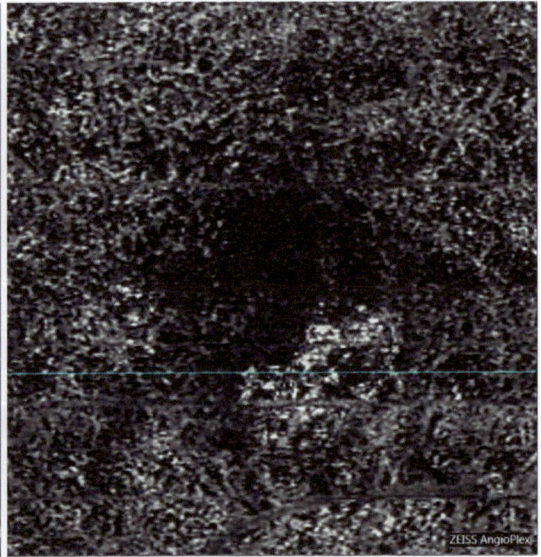
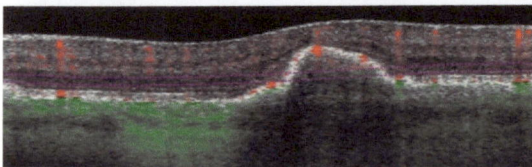
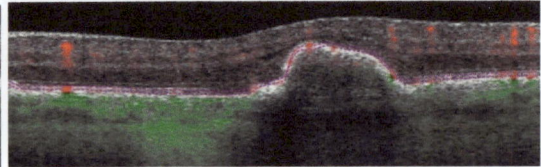

C3

C4

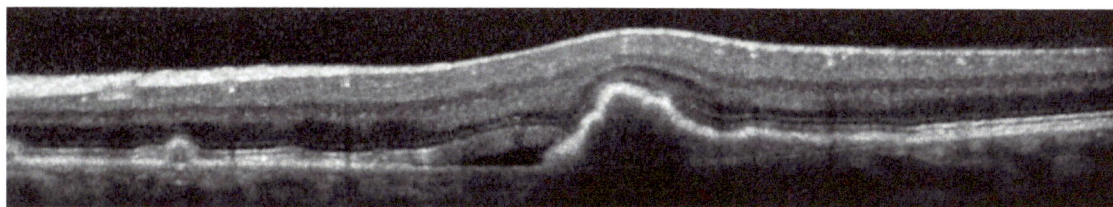

D1

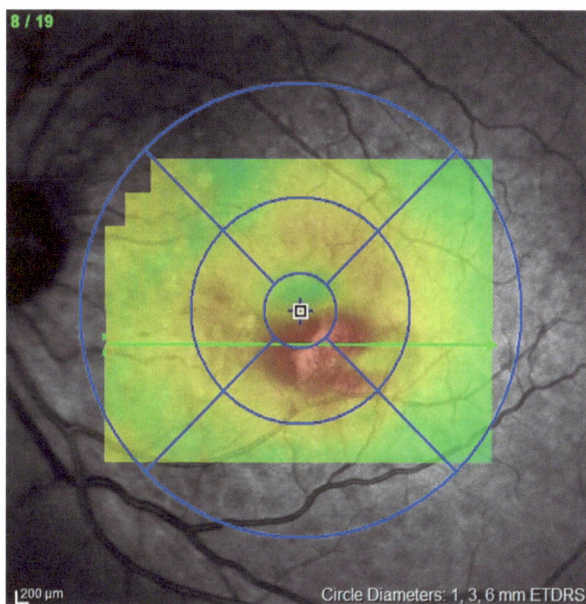

D2

Case 33: *Exudative Macular Degeneration*

Clinical Summary

92-year-old healthy white male presents with complaints of blurry vision OS with metamorphopsia x 2 months. Vision OS is 20/50-.

Image Summary

A. Color Fundus: Shows a pale and cupped nerve. There is an area of RPE change in the macula.

B. Fluorescein Angiography: B1: Early to mid-phase fluorescein angiogram shows a hyperfluorescent lesion inferotemporal to the fovea. **B2**: Mid to late phase fluorescein angiogram shows increasing fluorescence intensity from the lesion and confirms the earlier findings.

C. ICG Angiography: C1: Early ICG shows CNV in the region of the lesion on FA and color images above. **C2**: Late ICG confirms the same findings with staining of a larger CNV complex surrounding the early appearing CNV.

D. OCT Angiography: D1: Depth encoded OCTA with corresponding B-scan shows a highly vascular complex in the macula. The color scheme on this and subsequent images is abnormal due to a distorted retinal contour that is not detected by the automated segmentation scheme. Nevertheless, there is a neovascular complex in the fovea. **D2**: Full thickness retina composite OCTA with corresponding B-scan shows similar findings through another slab of the retina. **D3**: Avascular level OCTA with corresponding B-scan shows a large neovascular complex within the PED. **D4**: Choriocapillaris level OCTA with corresponding B-scan shows the further extent of the CNV **D5**: Choroidal level OCTA with corresponding B-scan shows even further extent of the CNV.

E. OCT: B-scan OCT shows a large PED with hyperreflective internal contents.

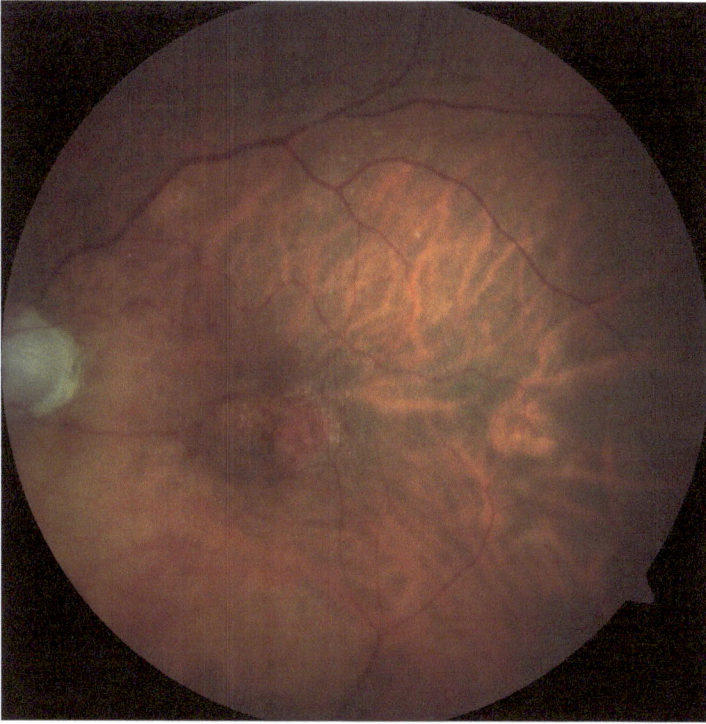

A

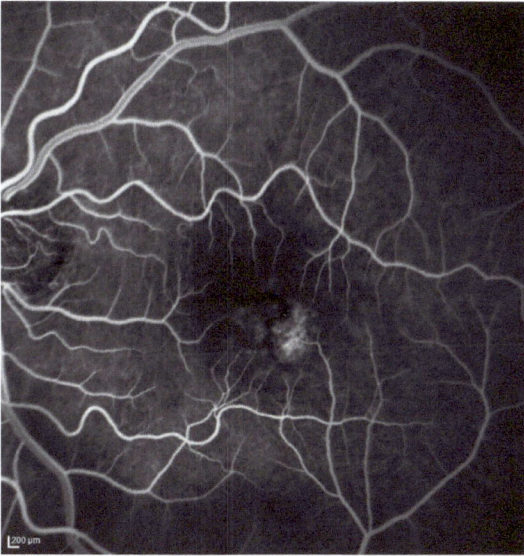

B1

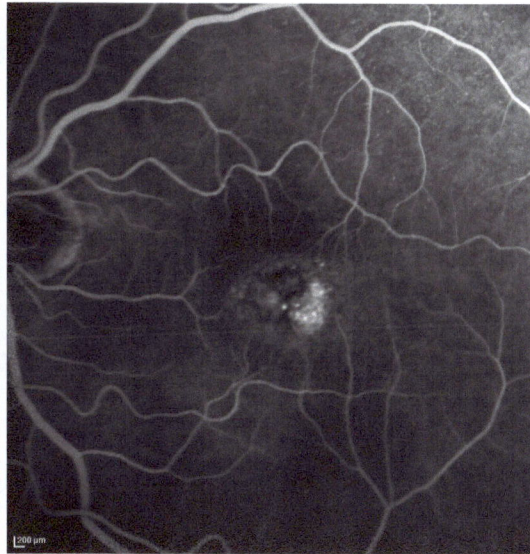

B2

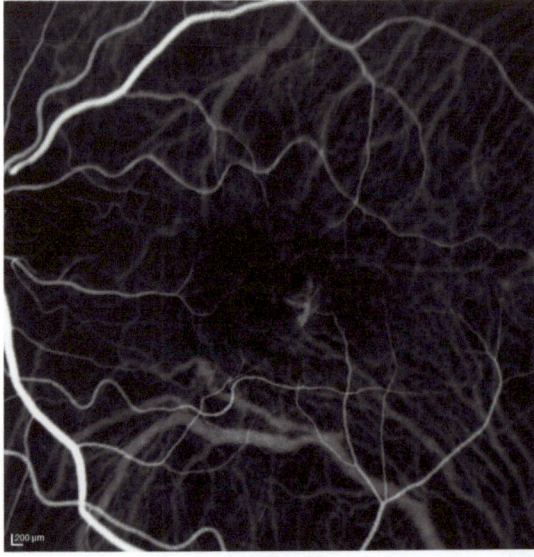
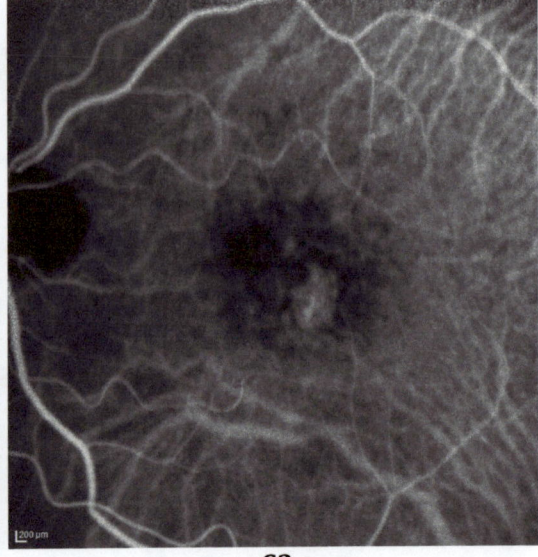

C1   **C2**

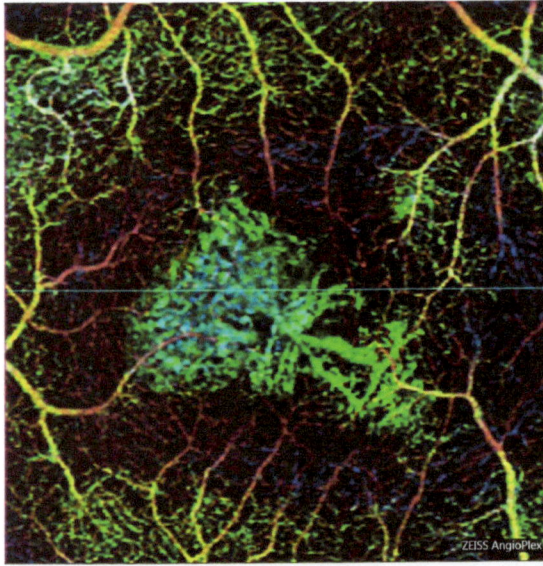
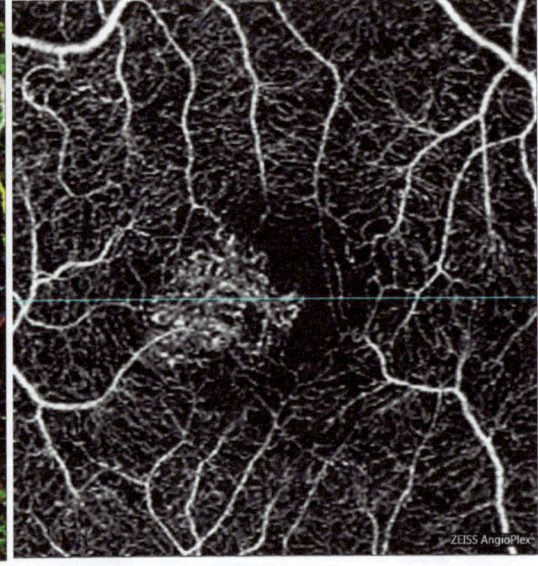

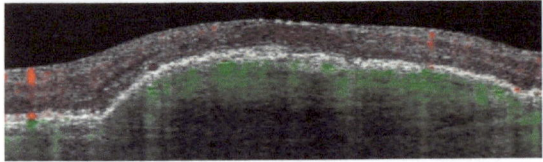
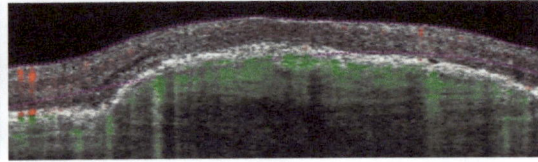

D1   **D2**

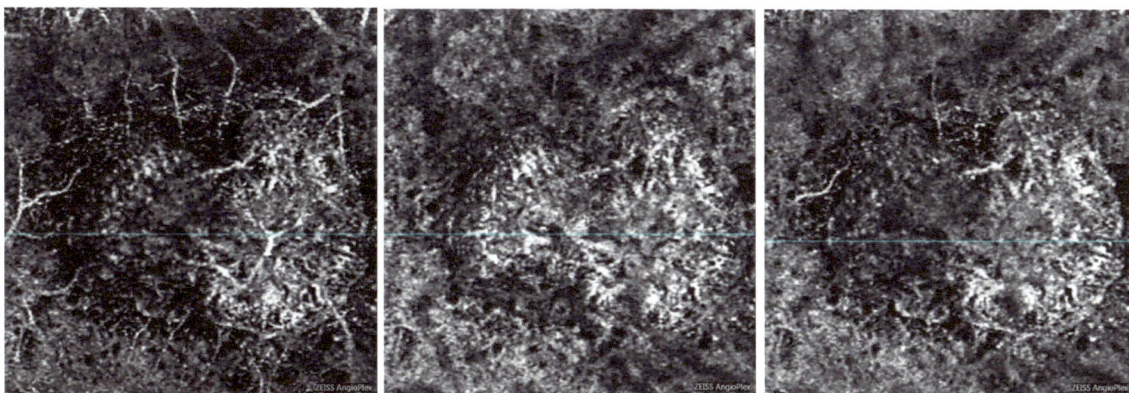

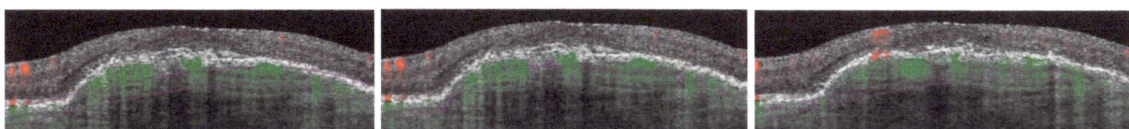

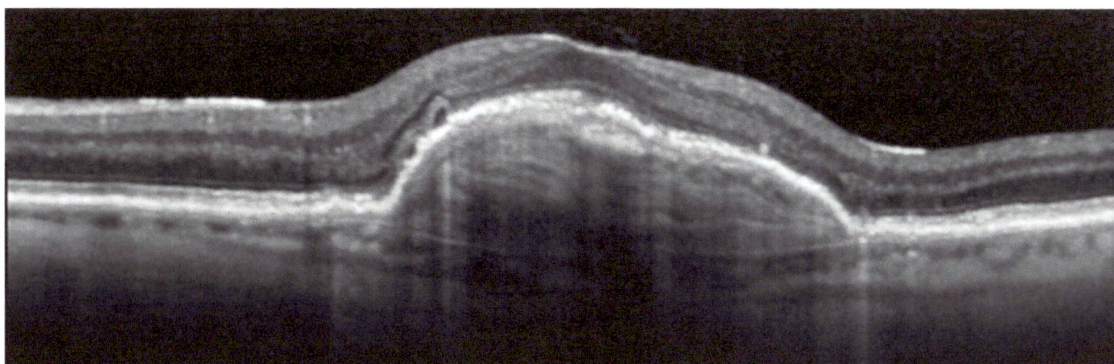

D3   D4   D5

E

Case 34: *Exudative Macular Degeneration With Follow Up After One Treatment*

Clinical Summary

66-year-old healthy white male presents with complaints of sudden blurred vision OS with metamorphopsia x 1 week. Vision was 20/200 initially. Patient was treated with intravitreal Ranibizumab and followed up one month later. At that visit, patient's vision was 20/70-.

Image Summary

A. Color Fundus: Shows subretinal hemorrhage surrounding a central lesion consistent with CNV.

B. Fluorescein Angiography: Mid to late phase fluorescein angiogram shows blockage from the hemorrhage and a hyperfluorescent lesion in the center of the hemorrhage corresponding to a CNV or RAP-like lesion.

C. OCT Angiography: C1: Depth encoded OCTA with corresponding B-scan shows a large neovascular complex superior to the fovea. The corresponding B-scan shows that there is a large subretinal lesion (PED) that has significant perfusion within it, consistent with CNV. The elevation of the retina by the lesion is not detected by the segmentation scheme in this image, and corresponding color scheme is not typical, so the reader has to carefully correlate the depth encoded image and the B-scans. The CNV lesion is much smaller on the follow-up visit. **C2**: Deep retinal plexus OCTA with corresponding B-scan confirm similar findings to those above. **C3**: Choriocapillaris level OCTA with corresponding B-scan shows the extent of the impaired perfusion around the CNV and the decrease in size of the CNV after treatment.

D. OCT: D1: B-scan OCT shows a large subretinal lesion with associated subretinal fluid.
D2: Volumetric OCT change analysis illustrates a decrease in central overall thickness of about 100 microns.

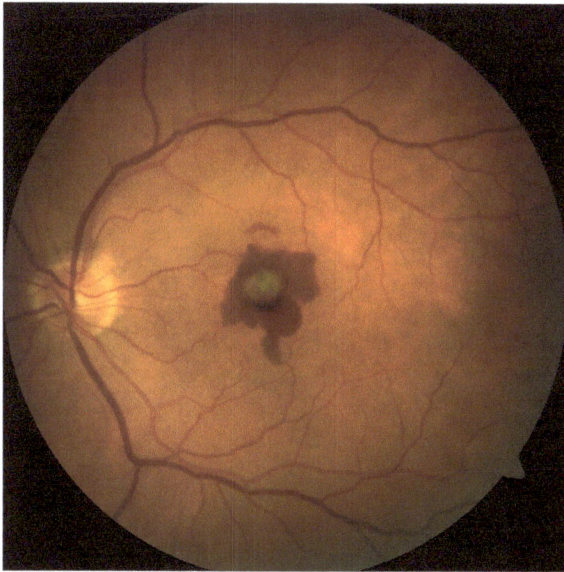

A

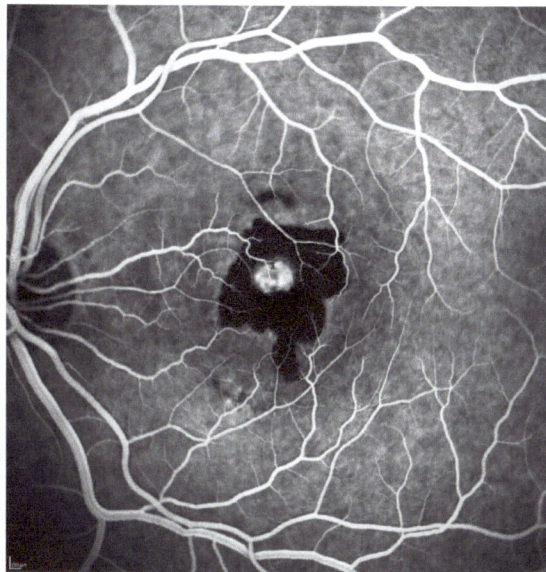

B

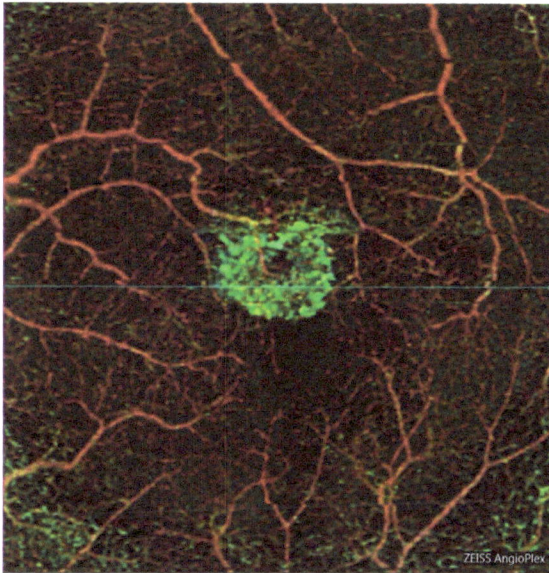

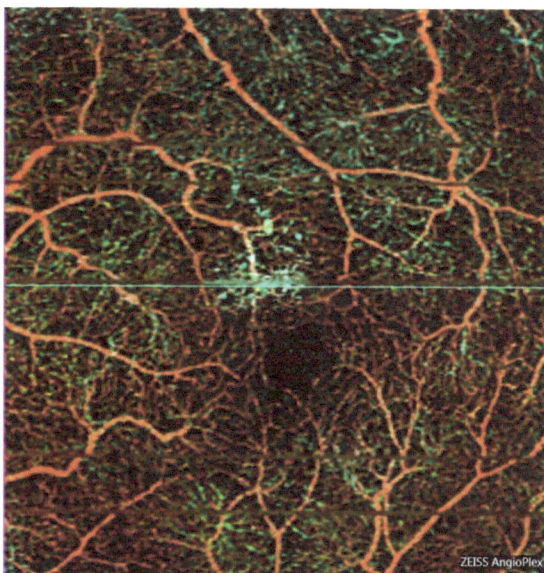

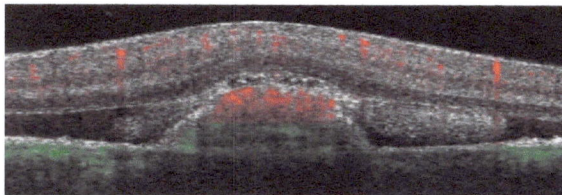

C1 Initial visit

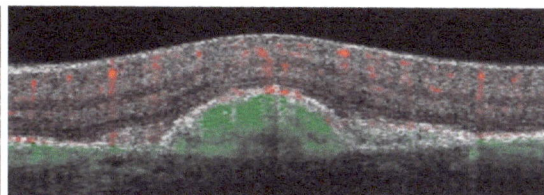

C1 Follow up

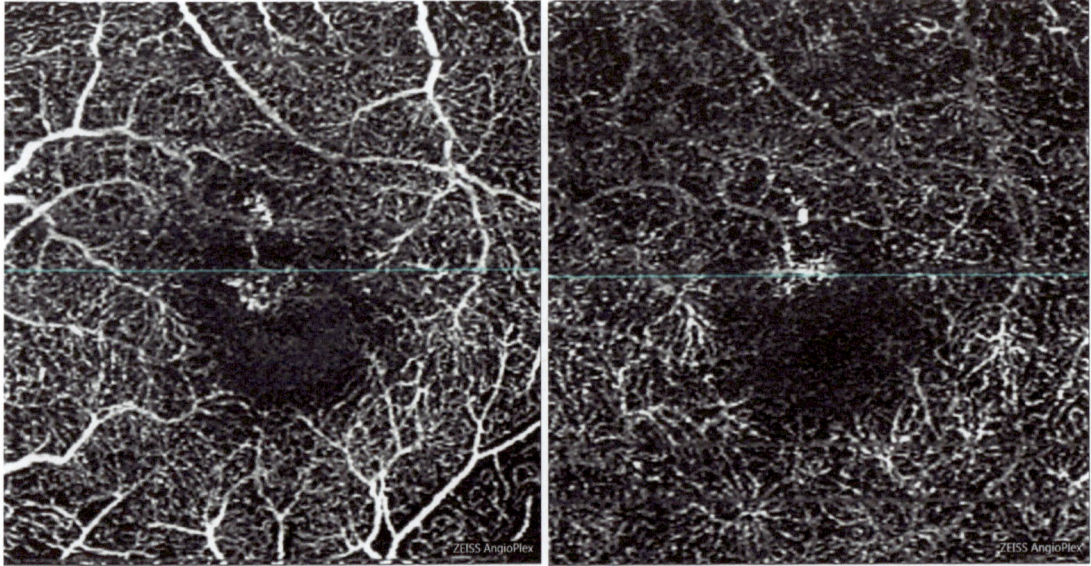

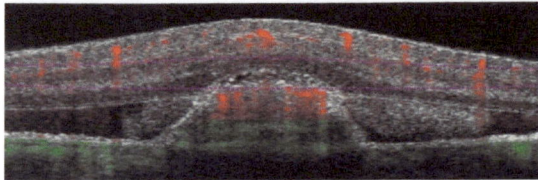

C2 Initial visit

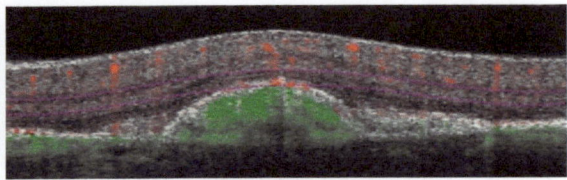

C2 Follow up

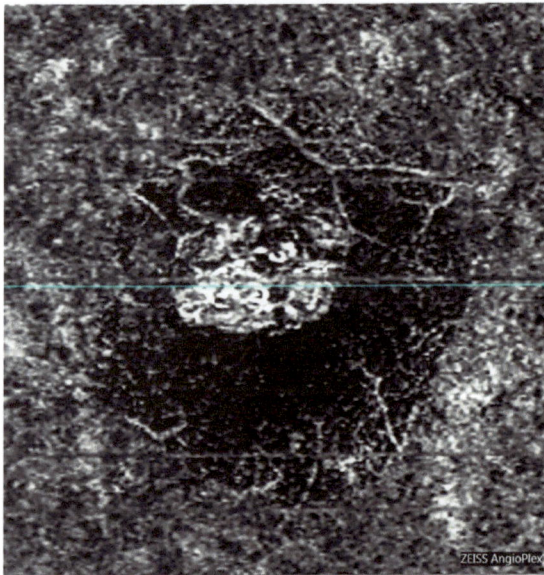

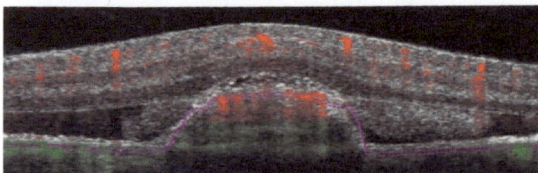

C3 Initial visit

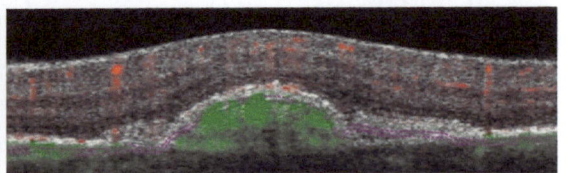

C3 Follow up

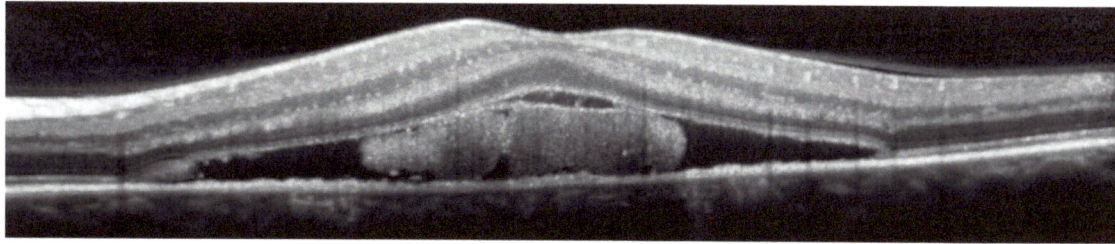

D1 Initial visit

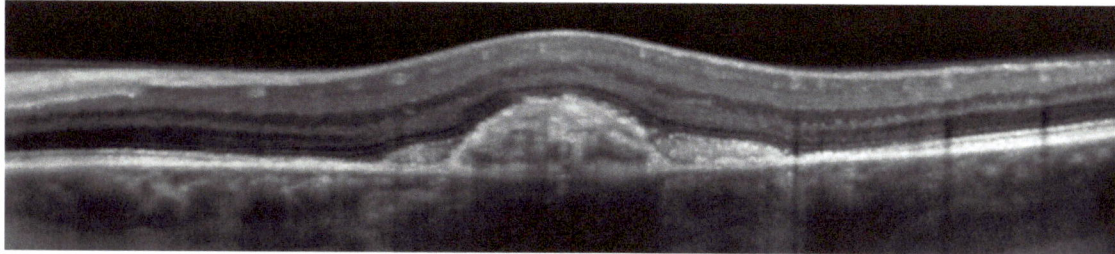

D1 Follow up

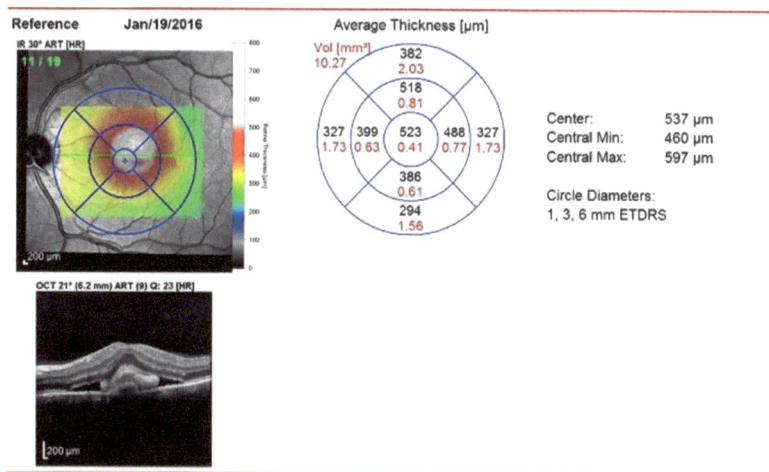

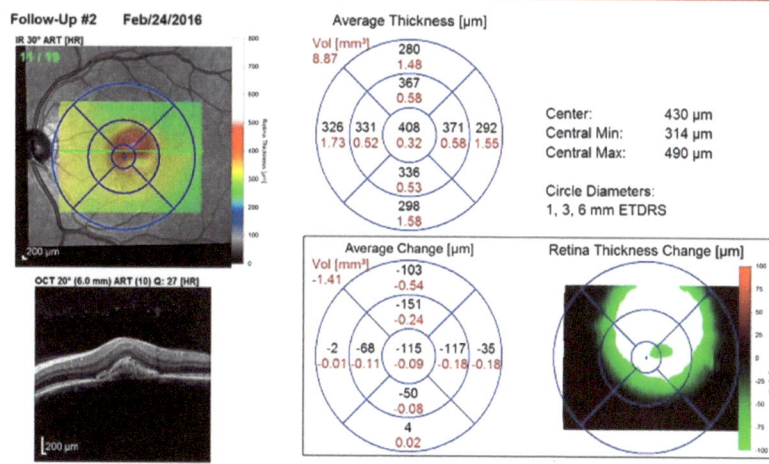

D2

Case 35: *Polypoidal Choroidal Vasculopathy*

Clinical Summary

92-year-old white female presents with complaints of blurred vision with mild metamorphopsia OS x 3 weeks. Vision is 20/60 OS.

Image Summary

A. Color Fundus: Shows several areas of RPE changes and a region of intraretinal hemorrhage that is inferior to the fovea.

B. Fluorescein Angiography: B1: Early to mid-phase fluorescein angiogram shows mild staining and hyperfluorescent spots superior to the fovea. **B2**: Late phase fluorescein angiogram shows increased staining in the region superior to the fovea and late staining of a lesion corresponding to the area with intraretinal hemorrhage on color image.

C. ICG Angiography: C1: Early ICG shows impaired perfusion in the central macula. **C2**: Late ICG shows impaired perfusion in the macula and several circular lesions consistent with polyps in the same region.

D. OCT: D1: B-scan OCT shows hyporeflectice PED with overlying subretinal fluid and intraretinal fluid. **D2**: Volumetric OCT illustrates the retinal thickening corresponding with the lesion seen on late fluorescein and intraretinal hemorrhage on color image.

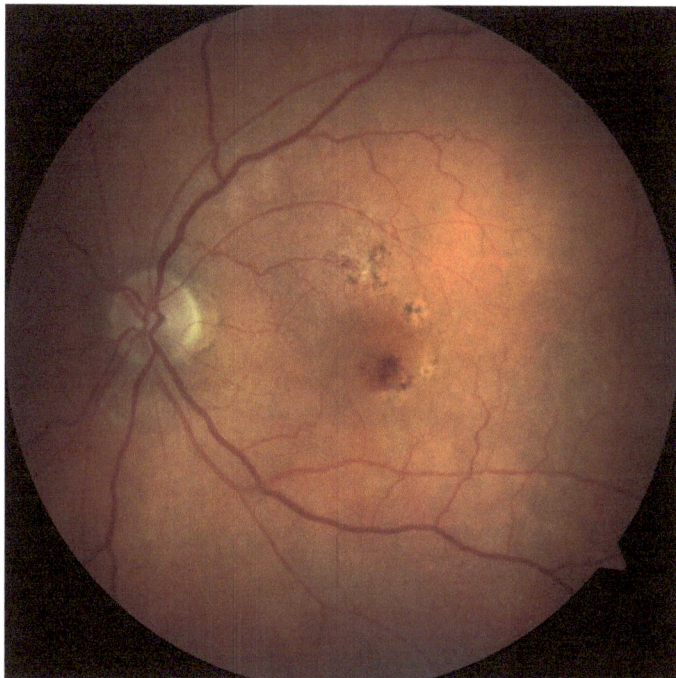

A

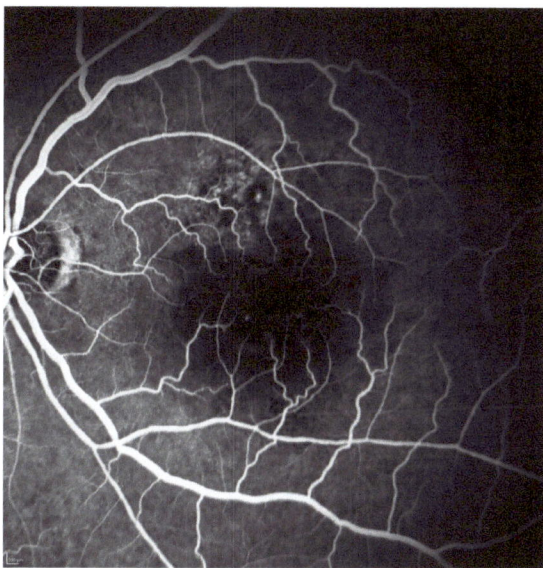

B1

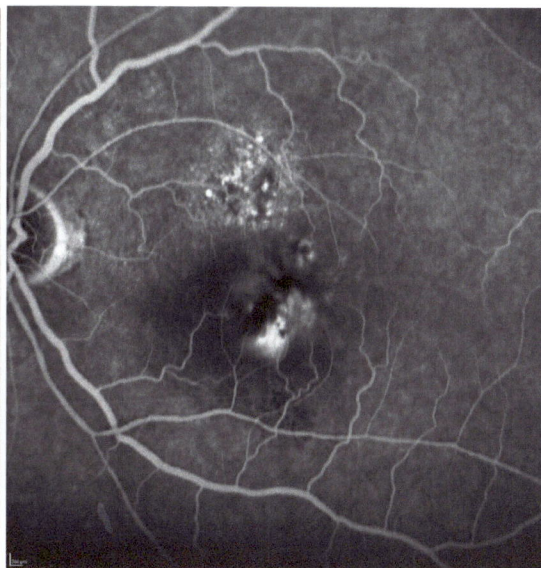

B2

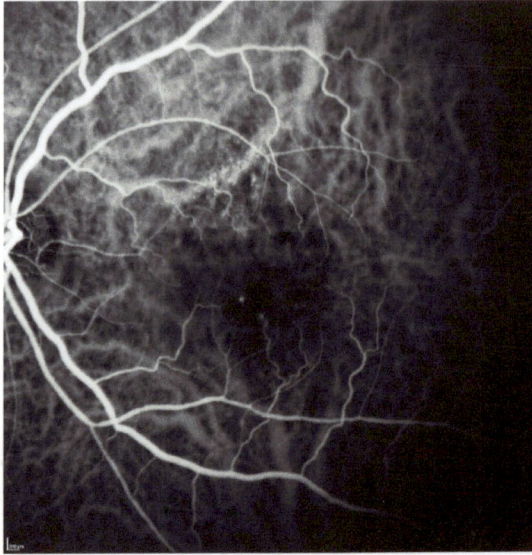

C1

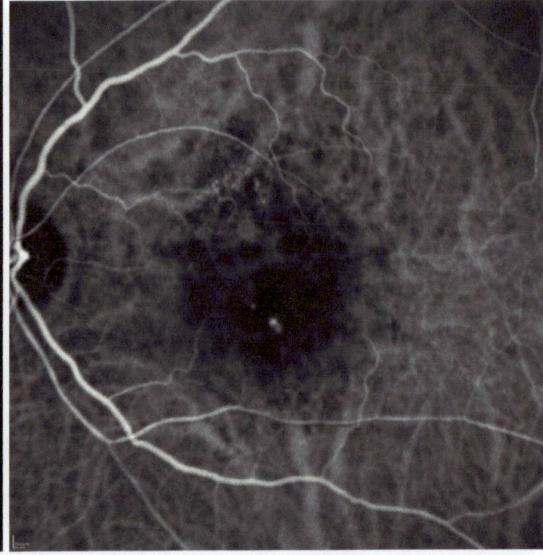

C2

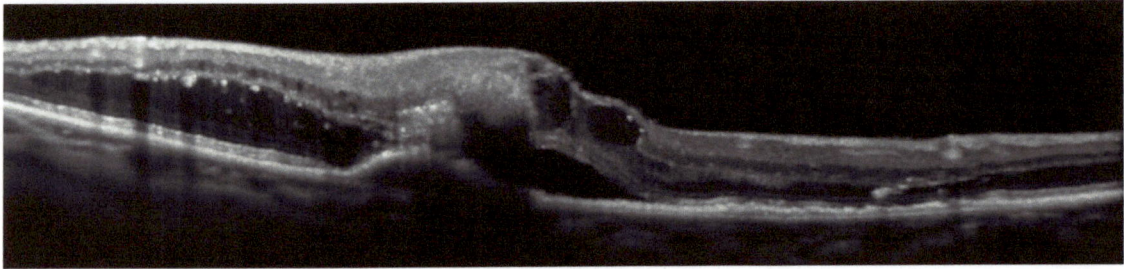

D1

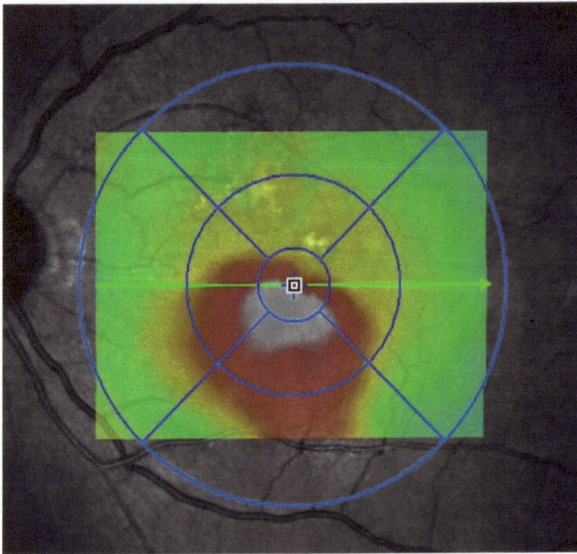

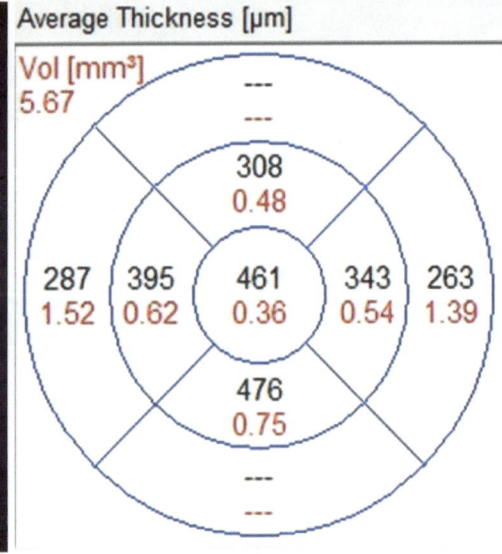

D2

Case 36: *Polypoidal Choroidal Vasculopathy*

Clinical Summary

93-year-old white female with history of NIDDM, hypothyroidism, hypertension, and CVA complains of metamorphopsia OD x 1 year. Vision OD is 20/80.

Image Summary

A. Color Fundus: Shows yellow deposits in the inferonasal macula and peripapillary subretinal hemorrhage.

B. Fluorescein Angiography: B1: Early phase fluorescein angiogram shows blockage of fluorescence in the region of the peripapillary hemorrhage **B2**: Late phase fluorescein angiogram shows intense fluorescence (leakage) along the superior aspect of the hemorrhage consistent with possible peripapillary CNV.

C. ICG Angiography: C1: Early ICG confirms the CNV in the hemorrhage. **C2**: Late ICG confirms the CNV in the hemorrhage. The area superior to the hemorrhage does not appear to be CNV on the ICG.

D. OCT: D1: Horizontal B-scan OCT shows subretinal fluid and ERM. There is a large subretinal lesion in the right of the image that is partially viewed. **D2**: Vertical B-scan OCT shows a large shallow area of subretinal fluid and ERM. **D3**: Volumetric OCT of the macula illustrates the extent of thickening nasal to and in the fovea. **D4**: Volumetric OCT of the disc confirms thickening parapapillary, corresponding to the extended fluid partially viewed on the horizontal B-scan.

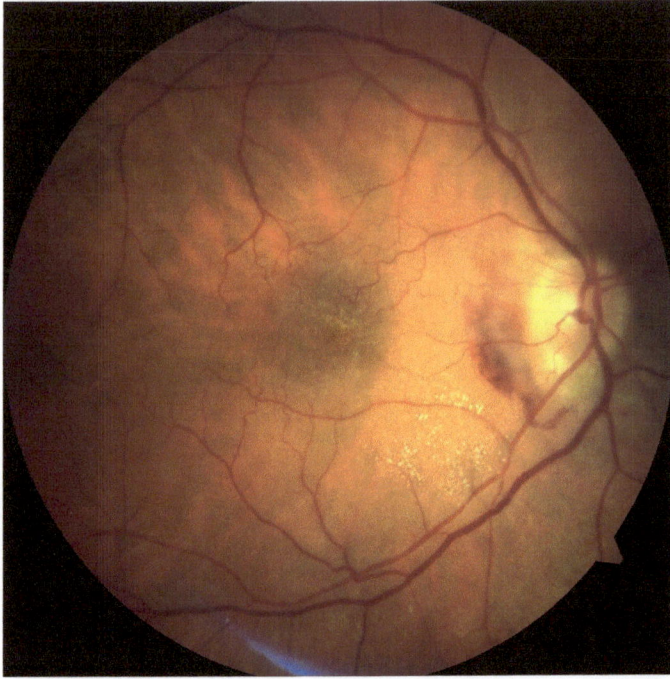

A

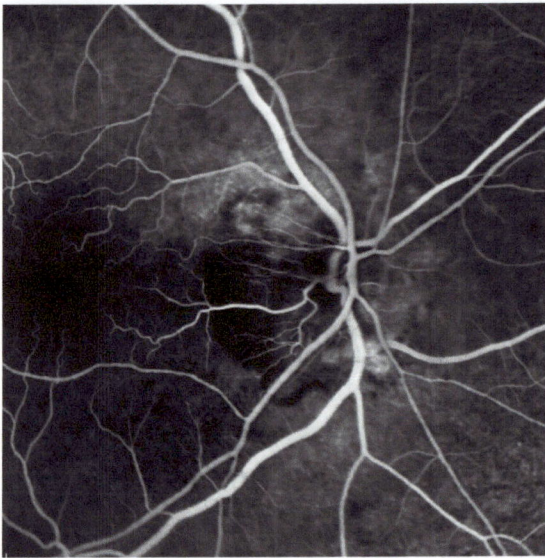

B1

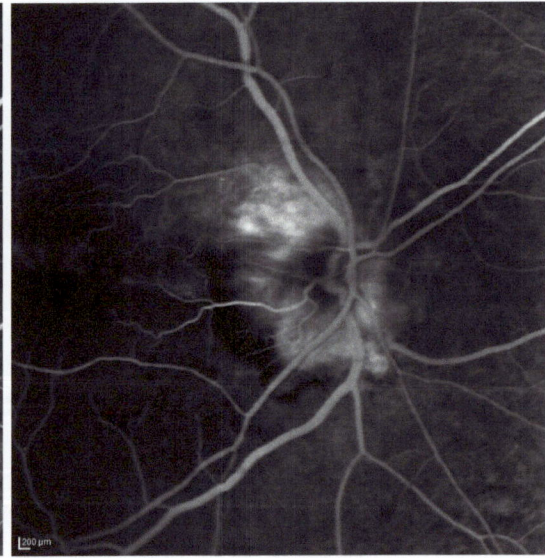

B2

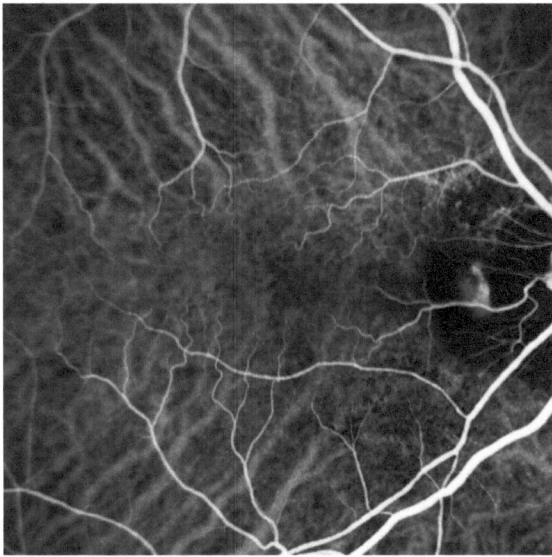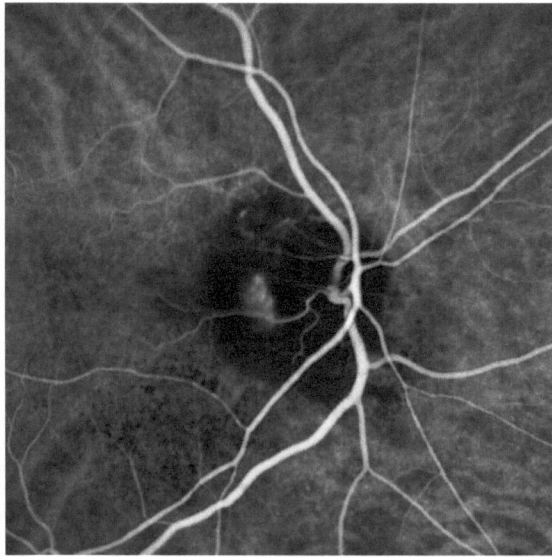

C1 **C2**

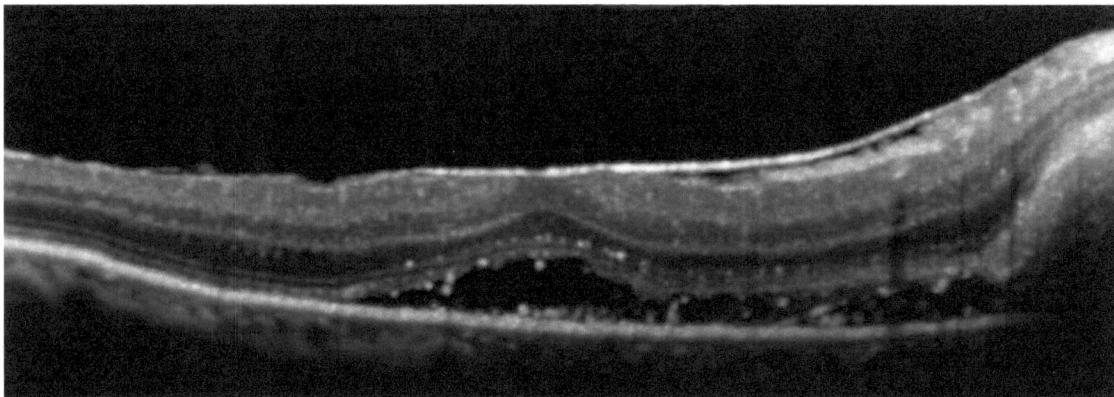

D1

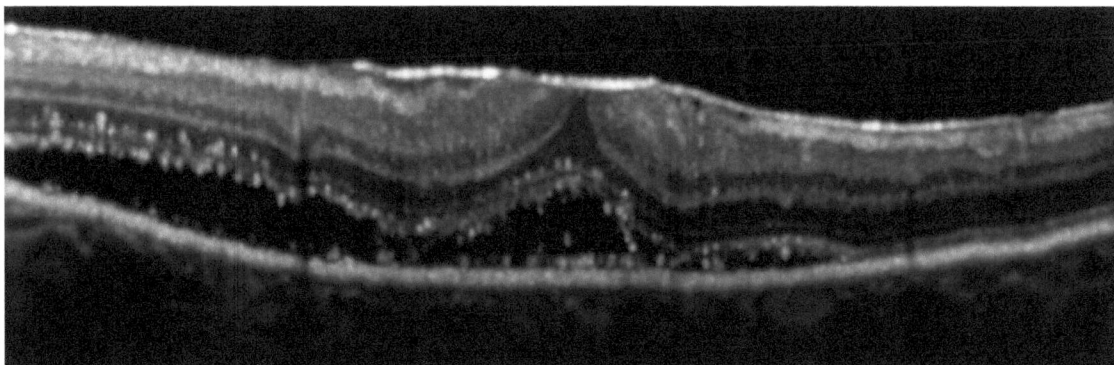

D2

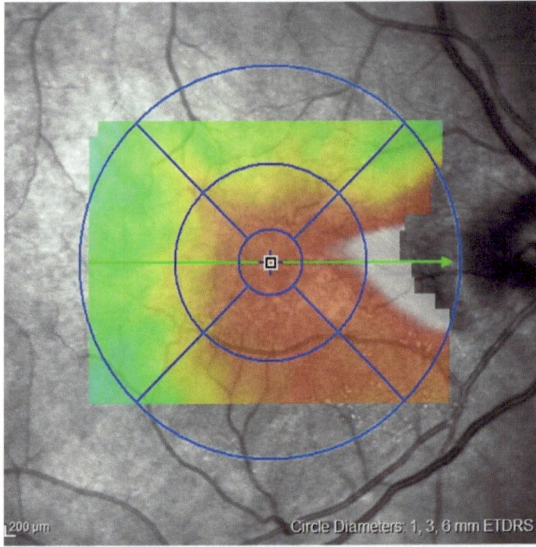

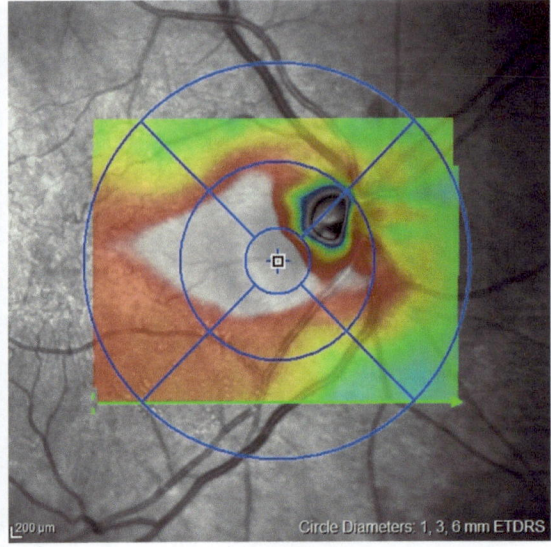

D3   **D4**

Case 37: *Polypoidal Choroidal Vasculopathy*

Clinical Summary

48-year-old healthy white male with complaints of slightly blurred vision OS x 3 weeks. Vision OS is 20/25-.

Image Summary

A. Color Fundus: Shows several orange, circular, subretinal lesions temporal to the disc and a larger lesion in the far temporal macula.

B. Fluorescein Angiography: B1: Early phase fluorescein angiogram shows multiple hyperfluorescent lesions in the nasal macula. **B2**: Late phase fluorescein angiogram shows progressive hyperfluorescence in the nasal macula lesions. There is mild but abnormal staining in the temporal macula.

C. ICG Angiography: C1: Early ICG shows some pinpoint hyperfluorescence in the same regions as the FA. **C2**: Late ICG shows late staining in the same regions.

D. OCT Angiography: D1: Choriocapillaris level OCTA shows a focal region of impaired perfusion in the same region as the earlier images nasal to the fovea. **D2**: Choriocapillaris level en face with corresponding B-scan. The B-scan shows subretinal fluid but no visible polyp. There is a slight elevation of the RPE under the SRF suggestive of shallow CNV.

E. OCT: B-scan OCT shows drusen with subretinal fluid and a very small serious PED.

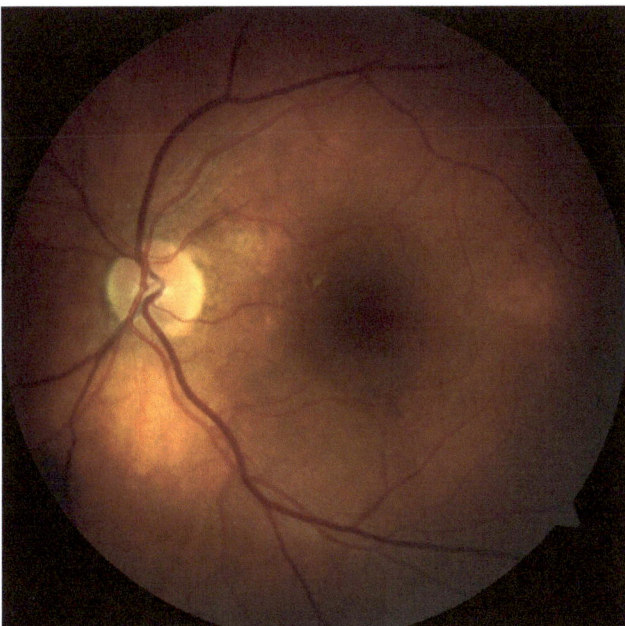

A

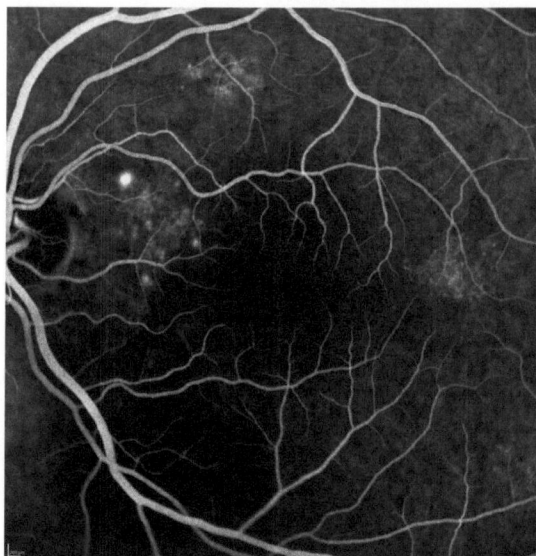
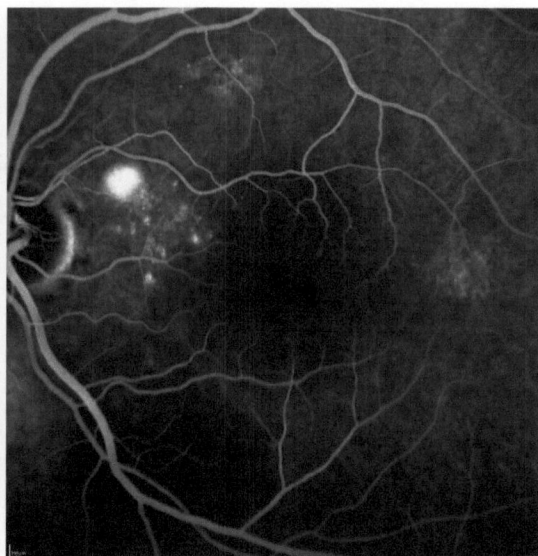

B1

B2

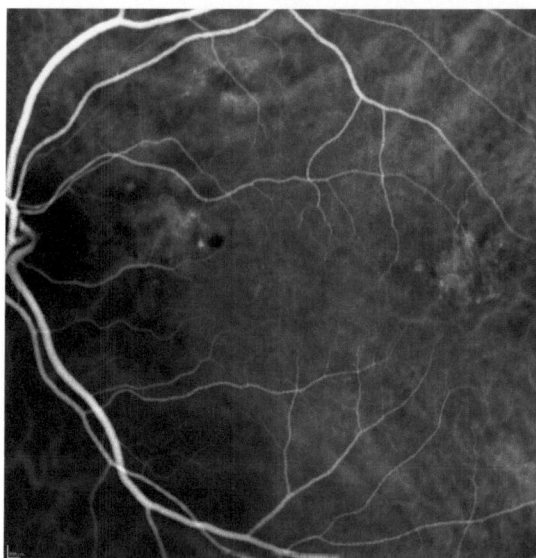
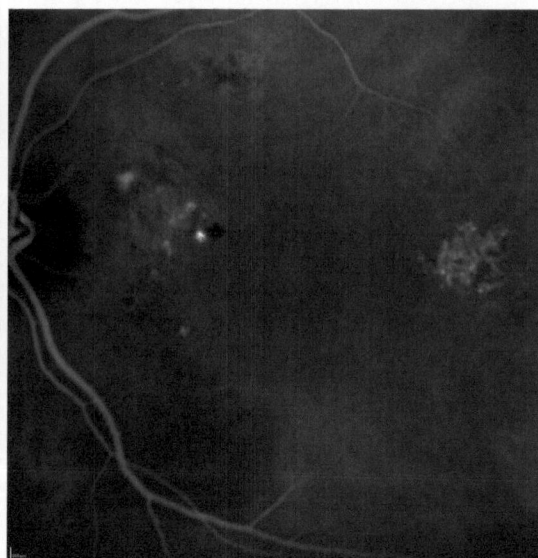

C1

C2

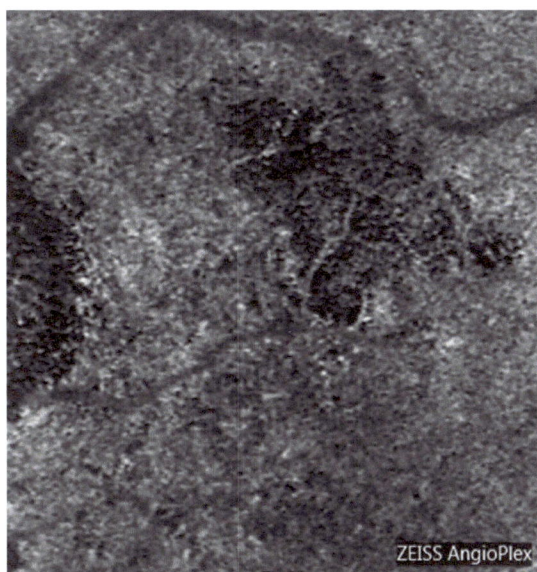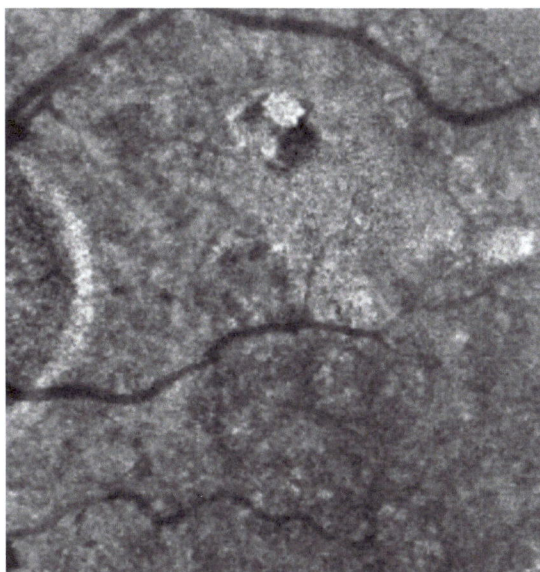

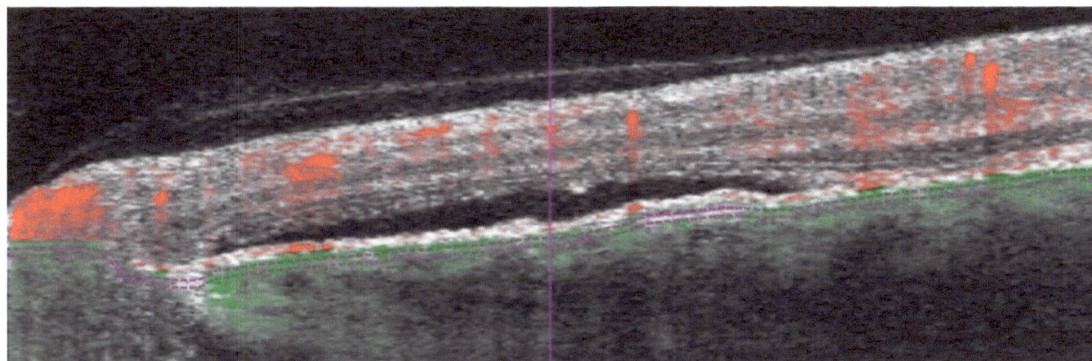

D1   **D2**

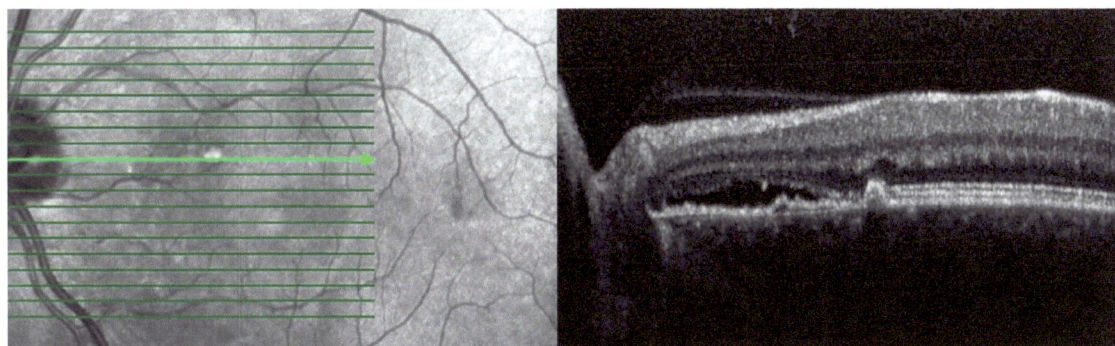

E

Case 38: *Retinal Angiomatous Proliferation- A 3 Visit Case*

Clinical Summary

78-year-old healthy white male with history of dry AMD, followed for drusen annually with vision stable at 20/30, presents with a complaint of sudden decrease in vision OD x 2 days. Vision OD is 20/200. Patient was given intravitreal ant-VEGF injection.

At 1-month follow-up, patient notes vision slightly better; measures 20/100 and another intravitreal anti-VEGF injection is given.

At 2-month follow-up, the patient states vision is much better, but still blurry. Vision measures 20/60 and another intravitreal anti-VEGF injection is given.

Image Summary

A. Color Fundus: Shows a discolored retina and numerous yellow deposits throughout the macula.

B. Fluorescein Angiography: B1: Early phase fluorescein angiogram shows a large area of impaired perfusion involving the central and temporal macula. There is a linear hyperfluorescent line that appears to originate from the choroid. **B2:** Late phase fluorescein angiogram shows diffuse staining of the inferotemporal macula with numerous hyperfluorescent spots. The whole lesion is consistent with a CNV.

C. ICG Angiography: C1: Early ICG shows hypofluorescence in the area of the lesion noted above and a chorioretinal anastomoses (yellow arrow). **C2:** Late ICG shows similar findings.

D-H. OCT Angiography: D1-3: Depth encoded OCTA with corresponding B-scan highlights the chorioretinal anastomosis (yellow arrow) which resolves over multiple injections.

E1-3: Deep retinal plexus OCTA with corresponding B-scan confirms the presence and location of the chorioretinal anastomosis. **F1-3:** Avascular level OCTA with corresponding B-scan further confirms the presence and location of the chorioretinal anastomosis. **G1-3:** Choriocapillaris level OCTA with corresponding B-scan confirms the presence and location of the chorioretinal anastomosis. **H1-3:** Choroid level OCTA with corresponding B-scan confirms the presence and location of the chorioretinal anastomosis.

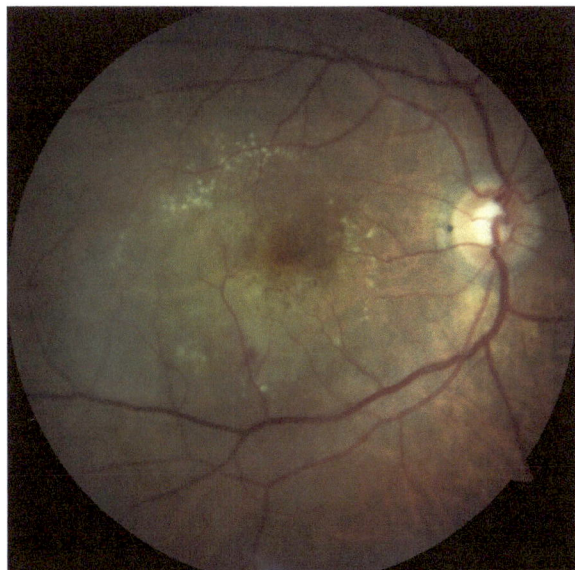

A

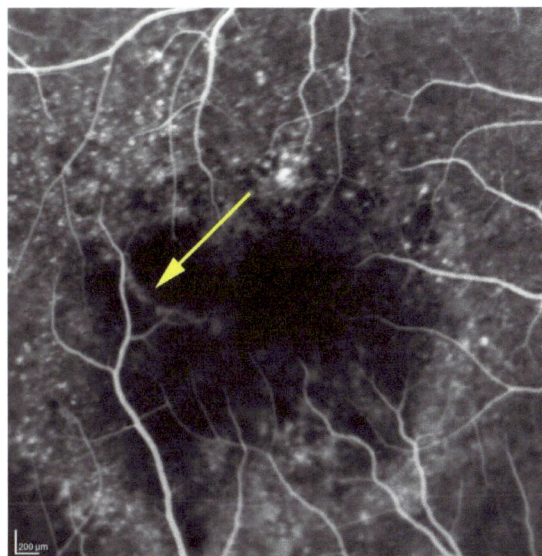

B1

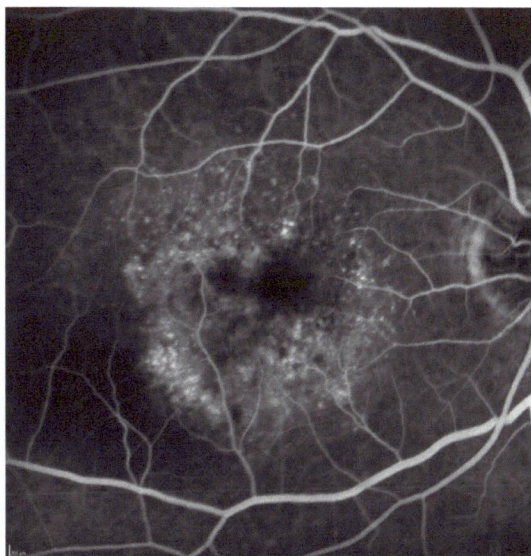

B2

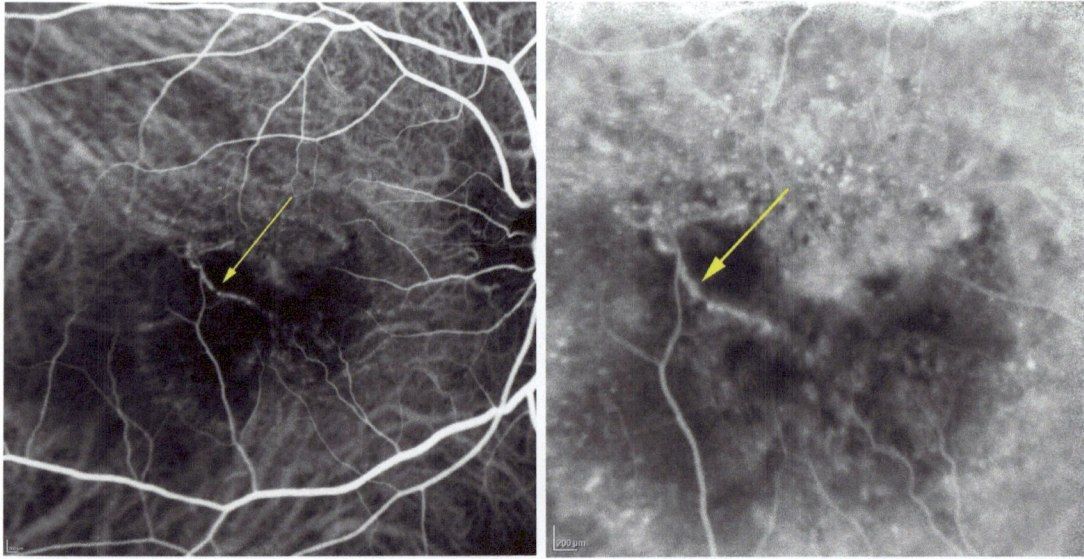

C1 C2

Initial visit 1 month 2 months

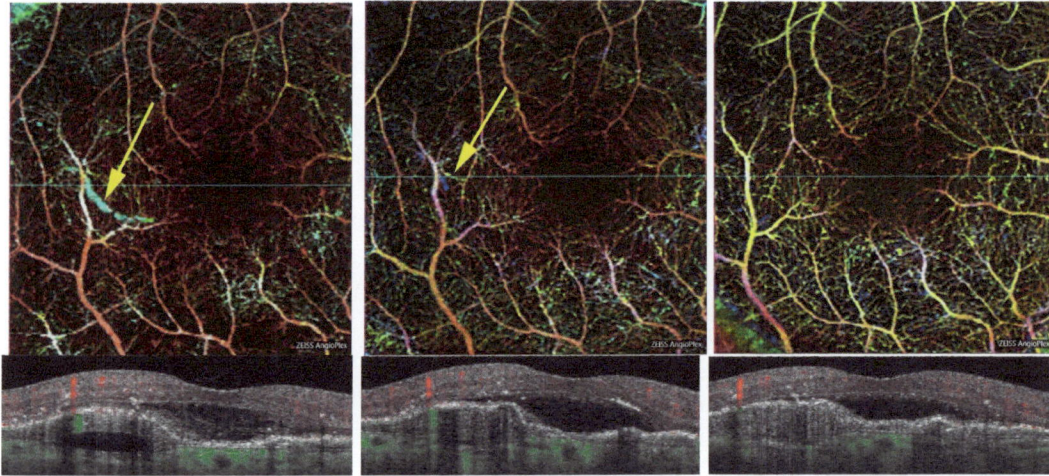

D1 D2 D3

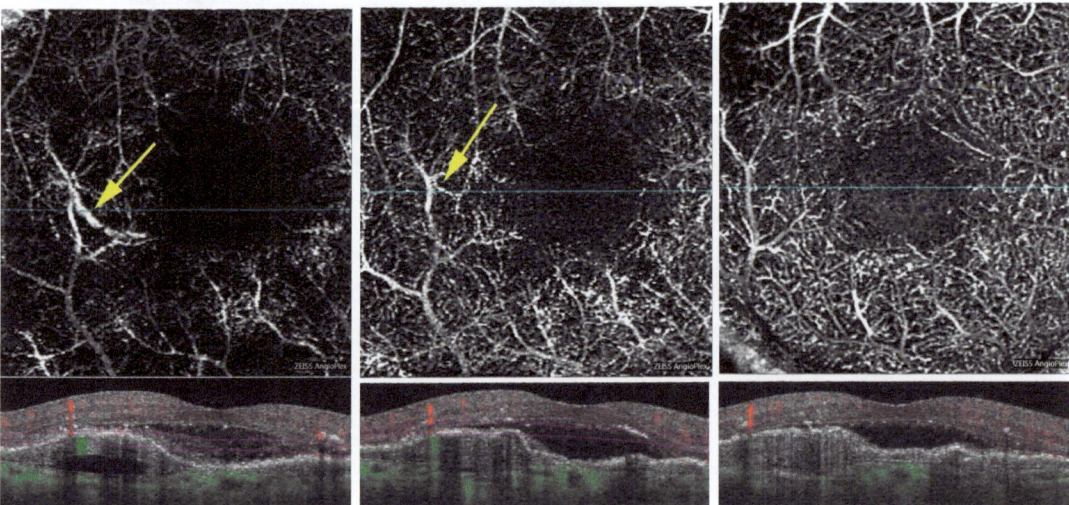

E1 E2 E3

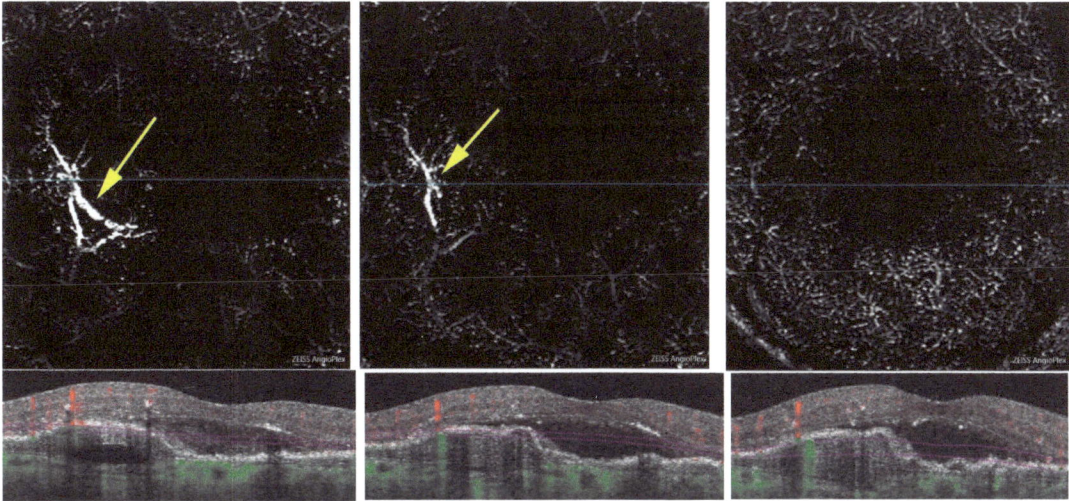

F1   **F2**   **F3**

Initial visit   **1 month**   **2 months**

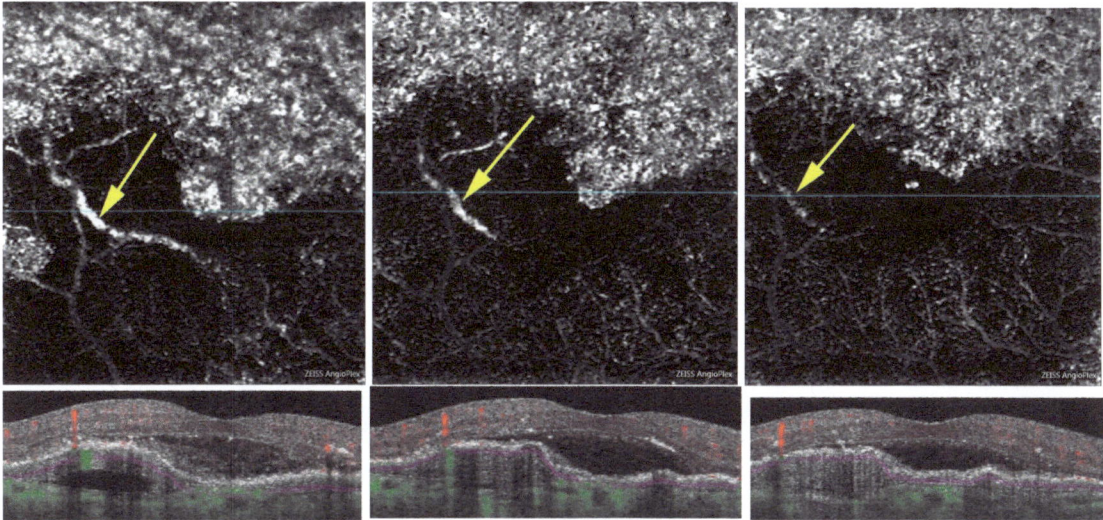

G1   **G2**   **G3**

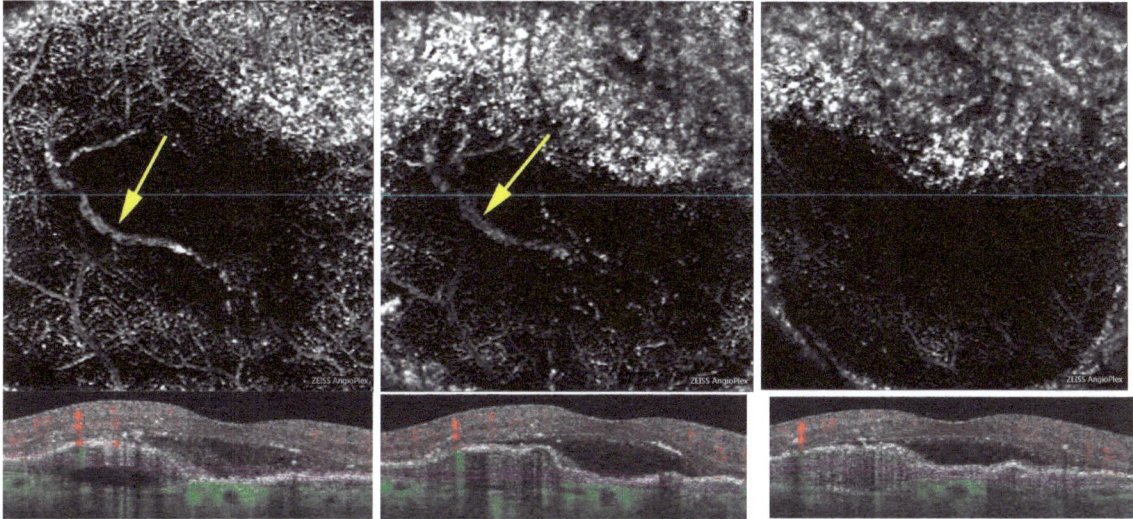

H1   **H2**   **H3**

Case 39: *Central Serous Chorioretinopathy*

Clinical Summary

35-year-old healthy white male with complaints of gradual blurriness OS x 1 month. Vision is 20/40 OS.

Image Summary

A. Color Fundus: Shows mild RPE changes in the fovea and peripapillary atrophy.

B. Fluorescein Angiography: B1: Early fluorescein angiogram is relatively unremarkable. **B2**: Late fluorescein angiogram shows peripapillary staining and a foveal hyperfluorescent spot inferonasal to the fovea.

C. OCT Angiography: C1: Depth encoded OCTA shows altered perfusion in the inferonasal foveal region. The corresponding B-scan shows minimal subretinal fluid. **C2**: Deep retinal plexus OCTA shows that the subretinal fluid is altering the retinal contour and the segmentation scheme.
C3: Choriocapillaris OCTA slab shows some mild decrease in perfusion signal in the region underlying the area of apparent perfusion abnormality. In this case the changes in retinal perfusion may be an artifact of the abnormal retinal contour and segmentation.

D. OCT: D1: B-scan OCT shows subretinal fluid and thickened choroid. **D2**: Volumetric OCT illustrates retinal thickening inferior to the fovea, corresponding to the hyperfluorescence seen in the late phase FA.

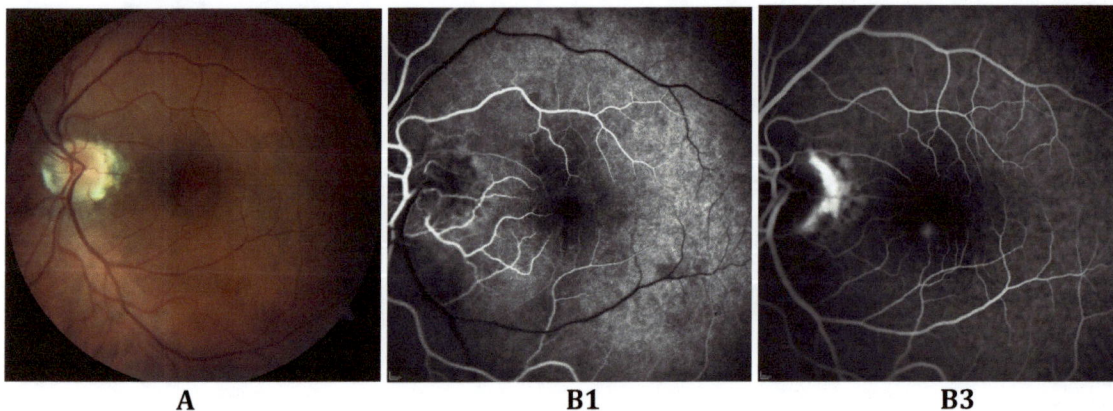

A   B1   B3

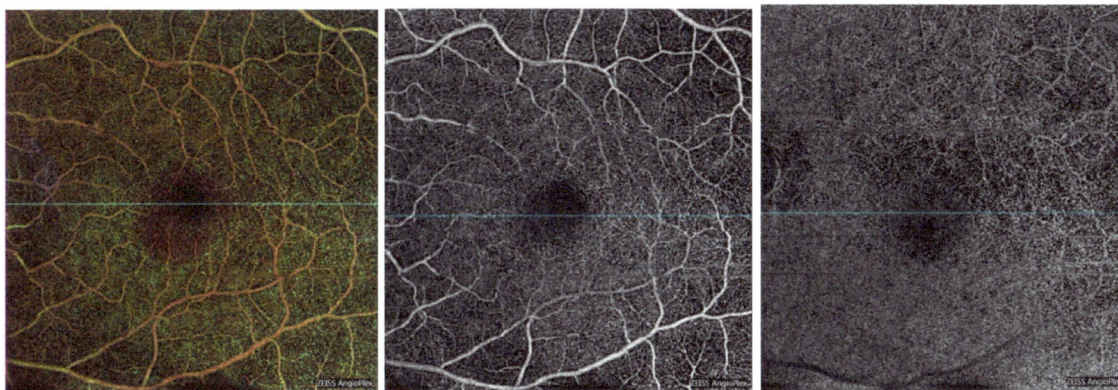

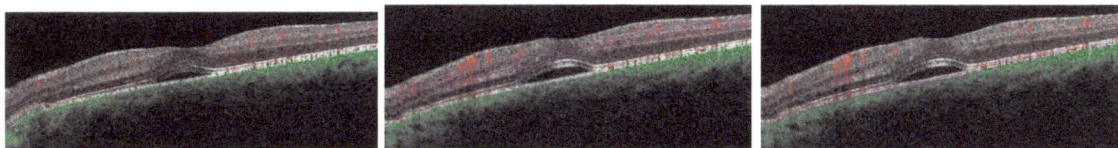

C1　　　　　　　　C2　　　　　　　　C3

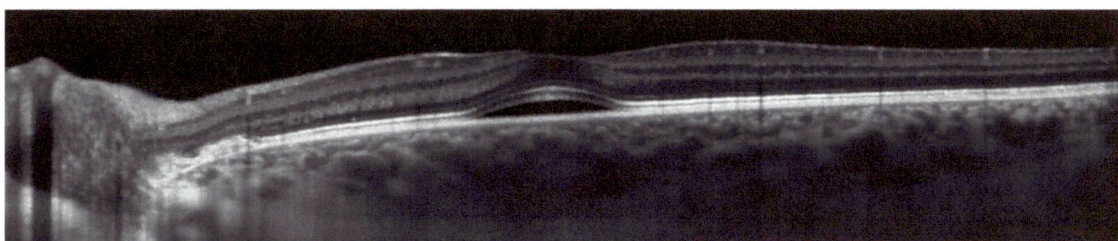

D1

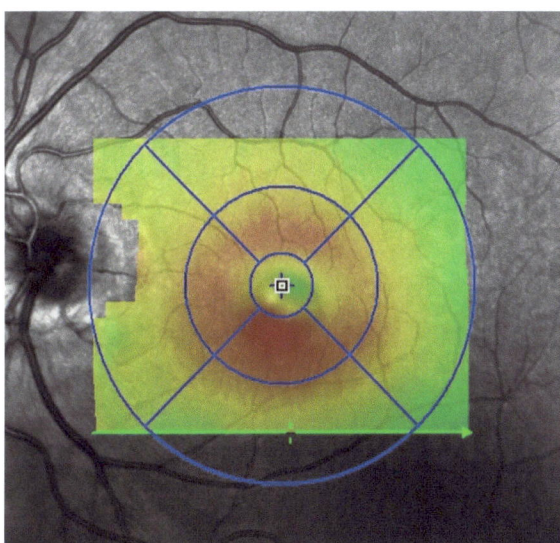

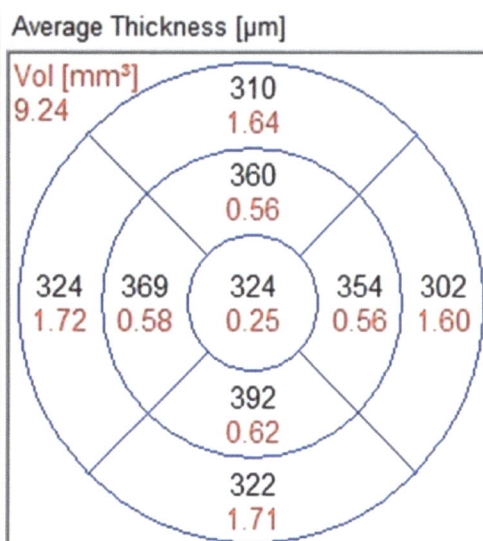

D2

Case 40: *Central Serous Chorioretinopathy*

Clinical Summary

61-year-old healthy white male with complaints of blurred central vision OS x 1 year. Vision OS is 20/40-.

Image Summary

A. Color Fundus: Shows mild RPE changes in the foveal region.

B. Fluorescein Angiography: B1: Mid phase fluorescein angiogram shows early staining in and around the fovea as well as in the superior macula. **B2**: Late phase fluorescein angiogram shows similar findings.

C. OCT Angiography: C1: Depth encoded OCTA with corresponding B-scan shows numerous floaters which appear as artifactual perfusion defects. **C2**: Deep retinal plexus OCTA with corresponding B-scan shows similar findings as depth encoded OCTA. **C3**: Choriocapillaris level OCTA with corresponding B-scan shows the early signs of a CNV process with surrounding impaired perfusion. The B-scans shows subretinal fluid with irregular and shallow PED that may contain the CNV.

D. OCT: D1: B-scan OCT subretinal fluid and irregular PED. Note the elongated outer segments that suggest a chronic process. **D2**: Volumetric OCT shows central foveal thickening.

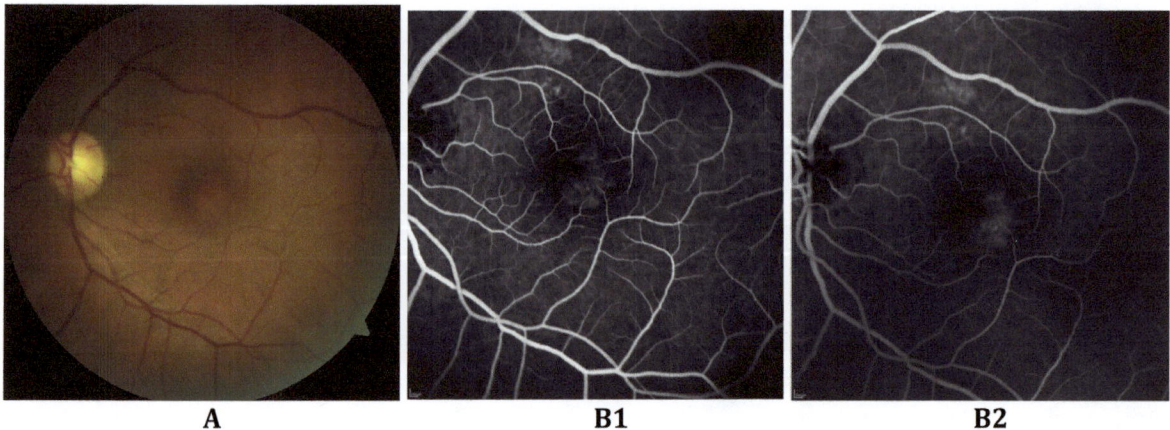

A　　　　　B1　　　　　B2

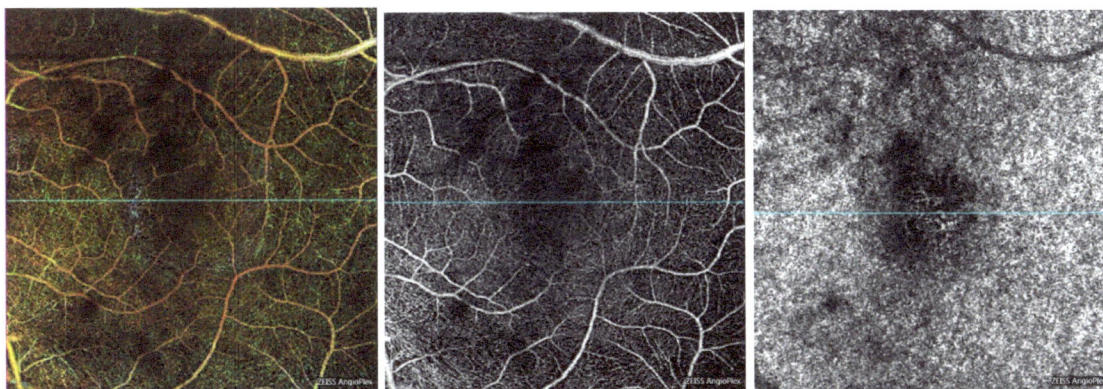

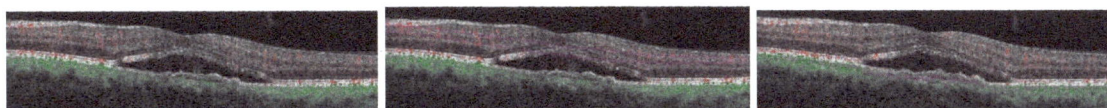

C1 **C2** **C3**

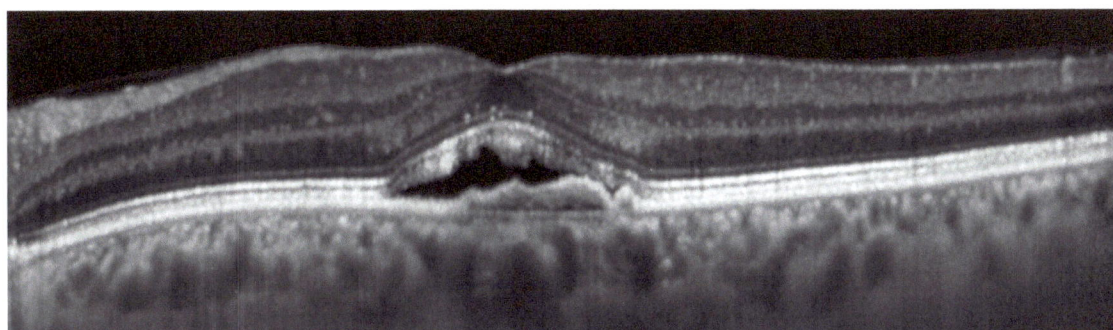

D1

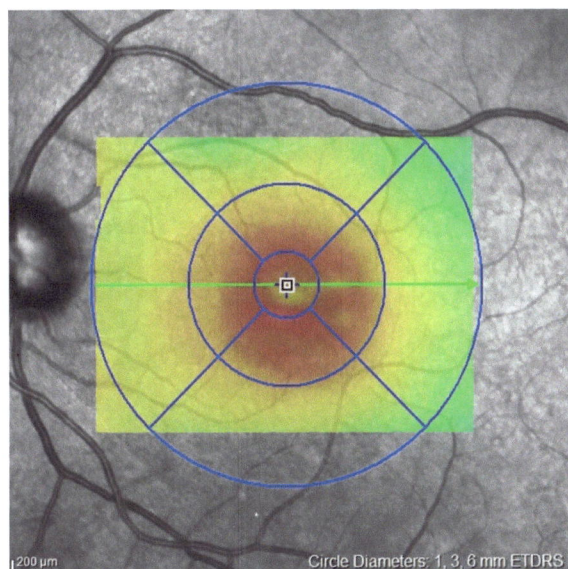

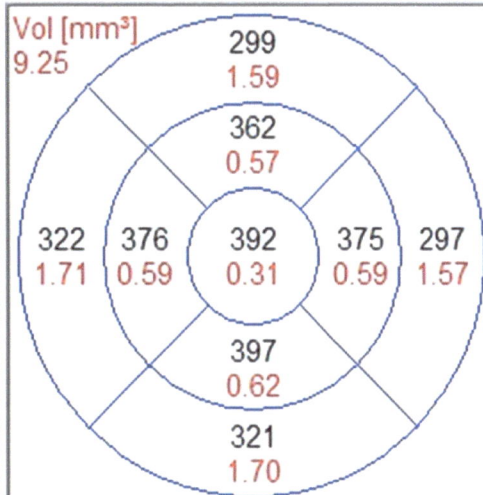

D2

Case 41: *Central Serous Chorioretinopathy*

Clinical Summary

52-year-old healthy white male presents with complaints blurred vision and metamorphopsia OS x 1 month. Vision OS is 20/200.

Image Summary

A. Color Fundus: Shows a region of subretinal fluid involving the fovea and most of the inferior macula.

B. Fluorescein Angiography: **B1**: Early phase fluorescein angiogram shows hypofluorescence from the region of subretinal fluid. **B2**: Late phase fluorescein angiogram shows a pinpoint hyperfluorescent lesion within the region of subretinal fluid and another hyperfluorescent lesion next to the disc.

C. ICG Angiography: C1: Early ICG shows hypofluorescence in the region of the subretinal fluid. **C2**: Late ICG shows similar findings.

D. OCT Angiography: D1: Depth encoded OCTA shows inferonasal retinal thickening corresponding to the hyperfluorescence seen on late FA. **D2**: Deep retinal plexus OCTA shows apparent lack of vessels, which are actually obscured by the retinal distortion induced by the subretinal fluid. **D3**: Deep retinal plexus en face illustrates the extent of fluid. **D4**: Depth encoded B-scan shows extent of fluid through the fovea.

E. OCT: Vertical B-scan EDI OCT shows subretinal fluid (note increased choroidal thickness under subretinal fluid). Note the elongated outer segments in the area of subretinal fluid suggesting a chronic process.

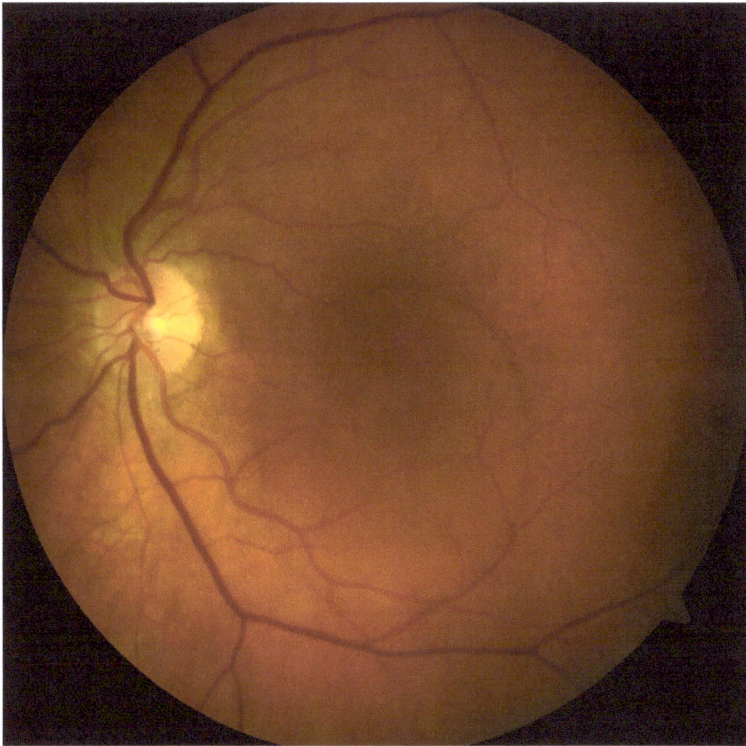

A

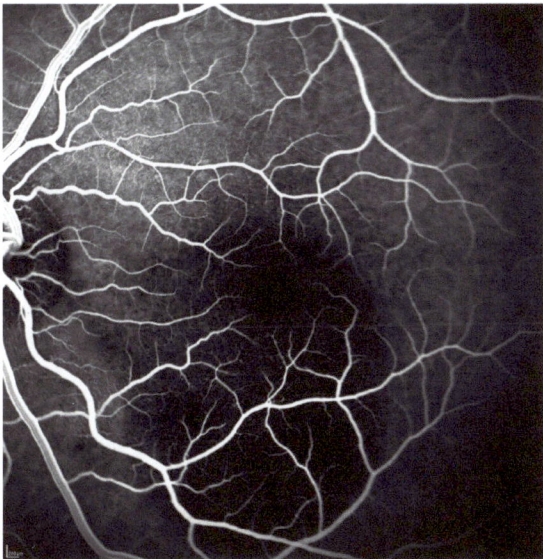

B1

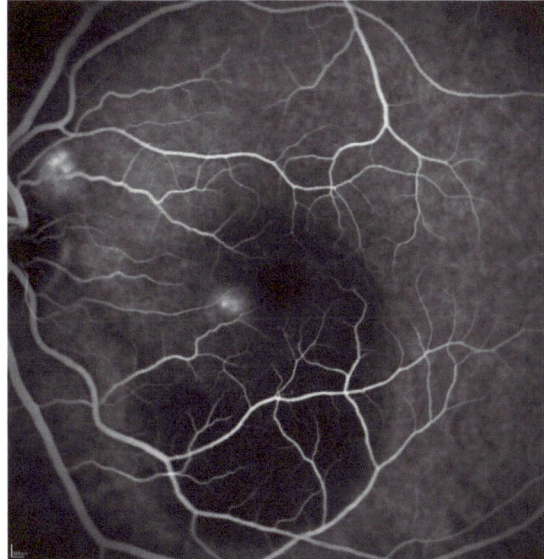

B2

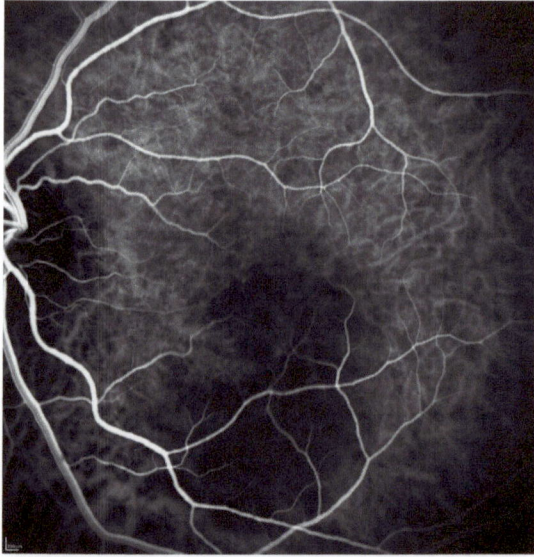

C1

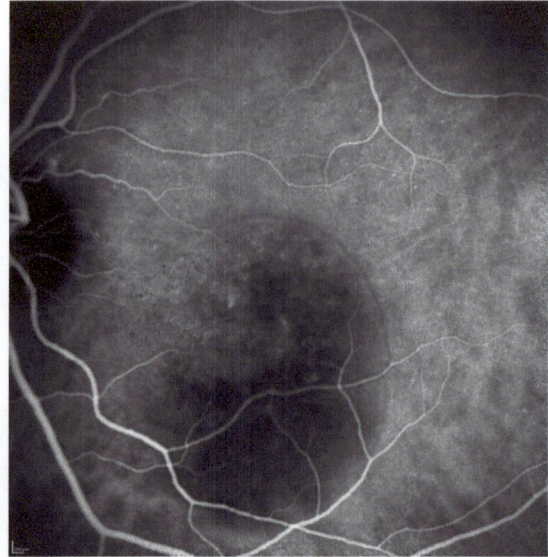

C2

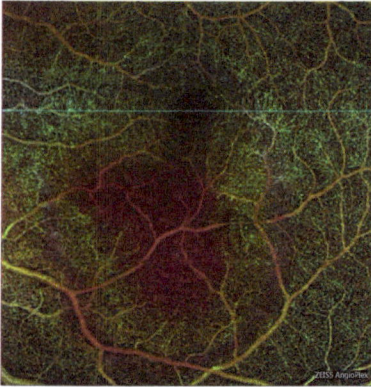

D1

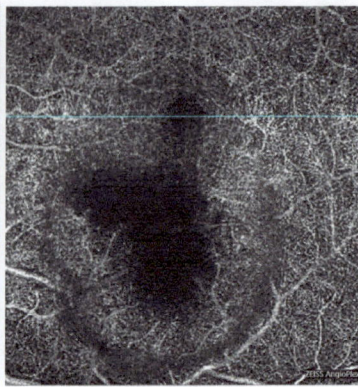

D2

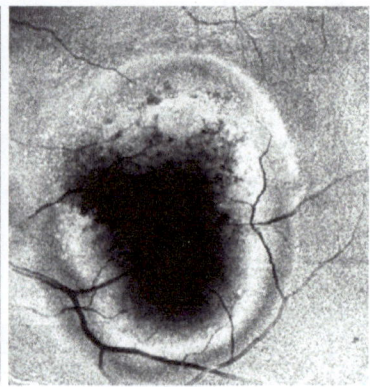

D3

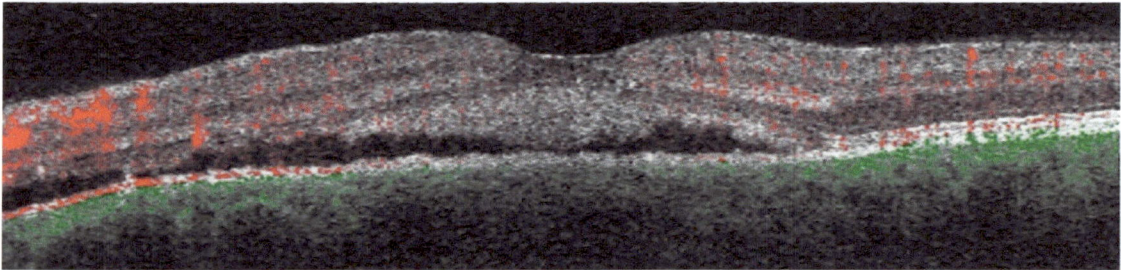

D4

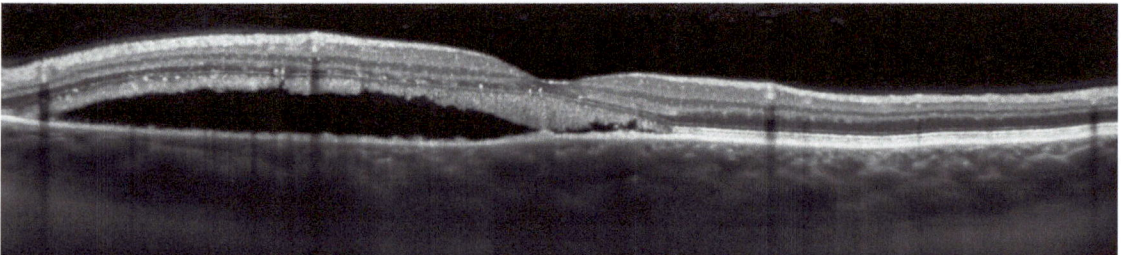

E

www.ingramcontent.com/pod-product-compliance
Lightning Source LLC
Chambersburg PA
CBHW041725210326
41598CB00008B/781